Emergency Nursing
at a Glance

This title is also available as an e-book.
For more details, please see
www.wiley.com/buy/9781118867679
or scan this QR code:

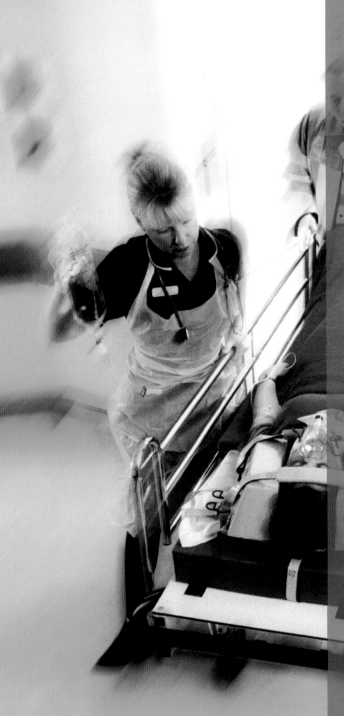

Emergency Nursing at a Glance

Edited by

Natalie Holbery
Lecturer/Practitioner Emergency Care
St George's University Hospitals NHS
Foundation Trust
Kingston University and St George's,
University of London
London

Paul Newcombe
Associate Professor
Kingston University and St George's,
University of London
London

Series editor: Ian Peate

WILEY Blackwell

Contents

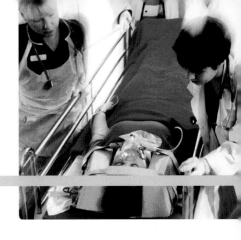

Contributors

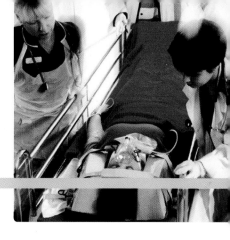

Jim Blair (Chapter 43)
Associate Professor (Hon)
Consultant Nurse Learning Disabilities
Great Ormond Street Hospital
London

Chris Brunker (Chapters 19, 20, 21 and 22)
Clinical Nurse Specialist
Neuro-Intensive Care
St George's University Hospitals NHS Foundation Trust
London

Claire Chinnock (Chapters 30, 31, 32 and 33)
Senior Lecturer Emergency Care
Kingston University and St George's,
University of London
London

Chris Hart (Chapters 39, 40 and 41)
Senior Lecturer Mental Health Nursing
Kingston University and St George's,
University of London
London

Caron Ireland (Chapters 44, 45, 46, 47, 48 and 49)
Paediatric Sister
Urgent and Emergency care
Sussex Community NHS Trust
Sussex

Heather Jarman (Chapters 65 and 66)
Clinical Director for Major Trauma
Consultant Nurse in Emergency Care
St George's University Hospitals NHS Foundation Trust
London

Emma Menzies-Gow (Chapters 15, 16 and 17)
Senior Lecturer Cardiac Nursing
Kingston University and St George's,
University of London
London

Matthew Parkes (Chapters 51, 52 and 54)
Matron
Urgent Care Centre
St George's University Hospitals NHS Foundation Trust
London

Nicola Shopland (Chapters 50, 53 and 54)
Divisional Chief Nurse of Medicine
Surrey and Sussex Healthcare NHS Trust
Surrey

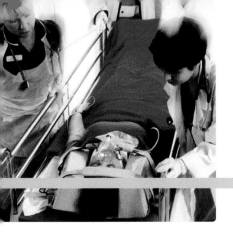

Preface

Demand for emergency care has risen in the UK in recent years, calling for a reshaping of the system. Innovative models of service provision and the development of new roles in urgent and emergency care are two initiatives to ensure that care is delivered to the right people in the right place at the right time. While it is an exciting time to be working in this specialty, it is not a job for the fainthearted! Emergency nursing is a rewarding yet sometimes challenging career that demands a broad knowledge base and commitment to lifelong learning.

This textbook offers up-to-date, peer-reviewed content that provides the reader with written and visual information relating to all aspects of emergency nursing. Chapters are organised into themes that reflect aspects of care or particular patient groups. Each chapter covers a clinical topic and includes background information, guidelines for assessment and care, and management of common clinical presentations. The text is accompanied by clear illustrations, photographs, diagrams and flow charts to further support learning. The 'At a Glance' format is perfect for student nurses or nurses new to emergency nursing because it allows quick reference to the diversity that is emergency nursing.

Acknowledgements

We would like to thank the contributors for dedicating their time and expertise to assist the development of this textbook. We would also like to thank Rosie Maundrill and Darrel Manuel for allowing us to use their work for the acute kidney injury chapter.

Thanks also to Oscar Cavero and Nichola Brown for posing as models in the neuro chapters, and to Sarah Yeomans, Chloe Yeomans, Drew Yeomans and Isla Qureshi for posing as models in the paediatric chapters.

We are very grateful to the team at Wiley for their direction in keeping us on track. Finally, we would like to thank our families for their support and encouragement, not merely during the writing of this book, but throughout our careers.

Natalie Holbery
Paul Newcombe

About the companion website

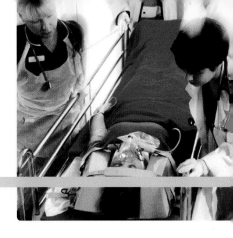

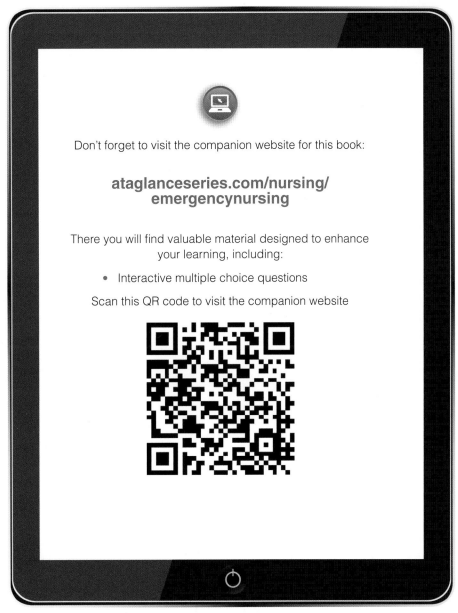

Don't forget to visit the companion website for this book:

**ataglanceseries.com/nursing/
emergencynursing**

There you will find valuable material designed to enhance
your learning, including:

- Interactive multiple choice questions

Scan this QR code to visit the companion website

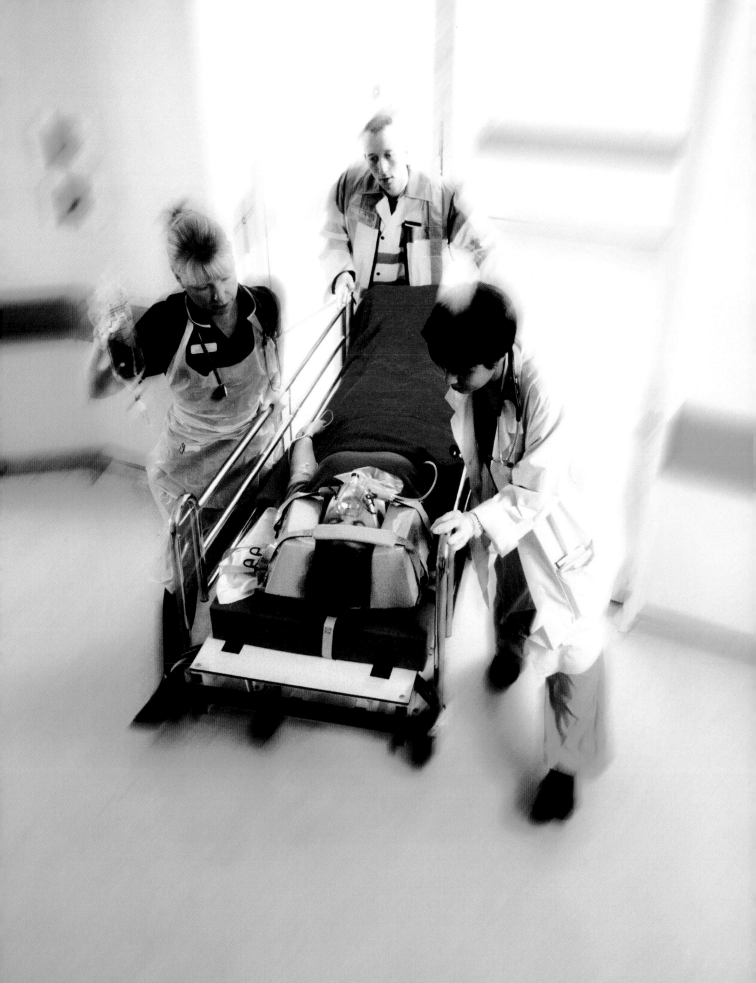

Initial patient assessment

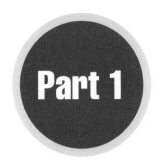

Part 1

Chapters

The context of emergency nursing

Figure 1.1 Emergency department nursing roles

Nurse consultant
- Clinical expert
- Leadership role
- Policy development
- Research engagement

Educator
- Facilitate clinical knowledge and skills
- Design, deliver and evaluate educational programmes

Matron
- Leadership
- Quality assurance
- Staff support

Emergency nurse practitioner (ENP)
- Autonomous, advanced role
- See, treat and discharge patients
- Prescribe medication

Registered nurse (RN)

Band 5 – Assess, plan, deliver and evaluate individual patient care

Band 6 – Assess, plan, deliver and evaluate individual patient care, manage areas of department and possibly shift lead

Band 7 – Assess, plan, deliver and evaluate individual patient care, manage areas of department, shift lead, manage a team of nurses, audit, clinical leadership

Figure 1.2 Areas within the emergency department

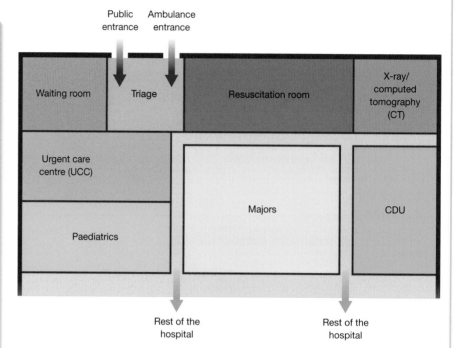

Emergency Nursing at a Glance, First Edition. Natalie Holbery and Paul Newcombe
© 2016 John Wiley & Sons, Ltd. Published 2016 by John Wiley & Sons, Ltd. Companion website: www.ataglanceseries.com/nursing/emergencynursing

The emergency department (ED) is a busy, fast-paced, unpredictable and often highly emotive place to work. ED nurses thrive on the pace, excitement and unpredictable nature of the environment. They need to be proficient in the assessment, recognition and care of patients across the lifespan with undiagnosed illness or injury. They are required to process large amounts of information to facilitate decision making, often in time-pressured situations. Violence and aggression towards ED staff has increased in recent years. Nurses therefore need to be adept at conflict resolution and proficient at communicating with all members of the public. Knowledge of legal and professional issues relating to consent, mental capacity, restraint, information sharing, forensics and end of life care is key to delivering safe and competent care. A number of core and advanced ED nursing roles exist in the UK (Figure 1.1) to ensure that care is delivered safely, efficiently and effectively.

Patients present to the ED day and night, every day of the year. They arrive at the ED in a number of ways (Chapter 2). Current health policy organises services to redirect people away from the ED whenever possible. In the UK, public education encourages individuals to choose the right option to meet their needs. The campaign advises people to access services beyond the ED such as a Pharmacist, a General Practitioner (GP) or a Walk in Centre (WIC) for non-emergency conditions. The majority of patients self-refer to the ED, however others may be referred by a telemedicine service (e.g. NHS 111), a GP, pharmacist or community nurse.

ED team

ED care is delivered by an inter-professional team of nurses, doctors and healthcare assistants. Current redesign of UK emergency and urgent care services has seen an increase in paramedics and physician associates working in EDs. Allied health professionals, such as speech and language therapists, physiotherapists, occupational therapists and dieticians, also work alongside ED nurses to address patients' physical and social needs as required.

4-hour target

A drive to reduce waiting times and expedite care saw the introduction of the 4-hour target in the UK. That is, most patients are to be seen, treated and discharged within 4 hours of arrival. Approximately 25% of patients in the UK are admitted to hospital from the ED, with the remainder discharged to their usual place of residence. To support the delivery of care within 4 hours, medical and (in some places) surgical units have been established across the UK. These are separate to EDs and have developed as specialties in their own right.

Areas within the ED

EDs vary in size but all are structured to accommodate a variety of urgent and emergency presentations (Figure 1.2).

Triage

Triage is a nurse-led area and usually the first point of contact for patients. It is also known as the 'front door' of the hospital. Triage nurses determine the severity of the illness or injury and allocate priority accordingly. Triage is covered in more detail in Chapter 3.

Resuscitation area

The resuscitation area, or 'resus', is designed for critically ill and injured patients with high acuity on a triage scale. Examples include trauma, cardiac arrest, stroke, respiratory distress, sepsis and altered conscious levels. This area should be staffed by experienced, specially trained ED nurses with appropriate knowledge, skills and competence.

Majors

'Majors' tends to be the core of the ED and is usually the largest part of the department. It accommodates acutely unwell patients with a wide variety of conditions or complaints. Examples include surgical (appendicitis, bowel obstruction, pancreatitis), gynaecological and obstetric (ectopic pregnancy, miscarriage, per vaginal [PV] bleed), oncology (neutropenic sepsis, generally unwell), medical (pneumonia, headache), urology (urinary retention) and mental health presentations. It is usually staffed by core ED nurses. In some departments, emergency advanced nurse practitioners see, treat and discharge patients from majors.

Minors/Urgent care centre (UCC)

'Minors' is a term that has been traditionally used to describe patients with lower acuity who are seen in the ED. Recent restructuring of emergency care led to the development of UCCs, some of which are attached to an ED. Regardless of the term used, patients seen in this area of an ED are lower acuity with minor injuries or minor health problems. Examples include limb injuries, epistaxis, cellulitis, eye conditions, back pain, ear, nose and throat conditions, and simple wounds. Minors is usually staffed by core ED nurses, emergency nurse practitioners and doctors.

Children

Children account for approximately 25% of emergency attendances. They and their families should have audio-visual separation from adult patients. This usually includes a separate triage area, waiting room and treatment area. Attention should also be paid to security and child-friendly facilities such as toilets, toys, and food and drink areas. A play specialist is recommended in departments that see more than 16,000 children a year. Registered children's nurses should be available to care for unwell or injured children. Registered adult nurses will also come into contact with children and their families in areas such as triage, resus and, occasionally, urgent care.

Observation area/Clinical decision unit (CDU)

The introduction of the 4-hour target led to the establishment of areas within EDs aimed at providing holistic care beyond 4 hours. These areas usually consist of hospital beds with single-sex amenities, food and drink facilities, and dedicated treatment areas. Patients who require allied health assessment or social care input benefit from these areas. Care is often pathway led and may also include patients with low-risk conditions who are waiting for serial blood tests or other investigations.

2 Pre-hospital care

Figure 2.1 Methods of pre-hospital transport

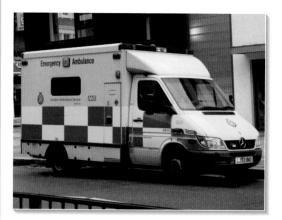

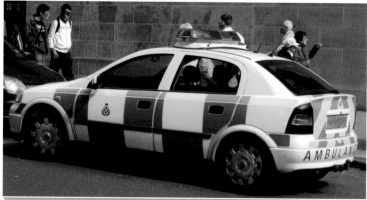

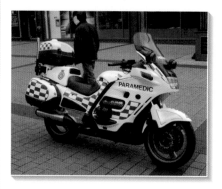

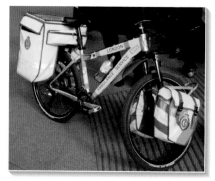

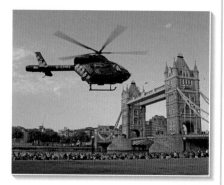

Figure 2.2 Pre-hospital environment: Scene assessment

- Dispatch information
- Safety
- Hazards
- Access
- Parking
- Weather
- Mechanism of injury
- Mode of illness
- Number of casualties
- Major incident
- Resources available
- Other emergency services

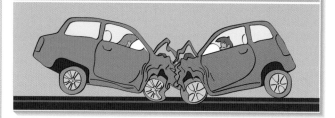

Figure 2.4 CASMEET

- **C**all sign
- **A**ge of patient
- **S**ex of patient
- **M**echanism of injury or mode of illness
- **E**xamination carried out
- **E**stimated time of arrival
- **T**reatment given

Figure 2.3 Care provision

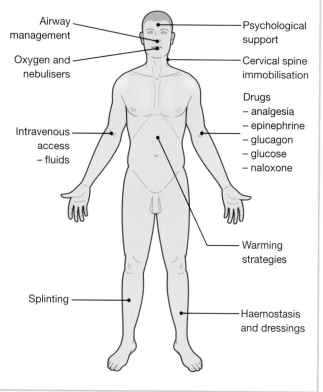

- Airway management
- Oxygen and nebulisers
- Intravenous access – fluids
- Splinting
- Psychological support
- Cervical spine immobilisation
- Drugs
  – analgesia
  – epinephrine
  – glucagon
  – glucose
  – naloxone
- Warming strategies
- Haemostasis and dressings

Emergency Nursing at a Glance, First Edition. Natalie Holbery and Paul Newcombe
© 2016 John Wiley & Sons, Ltd. Published 2016 by John Wiley & Sons, Ltd. Companion website: www.ataglanceseries.com/nursing/emergencynursing

Depending on the local services provided, pre-hospital care is delivered by a range of individuals using a variety of vehicles (Figure 2.1). Overall, about 25% of patients attend an emergency department (ED) via ambulance. Emergency ambulances are usually staffed by two qualified paramedics who can provide a range of advanced life support treatments. However, one or more crew members may be a technician with a more limited skill set. Support or transport crews may have skills limited to just basic life support. Some ambulances use volunteer personnel who have widely differing skills.

Many ambulance services have single responders using cars, motorcycles or bicycles. These are usually paramedics, although nurses and doctors may also be employed. They are able to attend quickly, start emergency treatment and decide whether an ambulance or transfer to hospital is required.

Finally, helicopter emergency medical services provide rapid critical care to carefully selected patients in large urban or rural areas. These are staffed by highly trained medics and paramedics, and often respond to major trauma and critical illness. These teams may also use fast-response cars.

Pre-hospital environment

All patients attending the ED have come from one of a variety of pre-hospital environments. This may be their home, work, school, residential care facility or public place. The environment will dictate the approach required by pre-hospital personnel. Whatever the environment an assessment of the scene takes place first (Figure 2.2). Scene assessment begins after the dispatch operator has provided information that will indicate whether the problem is an injury or illness, for example.

On arrival, pre-hospital personnel need to determine the safety of the scene, any hazards or risks, access, number of casualties, nature of the illness, mechanism of injury and the need for extra help. They will need to rapidly assess for and declare a major incident if appropriate. They frequently work alongside other emergency service personnel (e.g. police, firefighters). ED staff should remember that working in the pre-hospital environment is very different from working within the comfort, safety and support of an ED.

Patient assessment

As with patient assessment in an ED, pre-hospital patient assessment is a dynamic process. Using a structured approach, pre-hospital personnel need to quickly distinguish critical (or time-critical) illness or injury from less urgent problems.

History

Accurate history taking is an essential part of patient assessment (Chapter 3). A patient may be alone or accompanied by friends, relatives, bystanders, colleagues, carers or healthcare professionals. There may be varying levels of background information available. The quality of this information will ultimately have an impact on the quality of the handover between pre-hospital and ED staff.

Physical assessment

Pre-hospital personnel use an 'ABCDE' approach to patient assessment (Chapter 4). Paramedics have advanced physical assessment skills similar to those of a doctor or nurse practitioner. They also have a range of skills and equipment (e.g. electrocardiogram) for measuring vital signs, blood sugar level, etc.

Psychological assessment

A significant minority of individuals requiring pre-hospital care do so because of mental health problems. Pre-hospital personnel need to determine the risk of the individual to themselves or others, and the severity of the current crisis (Chapters 39–41).

Care provision

Because pre-hospital personnel need to make autonomous decisions regarding care provision, they formulate a working diagnosis based on their assessment. They use this to inform a plan of action, which may include:

- Further assessment
- Interventions
- Calling for further or more advanced help
- Following a care pathway
- Transfer to an ED or other service.

Interventions

Depending on the scope of the practitioner, available resources and local protocols, a range of emergency interventions are provided using an ABCDE approach (Figure 2.3). Specific examples include the provision of cardiopulmonary resuscitation (CPR) during cardiac arrest and the management of emergency childbirth.

Transfer to ED

Conveyance of a patient to an ED or other service is guided by protocols and care pathways, for example:

- Acute coronary syndrome (ACS)
- Acute stroke
- Major trauma.

Pre-hospital personnel triage the patient and determine whether a 'pre-alert call' is required to allow the ED to prepare for their arrival. The 'CASMEET' mnemonic is used to structure a pre-alert call (Figure 2.4). Blue-light transfer is used to minimise transfer time and patients are usually admitted directly to the resuscitation area. Most patients are not transferred to an ED by blue light.

Handover

Handover is a crucial point in the patient journey and requires good communication and documentation skills on the part of both groups of staff. Each ED has its own approach to receiving ambulances, but it should be carried out in a thorough and efficient manner. It should also be patient centred and protect patient dignity and privacy as far as possible. It is essential that all the relevant information is correctly received and recorded to ensure continuity and safety, and to maximise patient outcomes.

3 Triage

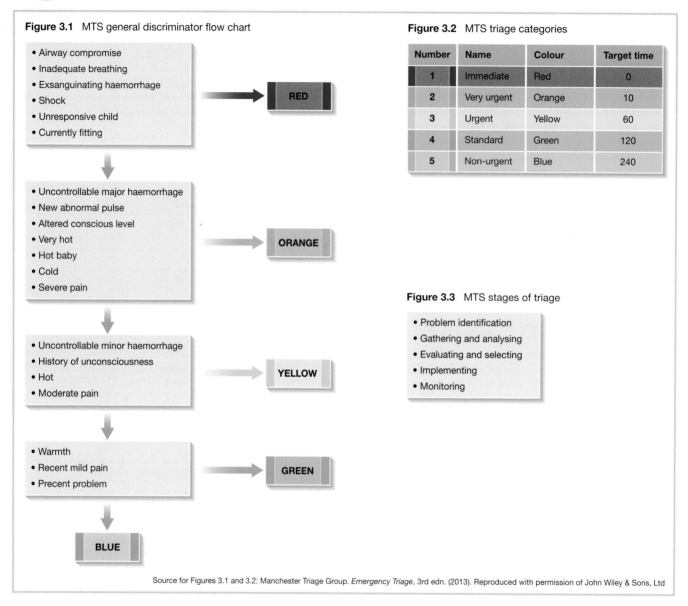

Figure 3.1 MTS general discriminator flow chart

- Airway compromise
- Inadequate breathing
- Exsanguinating haemorrhage
- Shock
- Unresponsive child
- Currently fitting

→ RED

- Uncontrollable major haemorrhage
- New abnormal pulse
- Altered conscious level
- Very hot
- Hot baby
- Cold
- Severe pain

→ ORANGE

- Uncontrollable minor haemorrhage
- History of unconsciousness
- Hot
- Moderate pain

→ YELLOW

- Warmth
- Recent mild pain
- Precent problem

→ GREEN

BLUE

Figure 3.2 MTS triage categories

Number	Name	Colour	Target time
1	Immediate	Red	0
2	Very urgent	Orange	10
3	Urgent	Yellow	60
4	Standard	Green	120
5	Non-urgent	Blue	240

Figure 3.3 MTS stages of triage

- Problem identification
- Gathering and analysing
- Evaluating and selecting
- Implementing
- Monitoring

Source for Figures 3.1 and 3.2: Manchester Triage Group. *Emergency Triage*, 3rd edn. (2013). Reproduced with permission of John Wiley & Sons, Ltd

Triage is a system used to sort patients into categories based on priority. Priority is determined by a focused initial assessment that identifies specific criteria. The priority category indicates the time the patient is deemed safe to wait before being seen by an appropriate decision maker, usually an emergency department (ED) doctor or nurse practitioner.

Triage originates from the development of battlefield medicine during the Napoleonic war. The word 'triage' comes from the French verb 'trier', which means 'to sort'. It was introduced into EDs in the 1980s, replacing what was essentially a 'first come, first served' system with ad hoc prioritisation.

Triage is the job of experienced, specially trained ED nurses. It is a high-risk activity and must be undertaken by those with the appropriate level of knowledge, skills and competence. Overestimating the severity of an illness or injury is less dangerous for patient care, but will have an impact on the smooth running of the ED. Underestimating the severity of illness or injury, and therefore creating a protracted waiting time, can have a significant impact on patient outcomes.

Manchester triage system (MTS)

MTS is the most commonly used triage system internationally. It is made up of the following components:

- Presentational flow charts
- Discriminators
  - General (Figure 3.1)
  - Specific.
- Triage categories (Figure 3.2).

MTS uses a reductionist approach: all patients start as a Priority 1 (P1). Priory decreases as the user moves down the flow chart. Triage requires patient assessment skills in collecting both subjective and objective data. Figure 3.3 shows the stages required.

Problem identification

The nature of the presenting problem may or may not be immediately obvious. It may be clearly described by the patient, someone accompanying them or another healthcare professional. The problem may be non-specific initially, such as 'unwell adult', but may become more specific after the initial assessment, such as 'diabetic emergency'.

Gathering and analysing

Subjective data (history taking)

Collecting an accurate focused history is the bedrock of effective triage. A funnelling process is used to encourage a patient to express the problem in their own words, but also to facilitate the efficient collection of relevant information. After greeting the patient, introducing themselves and gaining consent, the triage nurse should begin with an open question:

- How can I help you today?
- What is your reason for coming to hospital today?

Then a series of open and closed questions are used to clarify information and focus on areas that require further exploration:

- Can you tell me more about that?
- When did the problem begin?

Information gained will trigger a series of further questions or assessments. The MTS flow charts offer prompts for further questions to assess:

- Pain
- Chest pain
- Urinary symptoms
- Limb injury.

Finally, closed questions are used to ensure that all relevant information is collected:

- Past medical history?
- Any medications or allergies?

Objective data

Objective data are collected through patient observation. An 'ABCDE' approach should be used for unwell patients (Chapter 4). Observation should be used to corroborate the history:

- Does the patient look well or unwell?
- Are there any non-verbal signs of pain?
- Are they walking on the injured limb?

Vital signs are not necessary for every triage decision unless local protocols dictate otherwise. Specific examination or investigations may be indicated:

- Shortness of breath – peak expiratory flow rate
- Limb injury – neurovascular assessment
- Chest pain – electrocardiogram (ECG)
- Vaginal bleeding – pregnancy test.

Evaluating and selecting

The information collected should now enable a triage decision to be made using the MTS flow charts or equivalent. Certain factors may create an automatic triage category due to local protocols, including:

- Age (very young or very old)
- Care pathways (e.g. fractured neck of femur).

Implementing

The triage category should be clearly communicated to the patient and/or carer with an explanation of what it means and what will happen next. The triage decision should also be clearly documented including:

- Presentation
- Discriminator
- Category.

The category is communicated to other ED staff to ensure that appropriate actions are taken. The triage nurse may also be able to offer treatment or care to the patient while they are waiting, including:

- Analgesics (e.g. via a patient group direction [PGD])
- A bed, trolley or private room
- Dressings
- Splints
- Ice.

Some EDs may have a secondary assessment process in which more in-depth investigations are undertaken while the patient is waiting, including:

- Blood tests
- X-rays.

Monitoring

Triage is a dynamic process. The waiting room is a high-risk area and continuous monitoring is essential. If a patient's condition changes, reassessment should be undertaken and the triage category adjusted accordingly. Furthermore, if the waiting time changes, this should be communicated to the patient.

The 'ABCDE' approach

Figure 4.1 Causes of acute deterioration

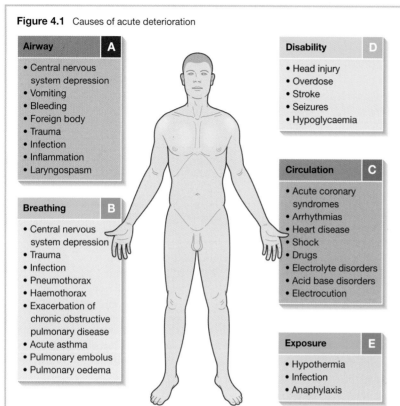

Airway **A**

- Central nervous system depression
- Vomiting
- Bleeding
- Foreign body
- Trauma
- Infection
- Inflammation
- Laryngospasm

Breathing **B**

- Central nervous system depression
- Trauma
- Infection
- Pneumothorax
- Haemothorax
- Exacerbation of chronic obstructive pulmonary disease
- Acute asthma
- Pulmonary embolus
- Pulmonary oedema

Disability **D**

- Head injury
- Overdose
- Stroke
- Seizures
- Hypoglycaemia

Circulation **C**

- Acute coronary syndromes
- Arrhythmias
- Heart disease
- Shock
- Drugs
- Electrolyte disorders
- Acid base disorders
- Electrocution

Exposure **E**

- Hypothermia
- Infection
- Anaphylaxis

Figure 4.2 Observation chart showing deterioration

Figure 4.3 ABCDE approach: Assessment

Airway	Breathing	Circulation
• Talking?	• Talking in sentences?	• Palpable pulse?
• Breathing?	• Complaining of difficulty in breathing/shortness of breath?	• Pale?
• Noisy breathing?		• Cool?
• Respiratory distress?	• RIPPAS:	• Sweaty?
• Obvious foreign body?	– Respiratory rate?	• Bleeding?
• Obvious facial injuries?	– tachypnoeic?	• Heart rate?
• Vomit/blood/secretions?	– bradypnoeic?	• Blood pressure?
• Swelling?	– Inspection	• Capillary refill time?
	– agitation?	• Urine output?
	– drowsy?	• Arrhythmias?
	– cyanosis?	
	– injuries?	**Disability**
	– equal chest expansion?	• AVPU (alert, voice, pain, unconscious)/GCS?
	– accessory muscle use?	• Pupils reacting?
	– Palpation	• Blood glucose?
	– tenderness?	• Recent drugs?
	– deformity?	
	– crepitus?	**Exposure**
	– surgical emphysema?	• Temperature?
	– tracheal deviation?	• Tenderness?
	– Percussion	• Wounds?
	– hyporesonance?	• Bleeding?
	– hyperresonance?	• Infection?
	– Auscultation	• Swelling?
	– breath sounds?	• Rashes?
	– equal air entry?	
	– wheezing?	
	– crackles?	
	– Saturations?	
	– hypoxic?	

Figure 4.4 ABCDE approach: Management

Airway

- Positioning
- Head-tilt/chin-lift
- Jaw-thrust
- Suction
- Oropharyngeal airway
- Nasopharyngeal airway
- Intubation

Breathing

- Oxygen
- Nebulisers
- Assisted ventilation

Circulation

- IV access
- Blood tests
- Fluid challenge
- Broad-spectrum antibiotics
- Stop bleeding

Disability

- Positioning
- IV glucose

Exposure

- Prevent heat loss
- Maintain dignity

Emergency Nursing at a Glance, First Edition. Natalie Holbery and Paul Newcombe
© 2016 John Wiley & Sons, Ltd. Published 2016 by John Wiley & Sons, Ltd. Companion website: www.ataglanceseries.com/nursing/emergencynursing

Most patients presenting to the emergency department (ED) are not critically ill or acutely deteriorating. However, many are. These patients need early identification, rapid assessment, appropriate initial management and establishment of a definitive plan.

Figure 4.1 shows common causes of acute deterioration. Factors that increase risk include:

- Very old or very young
- Comorbidities
- Significant acute illness or injury
- Shock
- Recent major surgery
- Failure to progress.

Patients who experience cardiac arrest often show signs of deterioration before the event (Figure 4.2). Those identified and treated early tend to have better outcomes, and cardiac arrest may be prevented. Early warning systems assist in identification and guiding appropriate actions (Chapter 5).

Using the ABCDE approach

Many systems of patient assessment exist. However, the ABCDE approach is recommended for the assessment (Figure 4.3) and management (Figure 4.4) of the deteriorating patient. It is an easy-to-remember mnemonic (Airway, Breathing, Circulation, Disability, Exposure), providing a standardised and efficient approach that can be used in all contexts. It allows the ED nurse to identify problems in order of priority (i.e. those that pose immediate threats to life). Problems should be addressed with simple interventions as they are identified. Constant reassessment to monitor progress is key. The ABCDE approach can be undertaken by an individual (as a linear, vertical approach) or as a team (as a simultaneous, horizontal approach), for example in cases of trauma or cardiac arrest. However, if alone, the ED nurse should have a low threshold for calling for help as soon as significant signs become apparent.

Airway

Airway obstruction is a medical emergency. Untreated, it leads to hypoxia, organ damage, respiratory or cardiac arrest and eventually death. A combination of lowered consciousness, vomiting and supine positioning is a common triad in critical illness and will quickly compromise airway patency. C-spine injury should always be suspected in trauma patients and considered during airway management (Chapter 7).

Basic airway assessment is performed by talking to the patient and seeking a verbal response. The patient who is talking can be assumed to have a patent airway. If the patient is not talking, then the presence of breathing should be quickly confirmed. In the absence of breathing, the advanced life support (ALS) algorithm should be followed (Chapter 18). Further airway assessment may reveal visible or audible signs of obstruction.

Most airway problems can be resolved with simple interventions such as basic airway manoeuvres (head-tilt/chin-lift/jaw-thrust), suctioning, insertion of simple airway adjuncts (oropharyngeal or nasopharyngeal airways) and positioning (lateral). Patients with a reduced level of consciousness (Glasgow Coma Scale [GCS] <8) or those requiring ongoing airway support (e.g. toleration of an oropharyngeal airway) require definitive airway management. Call an anaesthetist and prepare for intubation.

Breathing

There are many causes of acute breathing problems. Again, left untreated, these will lead to hypoxic organ damage etc. Listening to what the patient is saying is essential. Are they complaining of dyspnoea? Are they talking in full sentences? Vital signs include respiratory rate and pulse oximetry. Pulse oximetry will indicate oxygen levels, but not carbon dioxide levels. Arterial blood gas (ABG) analysis is required to determine this. RIPPAS is a useful mnemonic for structuring respiratory assessment (Chapter 8). A chest X-ray is often indicated.

All critically ill patients require high concentration oxygen via a non-rebreathe mask at 10–15L/min. Those at risk of CO_2 retention (i.e. with chronic obstructive pulmonary disease [COPD]) should start at 28% via a venturi mask (Chapter 9). Depending on their condition, the patient may benefit from being sat upright to aid chest expansion. Specific respiratory interventions may be indicated, such as nebulisers, non-invasive ventilation, needle decompression and chest drain (Chapters 10, 17, 58). When there is absent or ineffective breathing, or if intubation has taken place, artificial ventilation will be required.

Circulation

Problems with circulation commonly arise from disruption to the circulating volume (shock) or because of a primary cardiac cause (acute coronary syndrome [ACS], arrhythmia). Poor perfusion will quickly lead to hypoxic organ failure and death.

Monitoring equipment should be used appropriately, but it is also important to touch the patient to palpate the quality of the pulse and feel the warmth of the skin (Chapter 12). Assessment focuses on looking for compensated shock (normal blood pressure [BP]) or decompensated shock (low BP) (Chapter 13). The presence of bleeding should also be identified. A 12-lead electrocardiogram (ECG) may be indicated (Chapter 14).

Management includes siting at least one large bore intravenous (IV) cannula. Draw blood for routine haematological, biochemical, coagulation and microbiological investigations, and cross-matching if required. Unless there is an obvious cardiac cause, give a rapid fluid challenge and reassess. Repeat if necessary and monitor for response and tolerance. Pressure should be applied to external bleeding (Chapter 12). Specific interventions may also be indicated.

Disability

Level of consciousness is usually determined early during assessment and constant monitoring is essential. The AVPU (Alert, Voice, Pain, Unresponsive) scale or GCS should be used and pupillary reaction assessed (Chapter 19). Consideration of recent drugs or medications may also provide clues. Blood sugar level must be measured and hypoglycaemia treated urgently with IV glucose. Hyperglycaemia may also be found (Chapter 28). CT scanning and urgent referral may be indicated (Chapter 20).

Exposure

Full exposure is essential to reveal any other obvious abnormal signs. Again, specific interventions may be indicated. Temperature should be measured to identify hypothermia or systemic infection. Cover the patient to avoid heat loss and protect dignity.

Ongoing management

Constant reassessment is essential. Findings should be clearly documented and communicated using a structured approach (ABCDE, National Early Warning Score [NEWS], SBAR [Situation, Background, Assessment, Recommendation, see Chapter 5]). Urgent referral should take place, ensuring that an appropriate definitive plan is established.

5 Track and trigger systems

Figure 5.1 National Early Warning Score (NEWS)

PHYSIOLOGICAL PARAMETERS	3	2	1	0	1	2	3
Respiration Rate	≤8		9 - 11	12 - 20		21 - 24	≥25
Oxygen Saturations	≤91	92 - 93	94 - 95	≥96			
Any Supplemental Oxygen		Yes		No			
Temperature	≤35.0		35.1 - 36.0	36.1 - 38.0	38.1 - 39.0	≥39.1	
Systolic BP	≤90	91 - 100	101 - 110	111 - 219			≥220
Heart Rate	≤40		41 - 50	51 - 90	91 - 110	111 - 130	≥131
Level of Consciousness				A			V, P, or U

*The NEWS initiative flowed from the Royal College of Physicians' NEWS Development and Implementation Group (NEWSDIG) report, and was jointly developed and funded in collaboration with the Royal College of Physicians, Royal College of Nursing, National Outreach Forum and NHS Training for Innovation.

Figure 5.2 NEWS chart

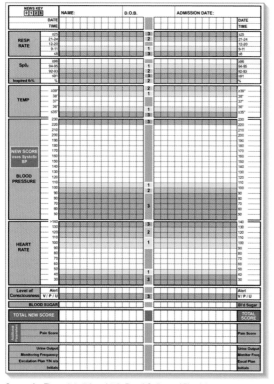

Figure 5.3 Clinical response to NEWS triggers

NEWS SCORE	FREQUENCY OF MONITORING	CLINICAL RESPONSE
0	Minimum 12 hourly	• Continue routine NEWS monitoring with every set of observations
Total: 1-4	Minimum 4-6 hourly	• Inform registered nurse who must assess the patient; • Registered nurse to decide if increased frequency of monitoring and / or escalation of clinical care is required;
Total: 5 or more or 3 in one parameter	Increased frequency to a minimum of 1 hourly	• Registered nurse to urgently inform the medical team caring for the patient; • Urgent assessment by a clinician with core competencies to assess acutely ill patients; • Clinical care in an environment with monitoring facilities;
Total: 7 or more	Continuous monitoring of vital signs	• Registered nurse to **immediately** inform the medical team caring for the patient – this should be at least at Specialist Registrar level; • Emergency assessment by a clinical team with critical care competencies, which also includes a practitioner/s with advanced airway skills; • Consider transfer of Clinical care to a level 2 or 3 care facility, i.e. higher dependency or ITU;

Source for Figure 5.1, 5.2 and 5.3: Royal College of Physicians

Emergency Nursing at a Glance, First Edition. Natalie Holbery and Paul Newcombe

© 2016 John Wiley & Sons, Ltd. Published 2016 by John Wiley & Sons, Ltd. Companion website: www.ataglanceseries.com/nursing/emergencynursing

'Track and trigger' systems, such as early warning scores (EWS), are advocated in the care of patients who present with acute illness or who are at risk of deterioration. A number of reports have highlighted the importance of these systems in identifying and successfully responding to these high-risk patient groups. Physiological track and trigger systems rely on periodic observation and recording of selected physiological signs (track) with clearly defined action criteria (trigger). Action typically results in increased frequency of monitoring and escalation of care.

EWS can help in determining appropriate allocation to clinical areas of the emergency department (ED) and triaging; assist in referral to specialist medical teams; support decision making for allocation to high dependency unit (HDU) or intensive care unit (ICU) beds; and provide evidence of patients who are unsafe to be transferred or who have been allocated to an inappropriate ward.

National Early Warning Score (NEWS)

Historically, within the UK, there were a number of track and trigger systems being used. Although they shared core principles, there was a lack of standardisation between them. The potential for misuse and misinterpretation when patients and staff moved between clinical areas defeated the object of a system that was designed to reduce risk. As a result, the Royal College of Physicians developed NEWS.

Using NEWS

NEWS (Figure 5.1) is a simple system in which a score is allocated to six standard physiological measurements commonly undertaken during patient assessment and monitoring in the ED:

- Respiratory rate
- Oxygen saturations
- Temperature
- Systolic blood pressure
- Pulse rate
- Level of consciousness.

Observations are recorded on the standardised NEWS chart (Figure 5.2). For each physiological parameter, a normal 'healthy' range is defined. Measured values outside this range are allocated a score that is weighted and colour-coded on the observation chart. The size of the score indicates how extreme the parameter varies from normal, and reflects the severity of the physiological disturbance. The individual scores are then added together. If supplemental oxygen is required to maintain oxygen saturations, two additional points are added to the total. The total score indicates the level of clinical risk, which is also colour-coded (Figure 5.3). A score of 0–4 indicates low risk (green), 5–6 medium risk (orange) and 7 or more high risk (red). A score of 3 in any individual parameter also indicates medium risk.

Low risk

Patients with a score of 0 should continue to have routine NEWS monitoring with every set of observations (minimum 12-hourly). A score of 1–4 requires a registered nurse to assess the patient (when other healthcare staff are involved in recording observations). The ED nurse must then decide if increased frequency of monitoring and/or escalation of clinical care is required. Junior staff should seek support with decision making if necessary. Frequency of observations should be a minimum of 4–6-hourly. ED patients will often have hourly observations undertaken anyway, but the 4–6-hourly frequency may be relevant in the clinical decision unit (CDU), or similar, where patient stay is longer.

Medium risk

A medium risk score (total of 5–6 or 3 in one parameter) requires the ED nurse to urgently inform the doctor or medical team caring for the patient. Urgent assessment by a clinician with core competencies to assess acutely ill patients is required. Additionally, clinical care should be provided in an environment with monitoring facilities. This may require the patient to be moved to a monitored cubicle in the major illness or resuscitation area of the ED. Frequency of observation should be increased to a minimum of 1-hourly if not already.

High risk

Patients with a score of 7 or more are considered those at greatest risk of deterioration. The ED nurse should immediately inform the doctor or medical team caring for the patient – this should be at least at specialist registrar level. Emergency assessment should be undertaken by a clinical team with critical care competencies that also includes a practitioner with advanced airway skills. All middle-grade and consultant ED medical staff should be able to provide this level of care, but other senior medical/ICU/anaesthetic staff may be called on. The patient should be considered for transfer to a level 2 or 3 care facility (i.e. higher dependency or ICU). They should be moved to the resuscitation area immediately, if not there already, in the interim. High-risk patients may include those in peri-arrest, and therefore activating a cardiac arrest call may be indicated depending on local protocols (Chapter 18). Some ED patients may have a high NEWS score, but an appropriate treatment plan and/or referral to HDU or ICU may already be in place to meet their needs.

SBAR (Situation, Background, Assessment, Recommendation)

Alongside track and trigger systems, a shared communication tool, such as SBAR, should be employed when seeking help with a deteriorating patient. The benefits of SBAR are that it is standardised, concise and easy to remember. Its key components include:

Situation

- Identify yourself and the site or unit you are calling from
- Identify the patient by name and the reason for your report
- Briefly describe your concern.

Background

- Give the patient's reason for admission
- Explain significant medical history
- Briefly describe relevant recent events.

Assessment

- Provide key vital signs
- Use ABCDE and NEWS
- Suggest your clinical impression.

Recommendation

- Explain what you need
- Be specific about request and time frame
- Make suggestions
- Clarify expectations.

6 Pain

Figure 6.1 Assessment of acute pain in the emergency department

	No pain Pain score: 0	Mild pain Pain score: 1–3	Moderate pain Pain score: 4–6	Severe pain Pain score: 7–10
Suggested route and type of analgesic	No action	Oral analgesic	Oral analgesic	IV opiates or rectal NSAID
Initial assessment	Within 20 mins of arrival	Within 20 mins of arrival	Within 20 mins of arrival	Within 20 mins of arrival
Re-evaluation	Within 60 mins of initial assessment	Within 60 mins of analgesic	Within 60 mins of analgesic	Within 30 mins of analgesic

Figure 6.2 Emergency department pain standards

1. Patients in severe pain (pain score 7–10) or moderate pain (pain score 4–6) receive appropriate analgesic
   (a) 75% within 30 mins of arrival
   (b) 100% within 60 mins of arrival
2. Patient group directives (PGDs) in place for nurse prescribing on arrival
3. Patients with severe pain or moderate pain – 90% should have documented evidence of re-evaluation and action within 120 minutes of the first dose of analgesic
4. If analgesic is not prescribed and the patient has moderate or severe pain, the reason should be documented in the notes

Figure 6.3 Triage category by pain score

Pain score	Description	Priority	Category
0	No pain	5	Non-urgent
1–3	Mild	4	Standard
4–6	Moderate	3	Urgent
7–10	Severe	2	Very urgent

Figure 6.4 Manchester Triage System Pain Assessment Ruler

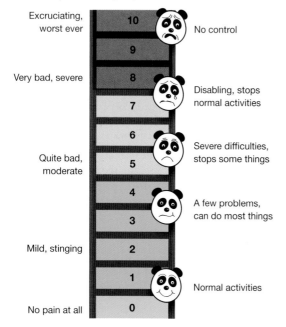

Figure 6.5 Algorithm for treatment of undifferentiated acute pain in the emergency department

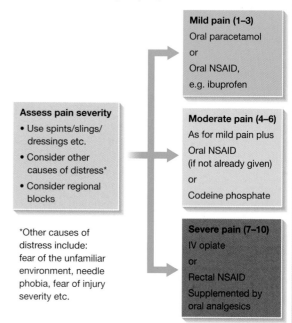

Source for Figures 6.1, 6.2 and 6.5: The College of Emergency Medicine. *Best Practice Guideline: Management of Pain in Adults*, December 2014. Reproduced with permission of The Royal College of Emergency Medicine

Source for Figure 6.4: Manchester Triage Group. *Emergency Triage*, 3rd edn. (2013). Reproduced with permission of John Wiley & Sons, Ltd

Emergency Nursing at a Glance, First Edition. Natalie Holbery and Paul Newcombe

Introduction

Pain is the single biggest reason for patients attending an emergency department (ED). As a result, early identification and relief of pain are key goals for ED nurses. This process should begin at triage, be continuously monitored throughout and end with effective pain management at or beyond discharge. Pain is often considered the fifth vital sign. However, pain management in EDs often falls below standard because of pain being under-recognised and under-treated, and treatment often delayed. This has a negative impact on patient satisfaction. It is for these reasons that there are clear guidelines (Figure 6.1) and standards (Figure 6.2) for ED pain assessment and management in the UK.

Pain assessment

Pain assessment and triage should be undertaken within 20 minutes of arrival in an ED. The Manchester Triage System (MTS) correlates pain scores with triage categories (Figure 6.3). Accurate pain assessment is a complex activity. Pain may be acute or chronic. Any pain assessment tool needs to be appropriate for the patient and clearly explained. Family or carers may be able to contribute. The MTS Pain Assessment Ruler (Figure 6.4) combines three pain assessment tools:

Verbal descriptor scale (VDS)

The most common example is a numerical scale of 0–10. Descriptive words are also used to identify severity, with mild, moderate and severe being the most commonly used terms. The VDS is quick and easy to use, but communication may be a barrier depending on language and cognitive level.

Visual analogue scale (VAS)

The VAS provides a visual representation of the 0–10 scale. This allows patients to identify where they think their pain is along the scale (a ruler in MTS). Faces with differing expressions are widely used in paediatrics and for those with cognitive impairment, such as dementia or intellectual (learning) difficulties.

Pain behaviour tool (PBT)

This uses the principle that patients who are in pain will exhibit certain behaviours and physiological changes. Those with minimal pain should be unrestricted, whereas patients with severe pain may be disabled by it. This tool is particularly useful for those with cognitive impairment or a reduced level of consciousness. Changes in behaviour or physiology may be key indicators. Non-verbal signs include agitation and grimacing, whereas physiological changes include tachycardia, tachypnoea and hypertension.

Other pain assessment tools

There are a wide range of tools that are specific to certain presentations, such as chest pain (Chapter 16) and abdominal pain (Chapter 24). Common elements include identifying the acuity, quality or nature (e.g. sharp versus dull), location (primary and any radiation), whether anything makes it better or worse (including any treatment) and also whether there are any associated symptoms (shortness of breath, dizziness etc.).

Pain management

Figure 6.5 is an algorithm for pain management in an ED. Those with no pain require no analgesia at this stage. Those with mild or moderate pain are given oral paracetamol; those with moderate pain are also given an oral non-steroidal anti-inflammatory drug (NSAID) or codeine phosphate. Those in severe pain are given an intravenous (IV) opiate or rectal NSAID. Inhaled nitrous oxide (entonox) is also effective for short-term pain relief. Regional anaesthesia may also be used. Non-pharmacological methods should always be considered, such as positioning, splints, slings and dressings, and providing reassurance.

In some situations patients decline analgesia. It is important to establish the reasons for decline because patients may be misinformed and this provides an opportunity to educate patients about pain management. They may fear addiction to analgesia or believe they need to be in pain for a correct diagnosis. If they continue to decline analgesia, this should be clearly documented.

Paracetamol

Paracetamol (acetaminophen in the US) is the most widely used analgesic and antipyretic. It is classified as a mild analgesic, but can be used in combination with other drugs for moderate and severe pain. It is generally safe at recommended doses, but very dangerous in overdose (Chapter 31). It comes in a wide variety of over-the-counter preparations and ED nurses should always check whether a patient has taken any before attending. It can be given orally, intravenously or rectally.

NSAIDs

NSAIDs are widely used for pain, inflammation and fever. They are available as oral, rectal, IV and intramuscular (IM) preparations. Examples include ibuprofen, naproxen and diclofenac. Although generally safe during short-term usage, there are a number of situations where NSAIDs should be avoided:

- Asthma (with previous reactions to NSAIDs)
- Peptic ulcer disease
- Renal impairment
- Older age
- Pregnancy.

Opiates

Opiates are strong analgesics that act on the central nervous system. They are available as oral, IM and IV preparations, and include codeine, morphine, diamorphine and tramadol (synthetic opioid). Opiates should be used with caution because they have a range of significant side effects, including:

- Sedation (and airway obstruction)
- Respiratory depression
- Nausea and vomiting
- Hypotension
- Pruritis (itching).

Doses should be titrated to achieve the desired response with minimal side effects. Anti-emetics are often given prophylactically, but should be reserved for those experiencing nausea or vomiting. Naloxone is used in overdose (Chapter 31). Opiate dependence is unlikely in short-term use.

Evaluation and documentation

Pain assessment, treatment and re-evaluation should be clearly documented. Further management should be considered when pain scores are still high.

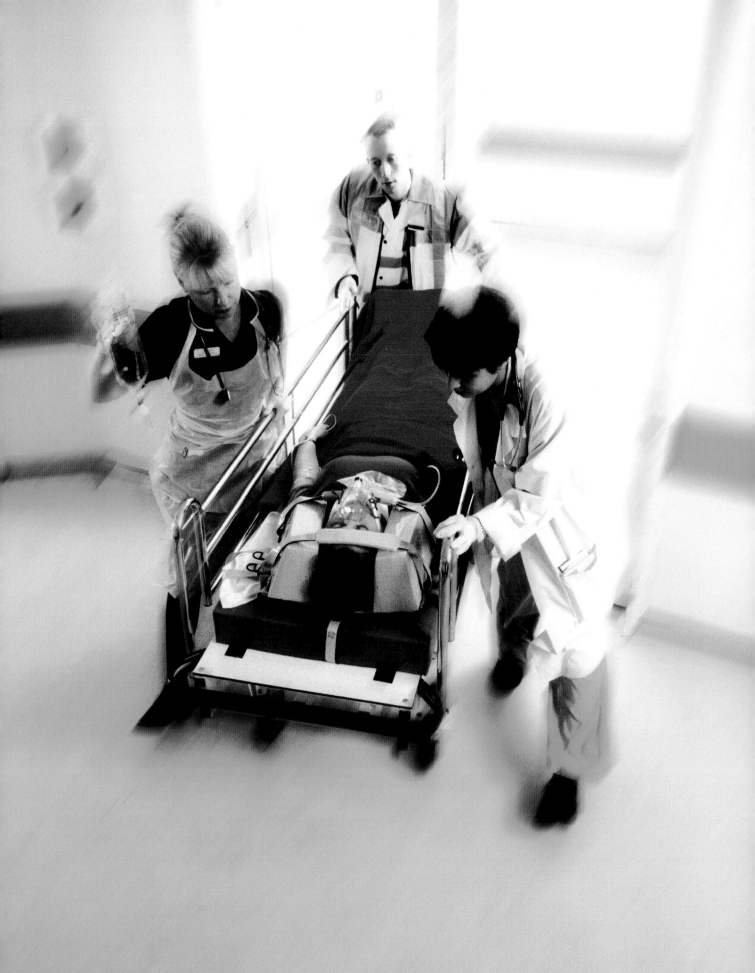

Airway and breathing

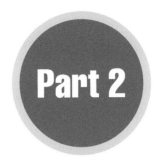

Part 2

Chapters

7

Airway assessment and management

Figure 7.1 Airway equipment

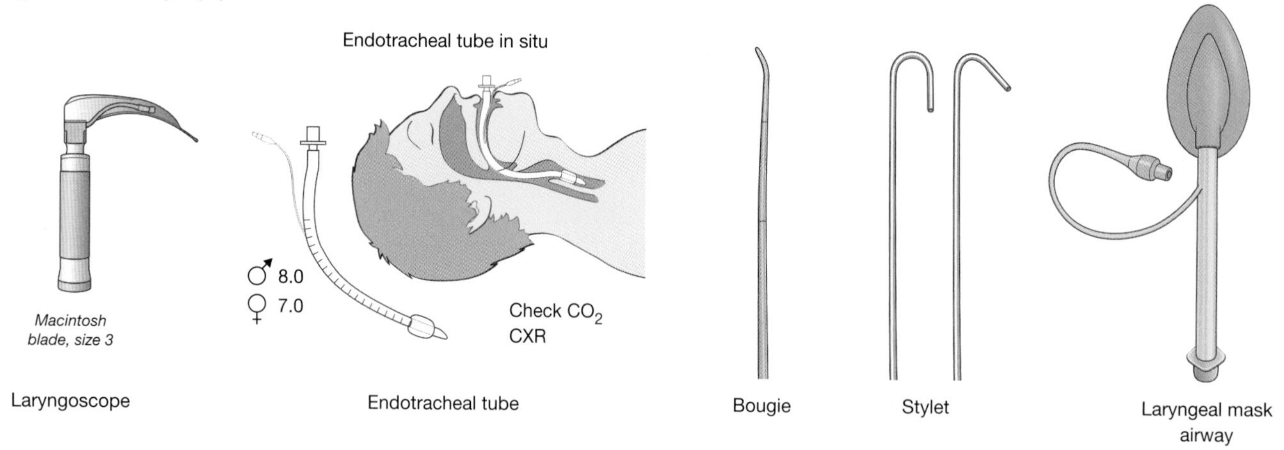

Endotracheal tube in situ

♂ 8.0
♀ 7.0

Check CO$_2$
CXR

Macintosh blade, size 3

Laryngoscope

Endotracheal tube

Bougie

Stylet

Laryngeal mask airway

Figure 7.2 Head-tilt and chin-lift

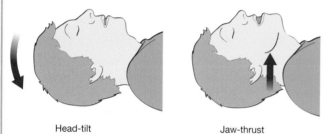

Head-tilt

Jaw-thrust

Figure 7.3 Oropharyngeal airway

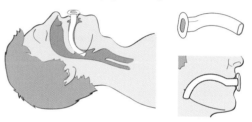

Measure from teeth to angle of jaw

Figure 7.4 Tilted nasopharyngeal airway

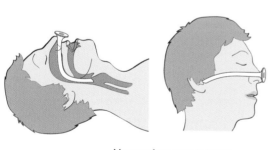

Measure from nose to tragus

Figure 7.5 Definitive airway

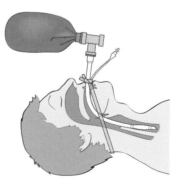

Figure 7.6 RSI equipment

- Suction (Yankauer)
- Laryngoscope
- Endotracheal tube
- Syringe
- Tube tie/securing device
- Stylet
- Bougie
- End-tidal carbon dioxide monitoring device
- Oxygen delivery device, e.g. mechanical ventilator

Source for Figures 7.1, 7.2, 7.3 and 7.4: Hughes T & Cruickshank J (2011) *Emergency Medicine at a Glance*. Reproduced with permission of Thomas Hughes and Jaycen Cruickshank

Emergency Nursing at a Glance, First Edition. Natalie Holbery and Paul Newcombe
© 2016 John Wiley & Sons, Ltd. Published 2016 by John Wiley & Sons, Ltd. Companion website: www.ataglanceseries.com/nursing/emergencynursing

Airway is the first step in the 'ABCDE' approach to the assessment and management of a patient (Chapter 4). Airway comes first in the approach because without a patent airway the patient will soon deteriorate. In an emergency department (ED), most patients have a patent airway and therefore this step is usually quick and simple.

Causes of airway problems

There are a number of conditions that can directly and indirectly cause a patient to have a partial or complete airway obstruction. Such conditions include depressed consciousness, facial trauma, anaphylaxis, burns, foreign bodies, epiglottitis, peritonsillar abscess and tumours. Not all these conditions will immediately cause an airway problem and in many cases the patient may initially be sitting up talking. However, airway obstruction can occur quickly and nurses need to perform regular airway assessment and notify a doctor of changes as soon as they become apparent. Nurses should also ensure emergency airway equipment is nearby and ready for use. Having a low threshold for providing a definitive airway is important, especially for patients with facial burns where oedema can rapidly progress, causing complete airway obstruction.

Airway assessment

Assessing airway patency initially involves seeking a verbal response from the patient. This is best achieved by using their name and asking an open-ended question such as 'How you are feeling?' or 'What happened to you today?' If the patient responds verbally, their airway is patent. It is important to note that airway assessment should be a dynamic process because the airway may become compromised if the patient deteriorates.

If the patient does not respond verbally, it must be assumed that the airway is not patent and potentially at risk. The nurse should attempt to rouse the patient by placing a hand on each of their shoulders and gently shaking them while asking loudly, 'Are you all right?' Further assessment involves listening for upper airway sounds such as gurgling or snoring. Gurgling may be due to blood, vomit or secretions. Snoring indicates a partial airway obstruction, usually caused by relaxation of the muscles around the oropharynx.

If the patient still does not respond, the nurse should call for help, usually by calling an ED colleague nearby or, if in an isolated area of the department, using the emergency bell. Although the patient's airway may be patent at this stage, it is considered to be compromised. The patient should be nursed on a 1:1 basis until help arrives.

Airway equipment

Basic airway equipment should be available in all areas of the ED, usually on a crash trolley. Such equipment includes suction, oropharyngeal airways and nasopharyngeal airways. More advanced equipment should also be available and includes laryngeal mask airways, endotracheal tubes, stylets, gum elastic bougies, curved and straight laryngoscope blades (various sizes), tube ties and end tidal carbon dioxide monitors (Figure 7.1). A difficult airway trolley should also be available and usually includes other equipment used for a surgical airway.

Airway management

Basic airway management involves the use of suction to remove any blood, vomit or secretions that may be causing a partial or complete airway obstruction. If the patient is gurgling, suction should be performed before the airway is opened, to avoid aspiration. Simple manoeuvres to open the airway involve a head-tilt and chin-lift (Figure 7.2). This should be avoided in trauma patients because of the risk of neck injury. In this situation a jaw-thrust is advised (Chapter 56). The goal of this manoeuvre is to lift the tongue away from the oropharynx, thereby opening the airway.

The next step in airway management is to consider the use of an oropharyngeal or nasopharyngeal airway. An oropharyngeal airway is used to lift the tongue away from the oropharynx and a nasopharyngeal airway creates an airway via the nasopharynx. Both should be measured before insertion.

The correct size of an oropharyngeal airway is established by measuring the length of the device from the tip of the incisors to the angle of the jaw (Figure 7.3). If a patient tolerates this, it indicates they are not conscious and require further airway support, usually a definitive airway.

Nasopharyngeal airway fit is estimated based on the patient's size. For example, size 6 for a small adult, size 7 for an average adult and size 8 for a large adult male (Figure 7.4). A conscious or semi-conscious patient will usually tolerate this airway. Some patients may require further airway support or to be cared for with a nasopharyngeal indefinitely, as is commonly seen with respiratory patients.

Definitive airway

If a patient's airway becomes obstructed or is at risk of obstruction, a definitive airway is often inserted in the ED. This is a high-risk procedure and requires a skilled and competent team. A definitive airway is defined as a cuffed tube inserted in the trachea, secured in place and attached to an oxygen source with assisted ventilation (Figure 7.5). Unlike in a planned setting, most definitive airways inserted in the ED are called rapid sequence induction (RSI). The main difference is that patients have not necessarily fasted in the ED and the risk of aspiration is greater.

If a patient is to have a RSI, the nurse should gather the equipment (Figure 7.6) and drugs. The doctor performing the RSI will usually have a preference for the medication used. As a general rule, the patient should be administered oxygen, an induction agent and a muscle relaxant. The nurse's role involves handing equipment to the doctor, administering medication, monitoring the patient's response and vital signs, documentation and caring for the family. In some EDs, operating department practitioners attend to assist this process.

8 Assessment of breathing

Figure 8.1 Causes of dyspnoea

- Exacerbation of COPD
- Acute asthma
- Pneumonia
- Pneumothorax
- Pulmonary embolus (PE)
- Pulmonary oedema
- Pleural effusion
- Rib fractures
- Anaemia
- Acute coronary syndrome (ACS)

Figure 8.2 History taking in dyspnoea

- Past medical history (PMH)
- Smoking
- Reduced exercise tolerance
- Usual medication ineffective
- Increased sputum production
- Fever
- Exposure to allergens
- Recent surgery
- History of trauma
- Chest pain

Figure 8.3 Signs of dyspnoea

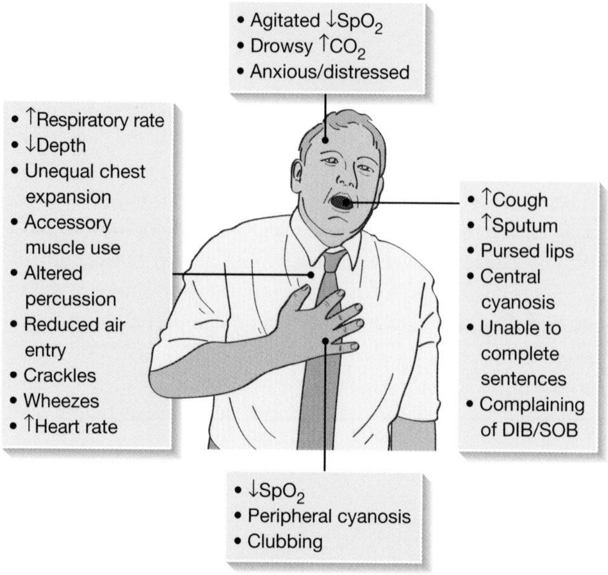

- Agitated ↓SpO$_2$
- Drowsy ↑CO$_2$
- Anxious/distressed

- ↑Respiratory rate
- ↓Depth
- Unequal chest expansion
- Accessory muscle use
- Altered percussion
- Reduced air entry
- Crackles
- Wheezes
- ↑Heart rate

- ↑Cough
- ↑Sputum
- Pursed lips
- Central cyanosis
- Unable to complete sentences
- Complaining of DIB/SOB

- ↓SpO$_2$
- Peripheral cyanosis
- Clubbing

Figure 8.4 ABG normal values

Value	Definition	Normal range
PaO$_2$	Partial pressure of oxygen	11.5–13.5 kPa
pH	Concentration of hydrogen (H$^+$) ions	7.35–7.45
PaCO$_2$	Partial pressure of carbon dioxide	4.6–6.0 kPa
HCO$_3^-$	Concentration of bicarbonate ions	22–26 mmol/L
Base excess	Amount of acid required to restore pH to normal	–2 to +2 mEq/L

Figure 8.5 Respiratory failure

Type I	Type II
PaO$_2$ low (<8 kPa)	PaO$_2$ low (<8 kPa)
PaCO$_2$ low or normal (<6 kPa)	PaCO$_2$ high (>6 kPa)
Causes: Asthma, pneumonia	**Causes:** COPD

Figure 8.6 Acid-base disorders

Disorder	Respiratory acidosis	Respiratory alkalosis	Metabolic acidosis	Metabolic alkalosis
Altered values	↓pH ↑PaCO$_2$	↑pH ↓PaCO$_2$	↓pH ↓HCO$_3^-$	↑pH ↑HCO$_3^-$
Cause	Hypoventilation	Hyperventilation	Excess acid or low alkaline	Low acid or excess alkaline
Examples	COPD, opiate overdose (OD)	Panic attack, asthma, pneumonia	Shock, diabetic ketoacidosis, diarrhoea	Vomiting, antacid OD

Figure 8.7 Normal CXR

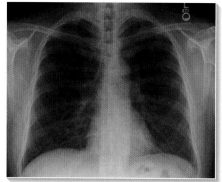

Source: By Stillwaterising [CC0 1.0] via Wikimedia Commons

Figure 8.8 Common abnormal findings on CXR

- Consolidation
- Collapse
- Pleural effusion
- Haemothorax
- Pneumothorax
- Tracheal deviation
- Hyperinflation

Figure 8.9 PEFR meter

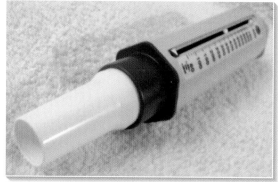

Source: Via Wikimedia Commons

Emergency Nursing at a Glance, First Edition. Natalie Holbery and Paul Newcombe.
© 2016 John Wiley & Sons, Ltd. Published 2016 by John Wiley & Sons, Ltd. Companion website: www.ataglanceseries.com/nursing/emergencynursing

Assessment of breathing is an integral component of patient assessment. Acute illness often has an impact on the respiratory system. A number of primary pulmonary and cardiovascular conditions result in presentations with dyspnoea (Figure 8.1), often referred to as difficulty in breathing (DIB) or shortness of breath (SOB).

History

The emergency department (ED) nurse should be mindful of underlying pathophysiology when undertaking assessment. Features of common respiratory conditions are discussed in Chapter 10. Prompts for history taking are shown in Figure 8.2. The patient with a known long-term condition (e.g. chronic obstructive pulmonary disease [COPD]) should be able to provide a good history. Comparing their current symptoms with normal is a good starting point.

Structured assessment

RIPPAS is a useful mnemonic for structuring respiratory assessment. Talking to the patient is vital and will determine their ability to complete sentences in one breath – a key indicator of respiratory function. Figure 8.3 shows other signs of dyspnoea.

Respiratory rate

Normal respiratory rate is 12–20/min (although >18/min might be high for healthy adults). Tachypnoea is common in acute respiratory conditions, but may also occur because of shock, pain or anxiety. Patients with COPD may be tachypnoeic normally. Bradypnoea is a cardinal sign of acute deterioration as a patient tires, and may indicate peri-arrest. Other causes include CNS (central nervous system) depression and opiate overdose.

Inspection

Observe the general condition of the patient. Do they look well or unwell? Are there any signs of chronic illness? Are there any chest injuries (Chapter 58)? Are they alert? Hypoxia causes agitation initially, whereas hypercapnia (raised CO_2) causes drowsiness. Cyanosis (blueness) is a late sign of hypoxia but should be noted peripherally around the digits and centrally around the mouth or nose. Depth and symmetry of chest expansion should also be observed. The use of accessory muscles (those in the abdomen, neck and shoulders) indicates increased effort of breathing. Pursed-lip breathing reflects small airway collapse.

Palpation

Palpation uses the hands to feel for a number of signs: measuring chest expansion; feeling for tenderness, deformity or crepitus (moving bone fragments) in fractured ribs, for example; or feeling for tracheal deviation or surgical emphysema (air under the skin) in pneumothorax.

Percussion

Percussion involves tapping on the patient's chest to determine the composition of underlying tissues. Normal lung fields sound resonant. Hyporesonance (dullness, a low note) suggests fluid within the chest (e.g. pneumonia, pleural effusion, haemothorax), whereas hyperresonance (tympany, a high note) suggests too much air (e.g. pneumothorax, emphysema, air trapping).

Auscultation

Auscultation uses a stethoscope to listen to air moving through the airways on inspiration and expiration. Breath sounds are considered present, diminished or absent. The left and right lung fields are compared front and back. There are also a number of added sounds. Wheezing is a musical sound on expiration and indicates airway narrowing (bronchoconstriction). It is often associated with asthma. Crackles are non-musical sounds found on inspiration and indicate airway collapse and fluid. Crackles are associated with COPD, pneumonia and pulmonary oedema.

Saturations

Pulse oximetry is more reliable than subjectively assessing for clinical signs of hypoxia (e.g. cyanosis). Pulse oximetry measures the difference between saturated and unsaturated haemoglobin. Normal values are 94–98%. In patients at risk of hypercapnia, normal values are 88–92%. Pulse oximetry has a number of limitations. It will only indicate oxygen levels, not carbon dioxide levels. False high readings occur in anaemia and carbon monoxide poisoning. Readings may be difficult with poor peripheral perfusion, arrhythmias and agitation.

Investigations

Arterial blood gas (ABG)

ABG analysis is the gold-standard method of assessing the efficacy of ventilation. Blood is taken from the radial or femoral artery or an arterial line. ABG analysis provides data on oxygenation, carbon dioxide, acid-base balance and a range of other blood levels. Normal ranges are shown in Figure 8.4.

Oxygenation

PaO_2 values assume the patient is breathing room air. The percentage of inspired oxygen should be taken into consideration using the 'Rule of 10'. For example, if someone is breathing 60% oxygen, their PaO_2 should be about 50kPa (60–10=50). Anything significantly less suggests impaired ventilation. PaO_2 less than 8kPa on room air indicates respiratory failure (Figure 8.5).

Acid-base balance

By comparing values for pH, $PaCO_2$ and HCO_3^- (or base excess), it is possible to determine whether an acid-base disorder exists and is caused by a respiratory or metabolic problem, or both. Figure 8.6 shows the four primary acid-base disorders and common causes. Identifying compensation is more complicated, but essentially the body tries to create the opposite disorder to return the pH to normal. For example, a metabolic acidosis produces hyperventilation as the body tries to blow off CO_2 and produces a respiratory alkalosis. Respiratory compensation is rapid, metabolic compensation is slow. Mixed disorders also occur and the pH may be normal in chronic compensation (e.g. COPD).

Chest X-ray (CXR)

A CXR is usually requested after chest examination and may aid diagnosis. A normal CXR is shown in Figure 8.7 along with a list of common findings in Figure 8.8.

Peak expiratory flow rate (PEFR)

PEFR is the maximum speed of expiration, as measured with a peak flow meter (Figure 8.9). It measures airflow through the bronchi and therefore reflects airway calibre or degree of obstruction. The best of three readings is compared with the normal or expected normal for the patient. PEFR is mainly used in asthma and indicates response to treatment (Chapter 10). Spirometry is more useful in COPD.

Oxygen therapy

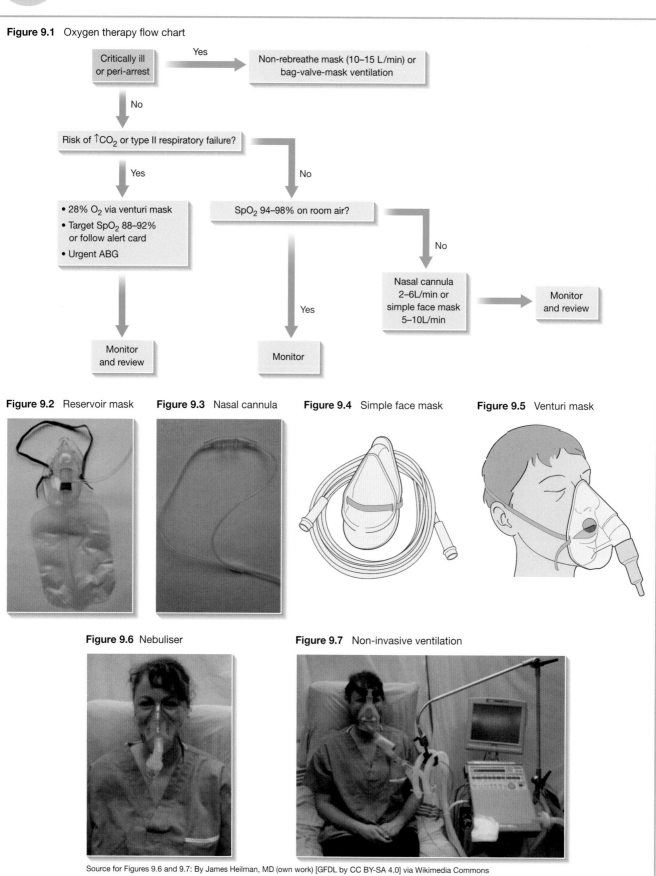

Figure 9.1 Oxygen therapy flow chart

Critically ill or peri-arrest → Yes → Non-rebreathe mask (10–15 L/min) or bag-valve-mask ventilation

No

Risk of ↑CO_2 or type II respiratory failure?

Yes →
- 28% O_2 via venturi mask
- Target SpO_2 88–92% or follow alert card
- Urgent ABG
→ Monitor and review

No → SpO_2 94–98% on room air?
- Yes → Monitor
- No → Nasal cannula 2–6L/min or simple face mask 5–10L/min → Monitor and review

Figure 9.2 Reservoir mask

Figure 9.3 Nasal cannula

Figure 9.4 Simple face mask

Figure 9.5 Venturi mask

Figure 9.6 Nebuliser

Figure 9.7 Non-invasive ventilation

Source for Figures 9.6 and 9.7: By James Heilman, MD (own work) [GFDL by CC BY-SA 4.0] via Wikimedia Commons

Emergency Nursing at a Glance, First Edition. Natalie Holbery and Paul Newcombe.

Many patients require supplementary oxygen in emergency departments (EDs). However, oxygen therapy is notoriously poorly understood by both doctors and nurses. Used inappropriately, it can be detrimental to patient care. The principles of the current guidelines for emergency oxygen use in adult patients are:

- Oxygen is a treatment for hypoxemia, not breathlessness.
- Oxygen should be given according to a target oxygen saturation range.
- Aim to achieve normal, or near-normal oxygen saturations for all patients except those at risk of hypercapnic (type II) respiratory failure, or those receiving end of life care.
- Emergency oxygen can be delivered without a prescription, but should be reviewed as soon as possible and prescribed accordingly.
- Both oxygen therapy and saturations should be recorded on the National Early Warning Score (NEWS) chart.
- Identify and treat the underlying cause.

A flow chart for the management of oxygen therapy is shown in Figure 9.1.

Critical illness

Critically ill patients are one exception to the first point above. High-concentration oxygen should be delivered via a non-rebreathe (reservoir) mask at 10–15L/min (Figure 9.2). Once stable, the oxygen dose is reduced and the target saturation 94–98% is used.

Examples of critical illness include:

- Peri-arrest
- Shock, including sepsis and anaphylaxis
- Major trauma
- Near drowning
- Carbon monoxide poisoning
- SpO_2 <85%.

Acute illness

Examples of acute illness are shown in Table 9.1. For patients experiencing serious illness that is not immediately life threatening, moderate levels of supplemental oxygen should only be given if the patient is hypoxaemic. Initial oxygen therapy should be provided via a nasal cannula (Figure 9.3) at 2–6L/min (preferably) or a simple face mask (Figure 9.4) at 5–10L/min unless otherwise stated. A tracheostomy mask can also be used in appropriate patients. The recommended initial oxygen saturation target range is 94–98%. If pulse oximetry is not available, give oxygen as above until pulse oximetry or blood gas results are available. Change to a reservoir mask if the desired saturation range cannot be maintained with a nasal cannula or simple face mask (and seek urgent medical review).

Chronic obstructive pulmonary disease (COPD) and patients at risk of hypercapnia

Some patients are at high risk of CO_2 retention and subsequent respiratory acidosis. This is most commonly seen in COPD

Table 9.1 Examples of acute illness

- Acute asthma	- Pleural effusions
- Pneumonia	- Pneumothorax
- Lung cancer	- Severe anaemia
- Lung fibrosis	- Sickle cell crisis
- Acute heart failure	- Myocardial infarction/acute coronary syndrome
- Pulmonary embolism	- Obstetric emergencies

(Chapter 10), but may also include people with cystic fibrosis, chronic neuromuscular disorders, chest wall deformity or morbid obesity. The administration of uncontrolled high-concentration oxygen in these patients can lead to a further increase in CO_2 retention. Furthermore, if oxygen saturations are raised unnecessarily, this may mask the seriousness of the situation as CO_2 rises unnoticed.

Controlled oxygen therapy should be administered at 28% via a venturi mask (Figure 9.5) at 4L/min with target oxygen saturations of 88–92%. Those patients with previous episodes of respiratory acidosis may have an oxygen alert card with a pre-specified target saturation range. An urgent arterial blood gas (ABG) test should be done to assess $PaCO_2$. If $PaCO_2$ is normal and there is no history of previous respiratory failure, the target range 94–98% can then be used. The ABG should be rechecked after 30–60 minutes or sooner if required. If the $PaCO_2$ is raised but the patient is not acidotic, the percentage of oxygen can be titrated up and down using the venturi system and the target range of 88–92%. For patients with RR>30/min, the flow rate should be increased by 50%. Careful ongoing medical review and regular ABG analysis are required. If the patient is hypercapnic and acidotic, they may need non-invasive ventilation (NIV).

Maximising oxygenation

Supplemental oxygen is only one way of maximising oxygenation. As mentioned earlier, treatment of the underlying cause is essential. Other strategies include:

- Airway maintenance
- Upright positioning
- Reversing respiratory depressants (e.g. opiates)
- Bronchodilation (e.g. inhalers, nebulisers)
- Sputum clearance (e.g. coughing, suction)
- Invasive or non-invasive ventilation
- Increasing haemoglobin levels
- Increasing perfusion (e.g. fluid replacement).

Nebuliser delivery

For patients with asthma, nebuliser therapy (Figure 9.6) should be driven with oxygen at a flow rate of >6L/min. For patients with COPD and others at risk of hypercapnia, nebulisers should be driven by compressed air and, if necessary, supplementary oxygen can be given concurrently by nasal cannulae at 2–6L/min to maintain oxygen saturation of 88–92%. Once nebulised therapy is complete, the patient should be recommenced on their previous oxygen therapy.

Non-invasive ventilation (NIV)

For patients who continue to deteriorate despite oxygen therapy, ventilatory support may be necessary. Some may require intubation, a period of invasive ventilation and admission to the intensive care unit (ICU). For others, NIV may be considered, either with a view to preventing this or as a ceiling treatment if invasive ventilation is inappropriate. NIV is the provision of ventilatory support via the mouth and/or nose using a mask (Figure 9.7). It is indicated in hypercapnic (type II) respiratory failure with respiratory acidosis, and in the ED is most commonly used in COPD. Continuous positive airway pressure (CPAP) is similar to NIV, but it is not indicated for these patients because it may exacerbate hypercapnia. NIV uses bi-level pressure allowing CO_2 excretion on expiration. CPAP is particularly indicated in pulmonary oedema, but is also effective in pneumonia, sleep apnoea and chest wall trauma. Patients receiving NIV or CPAP require close monitoring in the resuscitation area.

10 Respiratory conditions

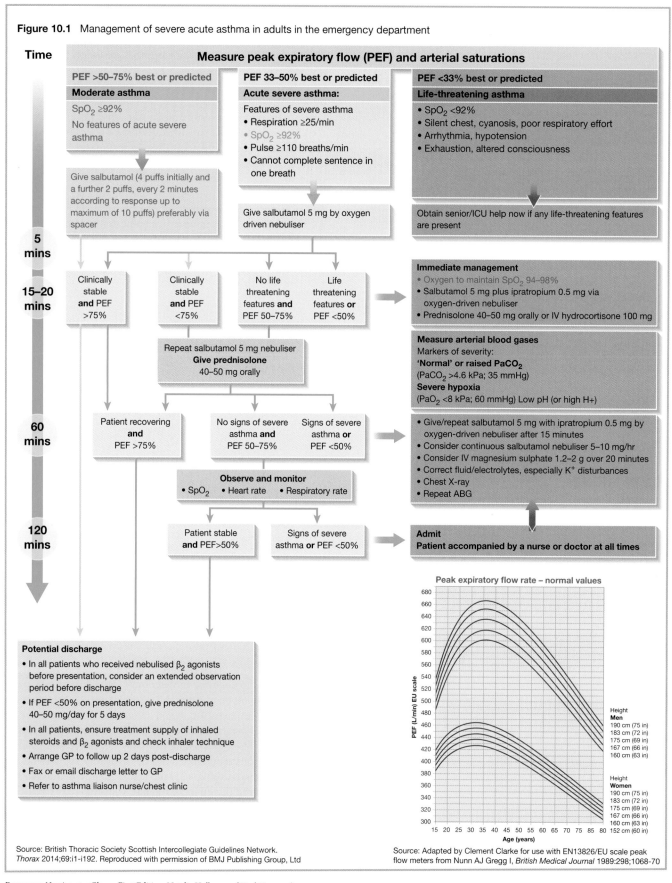

Figure 10.1 Management of severe acute asthma in adults in the emergency department

Time

Measure peak expiratory flow (PEF) and arterial saturations

PEF >50–75% best or predicted
Moderate asthma
SpO₂ ≥92%
No features of acute severe asthma

PEF 33–50% best or predicted
Acute severe asthma:
Features of severe asthma
• Respiration ≥25/min
• SpO₂ ≥92%
• Pulse ≥110 breaths/min
• Cannot complete sentence in one breath

PEF <33% best or predicted
Life-threatening asthma
• SpO₂ <92%
• Silent chest, cyanosis, poor respiratory effort
• Arrhythmia, hypotension
• Exhaustion, altered consciousness

Give salbutamol (4 puffs initially and a further 2 puffs, every 2 minutes according to response up to maximum of 10 puffs) preferably via spacer

Give salbutamol 5 mg by oxygen driven nebuliser

Obtain senior/ICU help now if any life-threatening features are present

5 mins

15–20 mins

Clinically stable **and** PEF >75%

Clinically stable **and** PEF <75%

No life threatening features **and** PEF 50–75%

Life threatening features **or** PEF <50%

Immediate management
• Oxygen to maintain SpO₂ 94–98%
• Salbutamol 5 mg plus ipratropium 0.5 mg via oxygen-driven nebuliser
• Prednisolone 40–50 mg orally or IV hydrocortisone 100 mg

Repeat salbutamol 5 mg nebuliser
Give prednisolone
40–50 mg orally

Measure arterial blood gases
Markers of severity:
'Normal' or raised PaCO₂
(PaCO₂ >4.6 kPa; 35 mmHg)
Severe hypoxia
(PaO₂ <8 kPa; 60 mmHg) Low pH (or high H+)

60 mins

Patient recovering **and** PEF >75%

No signs of severe asthma **and** PEF 50–75%

Signs of severe asthma **or** PEF <50%

• Give/repeat salbutamol 5 mg with ipratropium 0.5 mg by oxygen-driven nebuliser after 15 minutes
• Consider continuous salbutamol nebuliser 5–10 mg/hr
• Consider IV magnesium sulphate 1.2–2 g over 20 minutes
• Correct fluid/electrolytes, especially K⁺ disturbances
• Chest X-ray
• Repeat ABG

Observe and monitor
• SpO₂   • Heart rate   • Respiratory rate

120 mins

Patient stable **and** PEF>50%

Signs of severe asthma **or** PEF <50%

Admit
Patient accompanied by a nurse or doctor at all times

Potential discharge
• In all patients who received nebulised β₂ agonists before presentation, consider an extended observation period before discharge
• If PEF <50% on presentation, give prednisolone 40–50 mg/day for 5 days
• In all patients, ensure treatment supply of inhaled steroids and β₂ agonists and check inhaler technique
• Arrange GP to follow up 2 days post-discharge
• Fax or email discharge letter to GP
• Refer to asthma liaison nurse/chest clinic

Peak expiratory flow rate – normal values

PEF (L/min) EU scale

Age (years)

Height
Men
190 cm (75 in)
183 cm (72 in)
175 cm (69 in)
167 cm (66 in)
160 cm (63 in)

Height
Women
190 cm (75 in)
183 cm (72 in)
175 cm (69 in)
167 cm (66 in)
160 cm (63 in)
152 cm (60 in)

Source: British Thoracic Society Scottish Intercollegiate Guidelines Network.
Thorax 2014;69:i1-i192. Reproduced with permission of BMJ Publishing Group, Ltd

Source: Adapted by Clement Clarke for use with EN13826/EU scale peak flow meters from Nunn AJ Gregg I, *British Medical Journal* 1989;298;1068-70

Asthma

Asthma is a common chronic inflammatory condition of the airways characterised by reversible airflow limitation. Causes are genetic and environmental, resulting in bronchial inflammation, bronchospasm and mucous hypersecretion. Symptoms are recurring and variable, but include dyspnoea, wheezing, coughing and chest tightness. Asthma is most common in adolescents.

Assessment

Asthma presentations are categorised according to severity, so rapid, accurate assessment is essential. Patients often report worsening symptoms unresponsive to their usual inhaled medication. The onset may be over a few days or relatively sudden. There may be associated cold and flu symptoms or exposure to an allergen. History of emergency department (ED) attendances and hospital admissions are important clues, but particularly previous episodes requiring ventilation in an intensive care unit (ICU).

Management

See the ED asthma management flow chart (Figure 10.1).

Chronic obstructive pulmonary disease (COPD)

COPD is a common long-term condition characterised by persistent airflow limitation that is not fully reversible. Smoking is the predominant cause, resulting in an abnormal inflammatory response to noxious particles or gases due to airway and parenchymal damage (emphysema and fibrosis). This leads to reduced lung elastic recoil, airway collapse and air trapping. Gaseous exchange is altered and chronic hypoxia develops, with or without hypercapnia. COPD may not be diagnosed so should be considered in smokers with dyspnoea, chronic cough and sputum production. Symptoms are progressive, although there is little short-term variability. COPD is characterised by exacerbations.

Assessment

History often reveals symptoms worsening over a few days with reduced exercise tolerance and lack of response to usual treatment. Cold or flu symptoms may also be present. Incidence increases in the winter months. Increased effort of breathing is evident in the inability to complete sentences, accessory muscle use, pursed-lip breathing, cyanosis, reduced level of consciousness, etc. (Chapter 8). Chronic hypoxia and mild tachypnoea may be normal. Raised temperature and purulent sputum may suggest infection and a chest X-ray is indicated. Haemodynamic assessment should be undertaken to identify sepsis (Chapter 13). Peak expiratory flow (PEF) rate may be useful to demonstrate reversibility after treatment, but spirometry is more helpful in COPD. Sputum should be sent for microscopy, culture and sensitivity if purulent.

Management

Oxygen therapy in COPD requires careful management (Chapter 9). Usually, 28% via a venturi mask with target saturations of 88–92% is recommended initially, unless there is an alert card. An urgent arterial blood gas (ABG) test should be done to assess PaO_2, $PaCO_2$ and pH. Oxygen should then be titrated accordingly. Patients with type II respiratory failure and/or acidosis may require non-invasive ventilation (NIV). Other treatments include nebulised bronchodilators (salbutamol, ipratropium bromide – must be air driven), steroids, theophylline and antibiotics. The patient should be supported in an upright position and will require careful ongoing monitoring. Admission is usually required.

Pneumonia

Pneumonia is an acute inflammation of the lower respiratory tract, commonly due to bacterial or viral infection. Areas of alveolar tissue or whole lobes become colonised, inflamed and filled with fluid. Small airways collapse and result in impaired gaseous exchange. Pneumonia is classified as community acquired or hospital acquired. There may be comorbidity, such as asthma or COPD.

Assessment

Standard respiratory assessment should be undertaken (Chapter 8). Signs include dyspnoea, tachypnoea, productive cough, pleuritic chest pain and fever. Chest examination may reveal reduced air entry, crackles and dullness to percussion. Worrying signs include fatigue, confusion, reduced level of consciousness and cyanosis. Chest X-ray and sputum culture are usually required. ABG may be indicated with significant signs. As previously, signs of sepsis should be actively sought.

Management

Oxygen should be given if the patient is hypoxaemic. In severe cases, NIV, CPAP or invasive ventilation is indicated. Oral or intravenous (IV) antibiotics are given and admission may be required.

Pulmonary embolism (PE)

PE is a blood clot in the pulmonary artery caused by venous thromboembolism (VTE). It is most commonly a result of deep vein thrombosis (DVT) in the leg. Obstruction causes reduced blood flow through the lungs and increased pressure on the heart. The risk of PE is increased by immobility, surgery, cancer, pregnancy, obesity and smoking.

Assessment

PE causes dyspnoea, tachycardia, pleuritic chest pain, cough and dizziness. Massive PE is a cause of cardiac arrest. Signs of DVT should be actively sought. Positive D-dimer suggests evidence of thrombosis. An electrocardiogram (ECG) and chest X-ray (CXR) may show non-specific signs or other diagnoses. Computerised tomography pulmonary angiography (CTPA) is diagnostic.

Management

Anticoagulation is the main treatment for PE. Oxygen and analgesia may also be required. Thrombolysis is considered in massive PE and can be given during cardiac arrest.

Spontaneous pneumothorax

A pneumothorax is a collapsed lung and can occur due to trauma, surgery or lung disease. Spontaneous pneumothorax is more likely in tall, thin, young men and can recur.

Assessment

Signs include dyspnoea and pleuritic chest pain. Breath sounds may be reduced and percussion may be hyper-resonant. A CXR confirms the diagnosis.

Management

Management includes oxygen, analgesia and aspiration or chest drain insertion. Small pneumothoraces may resolve spontaneously.

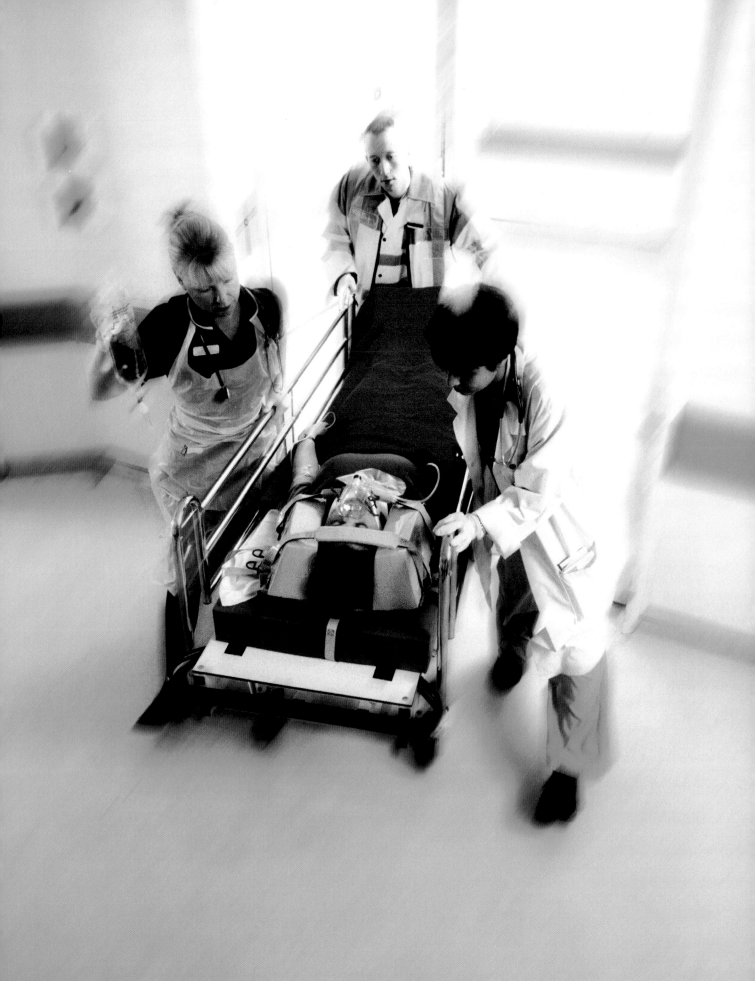

Circulation

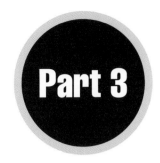

Part 3

Chapters

11 Assessment of circulation

Figure 11.1 Methods of haemodynamic assessment

Non-invasive haemodynamic assessment	Indicators of organ perfusion	Invasive haemodynamic assessment
Respiratory rate	Skin condition (capillary refill time)	Urine output
Heart rate	Level of consciousness	Arterial blood pressure
Blood pressure	Blood tests, e.g. lactate, ABG, U&E	Central venous pressure

Figure 11.2 Normal ranges

Parameter	Normal range	Abnormal range	Name of abnormality
Respiratory rate	12–20/min	<12/min	Bradypnoea
		>20/min	Tachypnoea
Heart rate	60–100/min	<60/min	Bradycardia
		>100/min	Tachycardia
Blood pressure	Systolic 90–140 mmHg	<90 mmHg	Hypotension
		>140 mmHg	Hypertension
	Diastolic 60–90 mmHg	<60 mm/Hg	Hypotension
		>90 mm/Hg	Hypertension
	MAP 70–100 mmHg	<70 mmHg	Hypotension
		>100 mmHg	Hypertension
Capillary refill time	<2 sec	>2 sec	Delayed capillary refill time
Urine output	>0.5 ml/kg/hr	<0.5 ml/kg/hr	Oliguria
Central venous pressure	2–6 mmHg	<2 mmHg	Low central venous pressure
		>2 mmHg	High central venous pressure

Figure 11.3 Relationship between blood pressure and cardiac output

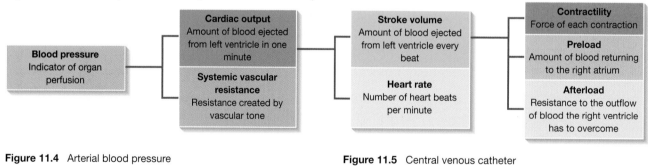

Blood pressure
Indicator of organ perfusion

Cardiac output
Amount of blood ejected from left ventricle in one minute

Systemic vascular resistance
Resistance created by vascular tone

Stroke volume
Amount of blood ejected from left ventricle every beat

Heart rate
Number of heart beats per minute

Contractility
Force of each contraction

Preload
Amount of blood returning to the right atrium

Afterload
Resistance to the outflow of blood the right ventricle has to overcome

Figure 11.4 Arterial blood pressure

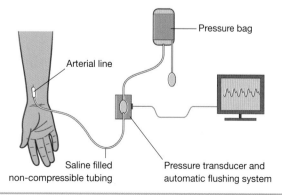

Pressure bag

Arterial line

Saline filled non-compressible tubing

Pressure transducer and automatic flushing system

Figure 11.5 Central venous catheter

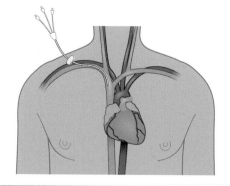

Emergency Nursing at a Glance, First Edition. Natalie Holbery and Paul Newcombe.
© 2016 John Wiley & Sons, Ltd. Published 2016 by John Wiley & Sons, Ltd. Companion website: www.ataglanceseries.com/nursing/emergencynursing

Assessment of circulation is a core element of patient evaluation and ongoing monitoring, regardless of whether there is a primary circulatory problem or not. Similarly, if there is a primary circulatory problem, this will have an impact on all aspects of vital function. Problems arise from disruption to the circulating volume (shock) or from a cardiac cause (acute coronary syndrome [ACS], arrhythmia). Poor perfusion leads to tissue hypoxia, organ failure and death (Chapter 13). Assessment focuses on measuring haemodynamic parameters and examining organ perfusion (Figure 11.1). Normal ranges are shown in Figure 11.2.

Non-invasive haemodynamic assessment

Respiratory rate (RR)

RR is one of the most sensitive indicators of impending cardiovascular problems. The respiratory centre in the medulla oblongata is triggered early in any potential demand for increased oxygen (e.g. after exercise or shock). In decompensated shock and other causes of metabolic acidosis, the respiratory centre responds to falling pH and increases breathing rate and depth to 'blow off' CO_2.

Heart rate (HR)

HR is also a sensitive indicator of cardiovascular problems. Terms like 'heart rate' and 'pulse' are used interchangeably, but may mean different things. HR may be measured from a manual pulse, from a pulse oximeter, from a cardiac monitor, from an electronic blood pressure machine, from invasive monitoring or from auscultating the heart. It is possible to record HR on a cardiac monitor, for example, but for the patient to have an absent pulse. This is called pulseless electrical activity (PEA) and is a cardiac arrest rhythm (Chapter 18). Therefore, palpating a manual pulse is essential, feeling for:

- Rate
- Rhythm – regular or irregular (an electrocardiograph [ECG] may be indicated)
- Amplitude – quality of the pulse.

Amplitude reflects stroke volume (SV) and therefore cardiac output and blood pressure (Figure 11.3). Findings include:

- Weak and thready
- Normal/good
- Bounding
- Palpable radial pulse = systolic blood pressure (BP) >90 mmHg
- Palpable brachial pulse = systolic BP >60 mmHg.

Blood pressure (BP)

BP is the pressure exerted by the blood on the arterial wall. It is determined by the amount of blood pumping out of the heart (CO) and the resistance created by the tone of the blood vessels (SVR). Systolic BP is the maximum pressure exerted when the heart is contracting, whereas diastolic BP is the minimum pressure when the heart is at rest.

There are a large number of factors that influence a person's BP, such as age, sex, weight and lifestyle, so it is important to compare current measurements with the patient's normal or predicted normal readings. There are many different manual and electronic devices used for non-invasive BP measurement and all have the potential to provide inaccurate readings. Factors such as cuff size and arm position will also affect accuracy.

Pulse pressure (PP) is the difference between systolic and diastolic BP and indicates vascular tone.

- Narrow PP (<30 mmHg) indicates vasoconstriction
- Wide PP (>50 mmHg) indicates poor arterial compliance or vasodilation.

Indicators of organ perfusion

Skin condition

The skin is an important indicator of tissue perfusion. Vasoconstriction during compensation reduces peripheral blood supply and the skin becomes pale, cool and sweaty.

Capillary refill time (CRT) is a measurement of skin perfusion. It is the amount of time taken for blanched peripheral tissue to re-perfuse. It is undertaken by holding the hand above the level of the heart and pressing on the nail bed for five seconds. Alternatively, digital pressure can be applied to the sternum. The amount of time taken for a pink colour to return to the skin is the CRT. Age, circulatory problems and ambient temperature can affect readings.

Level of consciousness (LOC)

The brain is one of the last organs to lose its blood supply during compensation, so reduced LOC due to falling perfusion is a critical sign. Early signs include anxiety and confusion.

Blood tests

Blood tests that indicate organ perfusion include lactate, arterial blood gas (ABG) and urea and electrolytes (U&E).

Invasive haemodynamic assessment

Urine output (UO)

The kidneys are an essential window into organ perfusion, due to water conservation during compensation. Hourly UO needs to be measured invasively via a urinary catheter to ensure accuracy.

Arterial blood pressure (ABP)

Invasive ABP is measured in critically ill patients by using a radial artery catheter and electronic transducer (Figure 11.4). It is more accurate than non-invasive BP measurement and provides continuous readings for systolic, diastolic and mean arterial pressure (MAP). MAP is an average value derived from systolic and diastolic readings and considered to be a more accurate indicator of end organ perfusion. Monitoring displays MAP as an arterial waveform. Risks include bleeding, infection and air bolus. Careful management is required to ensure reliable readings.

Central venous pressure (CVP)

CVP is measured using a central venous catheter (Figure 11.5) and either a water-filled manometer or, more commonly nowadays, an electronic transducer. It is the pressure measured in the vena cava just before it joins the right atrium, and it is therefore an indicator of preload. As a result, it is useful in assessing fluid replacement. It is influenced by a number of factors including body position, transducer height and intrathoracic pressure. Normal values vary and should be monitored as a trend. A waveform is displayed on the monitor.

12 Circulation interventions

Figure 12.1 Standard IV cannula

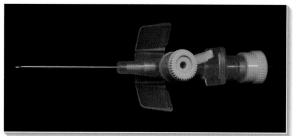

Source: By Fifo [GFDL by CC-BY-SA-2.5] via Wikimedia Commons

Figure 12.2 IV cannula flow rates

Size	Colour	Gauge	Flow rate (ml/min)
↑	Brown	14	300
	Grey	16	200
	Green	18	90
	Pink	20	61
	Blue	22	36

Figure 12.3 Determinants of cannula flow rate

Relationship between IV cannula, infusion and flow rate		Significance
Flow rate is directly proportional to...	Cannula diameter (bore or gauge)	• Wide bore cannulae offer fastest flow-rate • Use in combination with blood giving set which has a wider lumen than a standard infusion set
	Pressure gradient	• Pressure increased by raising height of the infusion fluids or applying pressure manually, via a pressure bag, or via an electronic device, e.g. rapid infuser
Flow rate is inversely proportional to...	Cannula length	• Short peripheral cannulae have a faster flow rate than long central lines
	Fluid viscosity	• Crystalloid and colloid are faster to give • Blood is slower to give because it is thicker

Figure 12.4 (a, b) Central venous catheter

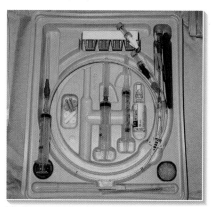

(a) Source: By Clinical Cases [GFDL by CC-BY-SA-2.5] via Wikimedia Commons

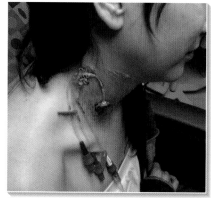

(b) Source: Via Wikimedia Commons

Figure 12.5 Intraosseus device

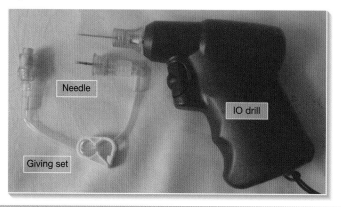

Emergency Nursing at a Glance, First Edition. Natalie Holbery and Paul Newcombe.
© 2016 John Wiley & Sons, Ltd. Published 2016 by John Wiley & Sons, Ltd. Companion website: www.ataglanceseries.com/nursing/emergencynursing

Most unwell patients presenting to an emergency department (ED) will receive interventions relating to circulation. These may be restricted to precautionary intravenous (IV) cannulation, but many patients will also require IV fluids, blood products, electrolytes and other interventions. Management should be based upon careful, accurate assessment that should consider the history, follow a thorough 'ABCDE' approach (Chapter 4) and include appropriate investigations. Evaluation of the effectiveness of these interventions through ongoing monitoring is essential.

Peripheral IV access

IV access is a common intervention in an ED. Many unwell patients will have blood tests taken and a peripheral IV cannula is usually inserted at the same time (Figure 12.1). IV cannulation should be undertaken by appropriately trained individuals, following local evidence-based standardised protocols. Consideration should include:

- Indications/contraindications
- Informed consent
- Equipment selection
- Site selection
- Infection control precautions
- Documentation.

The size and number of IV cannulae are dictated by the individual situation. Small cannulae are easier to insert, particularly with the very young, older patients and those with small or very fragile veins. However, they are difficult to draw blood from and have a slow infusion rate (Figure 12.2). A 14G (brown) cannula can deliver 1 litre of crystalloid in just over 3 minutes. IV cannula flow rate is influenced by a range of other factors (Figure 12.3), but for rapid fluid resuscitation two wide-bore cannulae are usually inserted in large, superficial peripheral veins (antecubital fossa).

Central venous catheter (CVC)

CVC line insertion is considered in a range of situations, but usually when the patient is critically ill. Other indications include:

- Peripheral IV cannulation impossible
- Haemodynamic monitoring
- Administration of drugs centrally
- Insertion of temporary pacemaker.

Femoral line insertion is usually the quickest and easiest to achieve, but is more suitable for short-term use. Access is gained in the groin with a single lumen catheter. A neck line, inserted in the internal jugular vein or subclavian vein takes more skill and time, but is more suitable for longer-term use (Figure 12.4). These are usually triple lumen catheters, which can have dedicated lines for different uses. Central line insertion carries a number of serious risks:

- Infection
- Haemorrhage
- Air embolism
- Thrombosis
- Arrhythmias
- Pneumothorax.

Intraosseus (IO) access

IO access is a rapid alternative to central venous access and other obsolete methods (such as venous cutdown), when emergency IV access is impossible. IO access is mainly used in children, but its use in adult trauma and cardiac arrest is increasing, particularly in the pre-hospital setting. A powered device is used to insert the needle (Figure 12.5). Recommended insertion sites include:

- Proximal tibia
- Distal tibia
- Proximal humerus.

Fluids require delivery using a pressure bag or 50 ml syringe.

Fluid challenge

A fluid challenge is a large volume of fluid given over a short period of time when fluid resuscitation is required (e.g. in shock). Specific protocols may differ but, as a guide, 500 ml crystalloid (e.g. 0.9% saline) is given over 15 minutes. The patient is reassessed for improvement in vital signs ($\downarrow$ respiratory rate [RR], $\downarrow$ heart rate [HR], $\uparrow$ blood pressure [BP], $\uparrow$ urine output (UO), $\uparrow$ central venous pressure [CVP]), but also to monitor for poor tolerance (evidence of pulmonary oedema – difficulty in breathing $\downarrow$ SpO$_2$). If required, a further fluid bolus of 250–500 ml is given followed by reassessment. This can be repeated up to 2,000 ml before expert help is sought. Large amounts of crystalloid increase the risk of complications, such as oedema, haemodilution and hypothermia (warmed fluids should be used).

Blood transfusion

Significant blood loss should ideally be replaced with blood products. However, blood is an expensive, finite resource that is also not risk free. Blood products include:

- Red cells
- Platelets
- Fresh frozen plasma (FFP)
- Cryoprecipitate (clotting factors).

Samples for blood grouping and crossmatching should be urgently sent to the laboratory. Blood for immediate use is usually available in the ED: O negative for women; O positive for men. ABO group-specific blood can be available within 10 minutes of a sample being received. Fully crossmatched blood takes 30–40 minutes. Many hospitals have a major haemorrhage protocol for significant blood loss. Indications include major trauma (Chapter 61), major obstetric haemorrhage and gastro-intestinal bleeding.

Other interventions

A range of other interventions are employed to correct problems with circulation. Early identification and management of the underlying cause is a key principle:

- Medical treatment (e.g. for diabetic ketoacidosis (DKA)
- Electrolyte replacement
- Cardioversion
- Inotropes
- Correct clotting (e.g. vitamin K, tranexamic acid)
- Positioning – lay flat, legs elevated
- Direct pressure (and elevation if appropriate) to obvious external haemorrhage
- Pressure dressings
- Reduce fractures (particularly long bones)
- Expedite to surgery.

Finally, it is essential that problems with airway and breathing are identified and corrected so that oxygen delivery to the tissues is maximised. Reassessment and careful ongoing monitoring are also essential.

(13) Shock

Figure 13.1 Classification of shock

Component	Problem	Type of shock	
Heart	Pump failure	Cardiogenic shock (also obstructive shock in some circumstances)	
Blood (or other body fluid)	Loss of circulating volume	Hypovolaemic shock (also haemorrhagic shock if caused by blood loss)	
Blood vessels (vasculature)	Loss of vascular tone (characterised by massive vasodilation)	Distributive shock	Septic shock
			Anaphylactic shock
			Neurogenic shock

Figure 13.2 Compensated versus decompensated shock

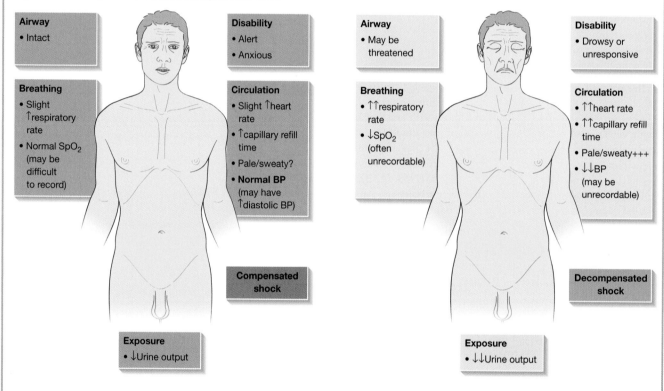

Airway
• Intact

Disability
• Alert
• Anxious

Breathing
• Slight ↑respiratory rate
• Normal SpO₂ (may be difficult to record)

Circulation
• Slight ↑heart rate
• ↑capillary refill time
• Pale/sweaty?
• **Normal BP** (may have ↑diastolic BP)

Compensated shock

Exposure
• ↓Urine output

Airway
• May be threatened

Disability
• Drowsy or unresponsive

Breathing
• ↑↑respiratory rate
• ↓SpO₂ (often unrecordable)

Circulation
• ↑↑heart rate
• ↑↑capillary refill time
• Pale/sweaty+++
• ↓↓BP (may be unrecordable)

Decompensated shock

Exposure
• ↓↓Urine output

Figure 13.3 Classification of sepsis

Systemic inflammatory response syndrome (SIRS) (two or more of the following features)	
Temperature	Hyperthermia (>38°C) or hypothermia (<36°C)
Heart rate	Tachycardia (>90/min)
Respiratory rate	Tachypnoea (>20/min or $PaCO_2$ <4.3 kPa)
White blood cells	High (>12 x 10⁹/L) or low (<4 x 10⁹/L)

Sepsis	SIRS plus clinical evidence of infection
Severe sepsis	Sepsis plus evidence of organ dysfunction: • Hypotension (SBP <90 mmHg or MAP <60 mmHg or reduction in patient's normal SBP by >40 mmHg) • Oliguria (urine output <0.5 ml/kg/hr) • Hypoxia (SpO_2 <93% or PaO_2 <9kPa) • Altered mental state • Metabolic acidosis • Lactate >2 mmol/L (hallmark of severe sepsis) • Coagulopathy (international normalised ratio [INR] >1.5 or activated partial thromboplastin time [APTT] >60 sec) • Bowel ileus (stasis) • Abnormal liver function tests
Septic shock	Severe sepsis with persistent hypotension despite adequate fluid volume replacement (1.5–2 L fluid)

Emergency Nursing at a Glance, First Edition. Natalie Holbery and Paul Newcombe.
© 2016 John Wiley & Sons, Ltd. Published 2016 by John Wiley & Sons, Ltd. Companion website: www.ataglanceseries.com/nursing/emergencynursing

Shock is a complex physiological state that results in an inability of the cardiovascular system to supply adequate oxygen and nutrients to the tissues. Cardiovascular dysfunction leads to poor tissue perfusion causing disrupted cellular metabolism, organ failure and eventually death. It is characterised by a problem with one or more component(s) of the cardiovascular system: heart, circulating volume or vascular tone. This reflects the type of shock seen (Figure 13.1). Hypovolaemic and septic shock are particularly common in the emergency department (ED), but anaphylactic and cardiogenic shock (Chapter 17) are also encountered. Obstructive shock is similar to cardiogenic shock, seen in tension pneumothorax, cardiac tamponade and pulmonary embolism. Neurogenic shock is mainly seen in cervical spinal cord injury and is uncommon.

Stages of shock

Shock is easiest to understand as either compensated or decompensated shock. The key difference is whether the systolic blood pressure (BP) is normal or not (Figure 13.2).

Compensated shock

During compensated shock, the body's compensatory mechanisms respond to the potential drop in blood pressure. This triggers a negative feedback response resulting in:

1 Raised heart rate and contractility
2 Vasoconstriction
3 Reduced urine output (conserving circulating volume).

The net result is maintenance of the patient's normal blood pressure. Respiratory rate and depth also increase to maximise oxygen availability. Compensated shock is easily missed because signs can be subtle. At this stage, shock is usually responsive to treatment.

Decompensated shock

Once systolic blood pressure drops, critical organ perfusion is no longer maintained and tissue damage occurs. Reduced oxygenation causes cells to switch to anaerobic metabolism, generating poor energy yields, excess lactic acid and metabolic acidosis. The cellular sodium/potassium pump fails, causing fluid and electrolyte shifts and cell death.

Decompensated shock may occur because of the size of the insult (e.g. significant blood loss), prolonged and untreated compensated shock, poor compensatory mechanisms (e.g. owing to increased age or comorbidities) or any combination of these. Shock may respond to treatment at this stage, but the outcome is more difficult to predict.

Hypovolaemic shock

Hypovolaemic shock is associated with the loss of blood (haemorrhagic shock) or other body fluid. Fluids may be lost either internally or externally (Table 13.1).

Previously healthy individuals can compensate for significant fluid volume losses (1.5L blood) before decompensation occurs and systolic blood pressure drops. Thorough cardiovascular assessment is undertaken (Chapter 11), looking in particular for subtle signs of compensation. Blood and other fluid losses should be actively identified. In trauma and surgery, consideration should be given to obvious external haemorrhage, but also significant hidden internal bleeding in body compartments, such as the chest and abdomen.

Management includes oxygen, intravenous (IV) access, fluid challenges, reassessment, ongoing monitoring and treating the cause, such as stopping the bleeding with surgery (Chapter 12).

Septic shock

Sepsis is a systemic inflammatory response to infection (often bacterial) and has a number of stages (Figure 13.3). The source

Table 13.1

Blood loss	Other fluid loss
Trauma	Diarrhoea and/or vomiting
Peri-/post-operatively	Excessive diuresis (e.g. diabetic
Gastro-intestinal (GI)	ketoacidosis [DKA])
bleeding (oral/per rectum)	Excessive sweating
Per vagina bleeding	Burns
Epistaxis	Pancreatitis

of infection is not always identified, but can be related to any body system. Chest, urinary and IV line infections are common. Sepsis is a complex inflammatory process resulting in poor tissue perfusion due to:

• Leaky capillaries
• Vasodilation
• Microthrombi.

Some patients may initially present with a hyperdynamic phase characterised by bounding pulses and warm, flushed skin. However, sepsis often presents with a classic shock picture: weak, thready pulses; hypotension; pallor/sweating.

Management of sepsis is focused on maximising oxygen delivery to the tissues while urgently treating the infection. Six key interventions have been shown to double the patient's chance of survival if delivered within the first hour of diagnosis. The 'Sepsis Six' are:

• High flow oxygen
• Take blood cultures
• IV broad-spectrum antibiotics
• IV fluid challenges
• Measure lactate and haemoglobin
• Measure hourly urine output.

The patient should be started on a sepsis care bundle and referred to the intensive care unit (ICU).

Anaphylactic shock

Anaphylaxis is a severe, life-threatening, generalised hypersensitivity reaction. The allergen is not always identified but includes:

• Stings
• Food: nuts, dairy, seafood
• Drugs: antibiotics, anaesthetics, contrast
• Latex.

Anaphylaxis is characterised by:

• Sudden onset and rapid progression of symptoms
• Life-threatening problems (airway, breathing, circulation)
• Skin/mucosal changes (flushing, urticaria, angioedema)
• GI symptoms (vomiting, abdominal pain).

Management of anaphylaxis includes:

• Lay patient flat with legs raised
• Remove trigger if possible (e.g. stop drug infusion)
• Intramuscular (IM) adrenaline (epinephrine) 0.5 mg (in adults)
• Airway support
• High-flow oxygen
• IV fluid challenge
• IM/IV antihistamine (e.g. chlorphenamine – Piriton®)
• IM/IV steroids (e.g. hydrocortisone)
• Ongoing monitoring – symptoms can recur.

14 12-lead electrocardiogram (ECG)

Figure 14.1 ECG calibration

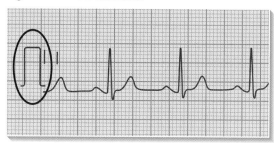

Figure 14.2 Limb electrode positions

Right arm limb lead (RA, red)	Right forearm, proximal to wrist
Left arm limb lead (LA, yellow)	Left forearm, proximal to wrist
Left leg limb lead (LL, green)	Left lower leg, proximal to ankle
Right leg limb lead (RL, black)	Right lower leg, proximal to ankle

Figure 14.3 Standard ECG chest electrode positions

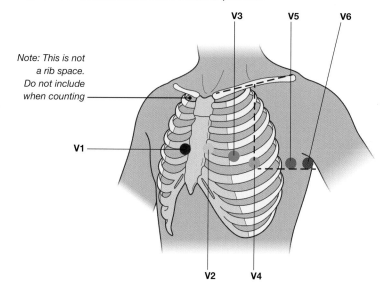

Note: This is not a rib space. Do not include when counting

V1 (C1)	Fourth intercostal space at the right sternal edge
V2 (C2)	Fourth intercostal space at the left sternal edge
V3 (C3)	Midway between V2 and V4
V4 (C4)	Fifth intercostal space in the mid-clavicular line
V5 (C5)	Left anterior axillary line at the same horizontal level as V4
V6 (C6)	Left mid-axillary line at the same horizontal level as V4 and V5

Figure 14.4 A normal 12-lead ECG

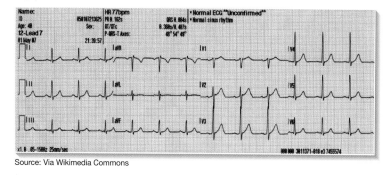

Source: Via Wikimedia Commons

Figure 14.5 12-lead ECG territories

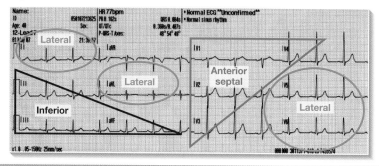

Emergency Nursing at a Glance, First Edition. Natalie Holbery and Paul Newcombe
© 2016 John Wiley & Sons, Ltd. Published 2016 by John Wiley & Sons, Ltd. Companion website: www.ataglanceseries.com/nursing/emergencynursing

Performing a 12-lead electrocardiogram (ECG) is one of the most common activities undertaken by nurses working in emergency care. It represents the heart's electrical activity and is used to confirm or rule out serious cardiac problems and other disease processes. Although used in conjunction with patient history, examination and other diagnostic tools, getting ECG recording correct is vital to aid diagnosis. This chapter outlines the correct procedure for recording an ECG and briefly explores basic ECG interpretation. To master ECG interpretation requires significant practice.

While it is termed a 12-lead ECG, there are only 10 leads that attach to the patient. The word 'lead' in this context is used interchangeably to refer to both the electrode that is attached to the patient and the view that is seen on the ECG recording.

Indications

There are a number of indications for performing an ECG in emergency care. The most common is chest pain; however, there are numerous other presentations and complaints that require an ECG. These may include, but are not limited to:

- Collapse
- Altered conscious level
- Shortness of breath
- Palpitations
- Abdominal pain
- Back pain.

Preparation

Before performing an ECG it is vital to prepare the patient. Verbal consent should be obtained. When consent is not possible, perhaps because a patient lacks capacity, it is deemed to be performed in the patient's best interest. The patient should be informed of the reasons for performing the ECG, that leads will be attached via adhesive clips, it requires them to remain still throughout the recording, it is painless and lasts a few minutes. The chest and legs need to be exposed so patient dignity needs to be assured. Uncovering only what is required, closing curtains or doors and placing a sign to prevent entry are recommended. For consistency, the patient should ideally be in a semi-recumbent position of approximately 45 degrees. Skin preparation may need to be undertaken to improve electrode adherence. Skin may be cleansed with either soap and water or alcohol wipes. Dry skin can be exfoliated with gentle abrasion. Chest hair may need to be removed with a clean disposable razor.

Before performing the ECG a couple of checks are required. First, the machine needs to be in good working order and within its service date. The leads should also be clean and intact. The voltage and paper speed should be checked to ensure they are calibrated as per standard. They should be set at a gain of 10 mm/mV (10 mm high = 1 mV) with a paper speed of 25 mm per second (5 mm wide = 0.2 seconds). This calibration can be seen on the ECG as small boxes at the beginning of the trace (Figure 14.1). If these settings are changed, the waves on the ECG will be misleading if the person interpreting the ECG has not checked this. For example, if the paper speed is set at 50 mm per second, the ECG trace may appear as a bradycardia.

Recording the ECG

In order to accurately record an ECG, the electrodes must be placed in the correct position. There are 4 limb leads and 6 chest leads. Limb electrodes should be placed on the wrists and ankles whenever possible (Figure 14.2). Moving them up the limbs will alter the appearance of the ECG. Attaching them to the torso should be avoided. The chest leads must be placed exactly as indicated in Figure 14.3. V1 and V2 are placed at the 4th intercostal space, either side of the sternum. Care should be taken to not count the small space between the clavicle and the first rib as the 1st intercostal space. Next, V4 is placed in the 5th intercostal space and in the mid-clavicular line. V3 should be placed between V2 and V4. V5 and V6 should be placed in horizontal alignment with V4. V5 is on the anterior axillary line and V6 on the mid-axillary line. V4, V5 and V6 should be placed under the left breast with female patients when necessary.

Before recording, the ECG filter should be switched off and only used if artefact on initial recordings makes interpretation impossible. When the patient is still and the trace on the screen is clear, the ECG can then be printed. A standard ECG will usually show a snapshot of 12 leads (Figure 14.4), plus or minus a rhythm strip (often lead II):

- I, II, III
- aVR, aVL, aVF
- V1–V6 (or C1–C6).

Once the ECG has been recorded, it is imperative that it is labelled correctly. Patient information should include their full name, date of birth and hospital number. Depending on local guidelines, these details may be programmed into the ECG before the recording. Often, however, this information is transcribed by the nurse once the ECG has been printed. If the ECG is part of a series, each one should also be numbered. In some cases, if the patient has chest pain the pain score may also be documented on the ECG. A senior clinician should then be asked to review and sign the ECG, documenting the findings on the ECG.

Basic interpretation

It is important to understand how the ECG relates to cardiac activity. Chapter 15 describes how the cardiac cycle relates to normal sinus rhythm and the variations seen in common cardiac arrhythmias. This is rhythm strip analysis. Chapter 16 discusses the use of the 12-lead ECG in helping to diagnose acute coronary syndrome (ACS). The focus here is on ST-segment changes. Figure 14.5 shows the groupings of ECG leads that reflect the different cardiac territories:

- V1–V4 (anterior/septal)
- V4, V5, I, aVL (lateral)
- II, III, aVF (inferior).

15 Cardiac arrhythmias

Figure 15.1 Cardiac conduction system

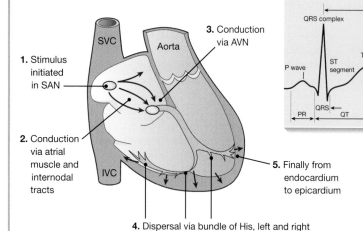

1. Stimulus initiated in SAN

2. Conduction via atrial muscle and internodal tracts

3. Conduction via AVN

4. Dispersal via bundle of His, left and right bundles, and Purkinje fibres to ventricular mass (4 m/s)

5. Finally from endocardium to epicardium

SVC

Aorta

IVC

Figure 15.2 Rapid rhythm analysis

1. Is the QRS rate fast or slow?
2. Are the QRS complexes regular or irregular?
3. Is the QRS complex wide or narrow?
4. Are P waves present?
5. Is there a P wave before each QRS complex?
6. What is the PR interval?

Figure 15.3 Sinus rhythm

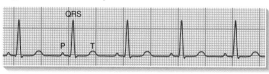

Figure 15.4 Ventricular ectopic

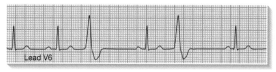

Figure 15.5 Atrial fibrillation

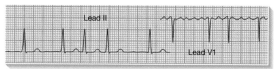

Figure 15.6 Atrial flutter

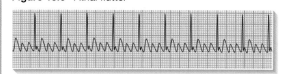

Figure 15.7 Supraventricular tachycardia

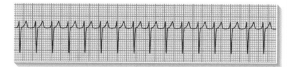

Figure 15.8 Ventricular tachycardia

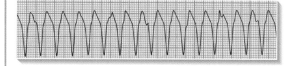

Figure 15.9 Ventricular fibrillation

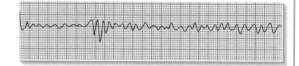

Figure 15.10 Heart blocks

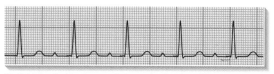

1° AV Block: Features of sinus rhythm but PR interval >0.2 secs

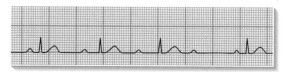

2° AV Block (Mobitz Type I, Wenkebach): PR interval lengthens until P wave is unconducted (i.e. no QRS)

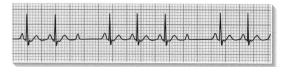

2° AV Block (Mobitz Type II): PR interval is fixed, occasional P waves are unconducted (i.e. no QRS)

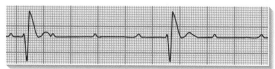

3° AV Block (complete heart block): P wave rate is regular, QRS rate is regular but there is no co-ordination between P waves and QRS complexes

Source for Figures 15.1, 15.3, 15.4, 15.5, 15.6, 15.7, 15.8, 15.9 and 15.10: Aaronson PI, Ward JPT & Connolly MJ (2012) *The Cardiovascular System at a Glance*, 4th edn. Reproduced with permission of John Wiley & Sons, Ltd

Emergency Nursing at a Glance, First Edition. Natalie Holbery and Paul Newcombe
© 2016 John Wiley & Sons, Ltd. Published 2016 by John Wiley & Sons, Ltd. Companion website: www.ataglanceseries.com/nursing/emergencynursing

Sinus rhythms

Sinus rhythm represents the electrical conduction associated with the normal cardiac cycle. The conduction system (Figure 15.1) controls the passage of an electrical impulse through the heart that is recorded on an electrocardiogram (ECG) as P waves (depolarisation of the atria); PR interval (transition through the atrioventricular [AV] node); the QRS complex (ventricular depolarisation) and T waves (ventricular repolarisation). The rate at which this sequence occurs is controlled by the autonomic nervous system to optimise cardiac output. Rhythm analysis can be undertaken using the approach outlined in Figure 15.2.

Sinus rhythm is present when P waves, PR interval, QRS and T waves are present, in sequence. The QRS rate will be regular, between 60 and 100/min (Figure 15.3).

Sinus bradycardia occurs when the regular QRS rate is less than 60/min. This occurs during sleep and is common among athletes.

Sinus tachycardia occurs when the regular QRS rate is greater than 100/min. This can occur on exertion but also in the presence of pain, hypovolaemia, pyrexia or hyperthyroidism, or with the use of drugs (e.g. salbutamol).

Sinus arrhythmia is the term used to describe a sinus rhythm with an irregular QRS rate. It is common in children and elderly people and is a normal variant.

Abnormal cardiac conduction

Arrhythmias occur due to disordered conduction of the myocardium and may affect cardiac output severely. They are caused predominantly by hypoxia, myocardial ischaemia/infarction and electrolyte imbalance, but they may also be associated with age-related degeneration of the conduction system, caffeine, alcohol, drugs and hypothermia. These issues change the homeostasis of myocytes, encouraging them to depolarise earlier than expected. This can give rise to atrial or ventricular ectopic beats (extra beats occurring earlier than expected) (Figure 15.4) or sustained arrhythmias, such as atrial fibrillation or ventricular tachycardia.

Atrial fibrillation (AF) occurs when the atria are stretched (e.g. heart failure) or irritated (e.g. excess caffeine intake) causing the myocytes to depolarise earlier than expected. This gives rise to fibrillating atria, rather than the coordinated contraction associated with sinus rhythm. Because the atria are not contracting, the risk of thrombus formation is high, often warranting anticoagulation therapy to prevent the occurrence of a cerebrovascular accident (CVA). The AV node allows some fibrillatory waves to pass to the ventricles, giving rise to a fast, irregular rhythm >100/min (Figure 15.5). If the AV node is damaged (e.g. in an elderly person), the ventricular response will be slow (e.g. 30–40/min). AF may be intermittent. This is known as paroxysmal AF (PAF).

Atrial flutter occurs when a single atrial cell fires at a rate faster than the sinoatrial nodal firing rate (approx. 300/min). This gives rise to characteristic 'flutter waves', which take a 'saw-tooth appearance' (Figure 15.6). There may be 1, 2, 3 or 4 flutter waves for each QRS (i.e. 1:1 conduction; 2:1 block; 3:1 block, etc.). Just like AF, atrial flutter carries the risk of thrombus formation in the atria.

Supraventricular tachycardia (SVT) occurs due to the presence of an extra pathway between the atria and the ventricles allowing a re-entry circuit to establish. The QRS will be normal (<0.1 sec) and regular with a fast rate between 140 and 250/min. Normally, no P waves are visible (Figure 15.7). Treatment involves vagal manoeuvres, adenosine or synchronised cardioversion to interrupt the circuit.

Ventricular tachycardia (VT) occurs when a single ventricular myocyte depolarises continuously, giving rise to a regular QRS rate between 100 and 250/min (Figure 15.8). The QRS will appear widened (>0.1 sec) as ventricular depolarisation is achieved using cell-to-cell conduction, rather than the rapid conduction system. This rhythm may be associated with cardiac arrest (Chapter 18). The most common cause of VT is myocardial ischaemia and may indicate the presence of an acute coronary syndrome (Chapter 16).

Ventricular fibrillation (VF) occurs when multiple ventricular myocytes are irritable and depolarise giving rise to disordered ventricular conduction and electrical chaos. This rhythm is associated with cardiac arrest (Figure 15.9).

Heart blocks occur most often due to age-related degeneration of the AV node but they can also be caused by ischaemia, electrolyte imbalance and, importantly, commonly used drugs such as beta-blockers, digoxin, amiodarone and some calcium channel blockers. Conduction of the P wave through the AV node is either slowed (1° AV block), intermittent (2° AV block) or absent (complete AV block) (Figure 15.10).

The patient

Patients presenting with arrhythmias have a variety of symptoms associated with reduced cardiac output, including dyspnoea, pre-syncope, syncope and chest pain. Some may present in cardiac arrest. Palpitations (awareness of the heart beating) are common. The nurse should use the 'ABCDE' approach (Chapter 4) to assess the patient, including palpation of the pulse, to establish the presence of arrhythmia. Blood pressure (BP) readings will identify if the patient is haemodynamically compromised.

Cardiac monitoring should be commenced at the earliest opportunity, viewing the rhythm strip in lead II. The monitor parameters should be set for the individual patient, to alert the nurse of any change in rate and haemodynamic status. Intravenous access should be established early and a urea and electrolytes (U&E) blood sample taken to assess for electrolyte imbalance. A 12-lead ECG should be recorded. The patient's respiratory rate, SpO_2, pulse and BP should be monitored at 5–15 minute intervals to assess for signs of deterioration.

If the patient is haemodynamically compromised, a tachyarrhythmia may require synchronised direct current cardioversion and/or anti-arrhythmic drugs (e.g. amiodarone, verapamil or adenosine). Bradyarrhythmias with haemodynamic compromise generally require cardiac pacing, although atropine may be useful in cases where the AV node is undamaged. It is vital that hypoxia and electrolyte imbalance (K^+ and Mg^{2+}) are corrected for all patients with arrhythmias to either stop the arrhythmia or to prevent reoccurrence.

16 Acute coronary syndromes (ACS)

Figure 16.1 Pathophysiology of ACS

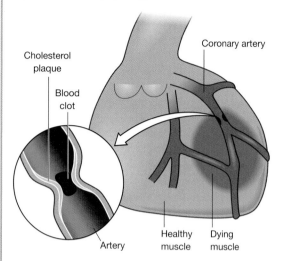

Coronary artery

Cholesterol plaque

Blood clot

Artery

Healthy muscle

Dying muscle

Figure 16.3 Classification of ACS

Suspected ACS

- ECG: ST depression/T wave inversion
  - Non-STEMI (+ve troponin at 12 hours)
  - Unstable angina (–ve troponin at 12 hours)
- ECG: ST elevation or new BBB
  - STEMI

Figure 16.5 ECG territories

ECG leads showing ST elevation/depression/T wave inversion	Territory of the left ventricle	Culprit coronary artery
V1–V4	Anterior wall, anterior septum	Left anterior descending (LAD)
V5–V6, I and aVL	Lateral wall	Circumflex (Cx)
II,III and aVF	Inferior wall	Right coronary artery (RCA)

Figure 16.2 OLDCARTS chest pain assessment tool

Onset	What were you doing when it started?
Location	Where do you feel any discomfort?
Duration	How long have you had the symptoms?
Character	What does it feel like?
Associated factors	Do you have any other symptoms, e.g. nausea, dyspnoea?
Relieving factors/	Does anything improve your symptoms?
Radiation	Do you have pain anywhere else?
Temporal factors	Have you ever had pain like this before?
Severity	Can you rate your pain out of 10?

Source: Seidel et al. (2011) *Mosby's Guide to Physical Examination*, 7th edn. Reproduced with permission of Elsevier

Figure 16.4 ACS on the 12-lead ECG

STEMI – regional ST elevation (2 or more adjacent leads) or new bundle branch block (BBB; not shown)

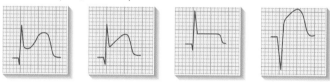

NSTEMI/UA

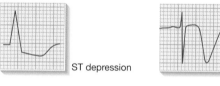

ST depression

or deep T wave inversion

Figure 16.6 Primary percutaneous coronary intervention

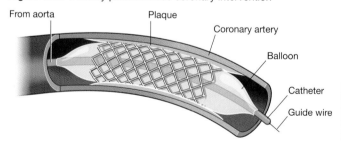

From aorta

Plaque

Coronary artery

Balloon

Catheter

Guide wire

Figure 16.7 ACS: Nursing care

Assess patient
- ABCDE assessment
- 12-lead ECG recording and urgent review
- Chest pain assessment and pain scoring
- Blood tests (U&Es, troponin, FBC, clotting screen)

Maintain patient safety
- Continuous cardiac monitoring
- Urgent cardiology review
- Bed rest, reassurance and brief information giving
- Give aspirin + P2Y$_{12}$ inhibitor (e.g. ticagrelor)
- 5–15 mins observation using NEWS chart
- Hourly BGs
- Contact next of kin
- If patient delayed in department, ensure other medications are prescribed and given (beta blocker, fondaparinux, etc.)

Commence treatment
- Oxygen therapy if SpO$_2$ is <94%
- IV access
- Pain relief – GTN /morphine
- Administer aspirin and ticagrelor
- Commence sliding scale insulin if BG >11 mmols/L
- Prepare for patient transfer for P-PCI

Emergency Nursing at a Glance, First Edition. Natalie Holbery and Paul Newcombe

'Acute coronary syndromes' (ACS) is an umbrella term used to describe three heart conditions: unstable angina (UA), non-ST elevation myocardial infarction (NSTEMI) and ST elevation myocardial infarction (STEMI). ACS occur when a coronary plaque ruptures, activating the clotting cascade, resulting in partial (UA/NSTEMI) or total occlusion of a coronary artery (STEMI) (Figure 16.1) and sometimes loss of myocardial function. The mortality rate associated with ACS is high. However, if the patient reaches hospital, their chance of survival improves significantly when they are promptly assessed and treated. This can reduce the severity of longer-term complications such as heart failure.

Presentation and triage

Chest pain is the most common symptom of ACS that brings patients to an emergency department (ED). The onset of pain typically occurs at rest but may be brought on by exertion. Importantly, the pain will not subside with rest or glyceryl trinitrate (GTN). The pain will typically be located behind the sternum and often radiates down the left arm or into the neck and jaw. It is frequently described as a 'tight band' around the chest or a 'dull ache'. Often, the pain can occur in the patient's neck, lower jaw or right arm and it is important to note that occasionally older adults and patients with diabetes in particular may not experience pain at all, known as a 'silent myocardial infarction (MI)'. Most patients will have associated symptoms such as nausea and/or vomiting, anxiety and have a grey pallor with cold, clammy skin.

Patients with suspected ACS require rapid triage and transfer to the resuscitation area where they should be assessed within 10 minutes of arrival, advised to remain on bed rest and given reassurance to reduce anxiety. The priorities of care are to treat the patient's pain, maintain their safety, prevent worsening of the condition and promptly commence treatment. If STEMI is suspected, paramedics will frequently transfer a patient directly to a heart attack centre for immediate treatment, bypassing the ED.

Rapid assessment

The nurse should use the 'ABCDE' approach (Chapter 4), remembering to explain each action and to reassure the patient. The patient's respiratory rate, oxygen saturation, pulse and blood pressure should be recorded on a National Early Warning Score (NEWS) chart and repeated every 5–15 minutes for the first hour or until the patient is stable .The nurse should commence O_2 therapy if SpO_2 is less than 94%, or less than 88% in patients known to retain CO_2. Cardiac monitoring should be commenced to observe for arrhythmias such as ventricular ectopic beats, heart blocks and ventricular tachycardia that may be caused by myocardial ischaemia (Chapter 15). A 12-lead electrocardiogram (ECG) should be recorded and promptly reviewed by a senior clinician and repeated regularly while the patient is in pain. Two cannulae should be inserted and used to take bloods, including urea and electrolytes (U&Es), troponin, blood glucose, clotting screen and full blood count (FBC). Blood glucose (BG)levels should be recorded hourly and an insulin sliding scale commenced if BG >11 mmols/L. A brief history should be obtained from the patient, including an assessment of the patient's pain using a systematic tool and a numerical rating scale (Figure 16.2), to explore their recent clinical history and likelihood of having coronary artery disease (e.g. age, risk factors, previous ACS).

The 12-lead ECG and cardiac troponins

The 12-lead ECG and cardiac troponin levels are used to identify the type of ACS (Figure 16.3). The presence of ST elevation, ST depression, or T wave inversion on the ECG is used to identify STEMI or NSTEMI/UA (Figure 16.4). It can also be used to identify the exact location of the ACS, including the culprit coronary artery (Figure 16.5). Serial ECGs should be recorded while the patient is experiencing their symptoms and then compared with previous ECGs (Chapter 14). The electrodes should remain in place on the patient's chest while they are experiencing pain but they will need to be replaced regularly if the patient's skin becomes clammy. An ECG should also be recorded once the patient is pain free. STEMI and NSTEMI will have an accompanying troponin rise 4–6 hours after onset. Troponins are released from the myocardium when it is damaged. No myocytes are damaged in UA and subsequently the troponin level will remain negative.

Priorities of care: The first hour

Treating a patient's pain is a key priority (Figure 16.6). The pain may be severe and distressing and will inevitably have an impact on myocardial work. The aim should be to eliminate the pain completely. Sublingual GTN, causing coronary vasodilation, is quick and easy to administer, although it is unlikely to resolve the pain completely. Intravenous (IV) morphine or diamorphine, with an accompanying anti-emetic, is most effective. It may be necessary to administer an IV GTN infusion should the pain continue, although careful monitoring is necessary to observe for hypotension.

The next priority is to minimise the damage to the myocardium by inhibiting the thrombotic process in the coronary artery and restoring blood flow. This is achieved by using a combination of primary percutaneous coronary intervention (P-PCI) and drug treatment (Figure 16.7). Patients diagnosed with STEMI require P-PCI within 120 minutes of presentation, which usually necessitates immediate transfer to a heart attack centre. Thrombolysis is indicated when P-PCI cannot be delivered within this time frame. Patients diagnosed with NSTEMI/UA require PCI within 72 hours.

Dual antiplatelet therapy (aspirin and a $P2Y_{12}$ inhibitor such as ticagrelor) should be administered at the earliest opportunity. Preventative medications should also be prescribed if the patient's stay in the ED is prolonged, including an antithrombin agent (e.g. fondaparinux), a beta-blocker (e.g. metoprolol), an angiotensin converting enzyme (ACE)-inhibitor (e.g. ramipril) and a 'statin' HMG-CoA reductase inhibitor (e.g. simvastatin).

17 Heart failure

Figure 17.1 The structurally normal heart and the heart with an enlarged left ventricle

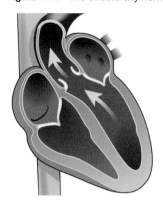
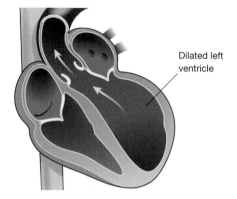

Dilated left ventricle

Figure 17.2 Peripheral oedema

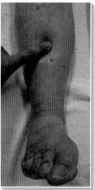
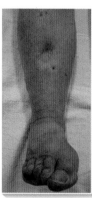

Source: By James Heilman, MD (own work) [GFDL by CC BY-SA 3.0] via Wikimedia Commons

Figure 17.4 A chest X-ray from a patient with left heart failure

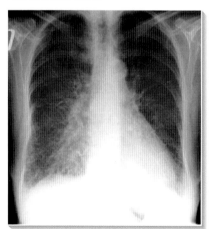

Source: Davey P (ed.) (2014) *Medicine at a Glance*, 4th edn. Reproduced with permission of Wiley

Figure 17.3 Common symptoms associated with heart failure

- Dyspnoea (>20 breaths/min)
- Wheezing
- Paroxysmal nocturnal dyspnoea
- Nocturnal cough
- Chronic fatigue
- Increased recovery time after exercise
- Peripheral oedema (e.g. ankle swelling)
- Elevated jugular venous pressure
- Weight gain (>2 kg/week)
- Weight loss (in advanced heart failure)
- Bloated feeling
- Loss of appetite
- Confusion (especially in elderly patients)
- Hepatomegaly
- Depression
- Ascites
- Tissue wasting (cachexia)

Figure 17.5 Symptoms and interventions for cardiogenic shock

Cardiogenic shock is a severe form of heart failure, diagnosed when the patient has sustained hypotension (SBP <90 mmHg) in the absence of hypovolaemia and poor organ perfusion

Symptoms:
- Laboured, rapid breathing
- Frothy, pink sputum
- Tachycardia with weak pulse
- Hypotension (SBP <90 mmHg >30 minutes)
- Inadequate urine output (<0.5 mls/kg/hr)
- Cold, clammy skin/cyanosis/cool extremities
- Reduced level of consciousness/confusion

Treatment:
- Intravenous inotropic support
- Intra-aortic balloon pump
- Percutaneous coronary intervention/coronary artery bypass graft surgery
- LV assist device

Emergency Nursing at a Glance, First Edition. Natalie Holbery and Paul Newcombe
© 2016 John Wiley & Sons, Ltd. Published 2016 by John Wiley & Sons, Ltd. Companion website: www.ataglanceseries.com/nursing/emergencynursing

Heart failure is a syndrome that occurs when the heart muscle is weak, limiting its ability to pump blood efficiently around the circulatory system. There are many causes of heart failure including myocardial infarction (MI), hypertension, cardiomyopathy and valvular heart disease. Rapid treatment of MI has significantly reduced the mortality associated with the condition but this has led to increasing numbers of people living with heart failure. There are several different types of heart failure but this chapter will focus on left ventricular systolic dysfunction (commonly called 'left ventricular failure').

Pathophysiology

The normal adult cardiac output (CO = HR × SV) is 4–7L/min and is a measurement of the volume of blood that leaves the left ventricle (LV; stroke volume) in 1 minute. Starling's Law dictates that the greater the degree of myocyte stretch during ventricular filling (diastole), the greater the force of myocardial contraction (systole). However, when myocytes are damaged, most commonly through MI, they lose the ability to forcibly contract, and the ability of the LV to create an adequate cardiac output will diminish as the walls stretch and dilate (Figure 17.1).

A fall in cardiac output and subsequent low blood pressure will trigger several compensatory mechanisms including tachycardia and vasoconstriction, to improve blood supply to key organs, and the renin-angiotensin-aldosterone system (RAAS), to increase circulating volume. These are usually effective short term and prevent the patient experiencing unpleasant symptoms. However, eventually these mechanisms will have a detrimental effect as they increase cardiac work, worsening LV enlargement and further diminishing its effectiveness as a pump.

Blood will become congested within the left side of the heart and eventually affect the pulmonary circulation, leading to dyspnoea particularly when lying flat (orthopnoea) or on exercise. The dyspnoea often causes the patient to wake at night (paroxysmal nocturnal dyspnoea). The congestion will eventually affect the right side of the heart and the venous circulation, resulting in peripheral oedema, typically affecting the ankles (Figure 17.2). Low cardiac output will inevitably cause the patient to experience other symptoms, including fatigue, depression, anxiety and loss of appetite (Figure 17.3).

Acute heart failure in the emergency department (ED)

Many people live with heart failure and manage their condition ably by monitoring their weight daily, taking regular drug treatment such as an angiotensin converting enzyme (ACE)-inhibitor, beta-blocker and diuretic, restricting their fluid intake and modifying their diet to avoid salt. Occasionally, patients will have an exacerbation of their condition, whereby excess blood volume leads to pulmonary oedema and acute dyspnoea, giving rise to many clinical signs associated with type I respiratory failure.

Patients are likely to have a fast respiratory rate and laboured, noisy breathing often associated with a cough and frothy, pink, blood-stained sputum, tachycardia, hypotension and occasionally chest pain, all causing considerable distress. This deterioration may be precipitated by another condition, such as an infection or new onset of atrial fibrillation (AF), by omitting to take their treatment or not adhering to fluid restriction. It may be a sign of their condition worsening. Occasionally, patients will present in a severe form of left ventricular failure, known as cardiogenic shock.

Nursing care

Patients should be systematically assessed using the 'ABCDE approach' (Chapter 4) and urgent medical attention sought as necessary. A patient may show signs of reduction in level of consciousness and therefore their airway should be closely monitored. High-flow oxygen therapy is usually administered to the patient via a non-rebreathe mask but with caution if chronic obstructive pulmonary disease (COPD) is suspected. Observations should be repeated at regular short intervals until the patient is haemodynamically stable, and continuous cardiac monitoring commenced to observe for arrhythmias such as AF, ventricular ectopic beats and ventricular tachycardia (VT).

Reassurance should be offered to the patient throughout this acute episode because it is likely to be a very frightening experience. Encouraging them to sit upright using supportive pillows is important to facilitate increased oxygenation and restrict blood pooling within the lungs.

Insertion of two intravenous (IV) cannulae is required for the administration of treatment and to take serum blood tests, including urea and electrolytes (U&Es), brain natriuretic peptide (BNP), troponin, blood glucose, clotting screen and full blood count (FBC). A chest X-ray (Figure 17.4) and arterial blood gas (ABG) should be assessed. Exposing the patient may reveal swollen ankles and legs and a raised jugular venous pressure (JVP) will give further indication of venous congestion. A 12-lead electrocardiogram (ECG) should be recorded and promptly reviewed by a senior clinician to identify if the patient has myocardial ischaemia or ST elevation myocardial infarction (STEMI). Consideration should also be given to identifying the cause of this exacerbation (e.g. pyrexia indicating sepsis).

Treatment

Urgent administration of IV diuretics and IV morphine should expedite a reduction in blood volume and alleviate anxiety resulting in haemodynamic stability. IV fluids are usually contraindicated because administration will worsen the cardiac congestion. The patient should have a urinary catheter inserted to monitor diuresis and a fluid chart commenced with fluid restriction applied. Weighing the patient daily is a further reliable measure of fluid balance. Their maintenance medications should be reviewed and administered at the earliest opportunity.

Observations should be repeated regularly until the patient is haemodynamically stable. However, if hypotension and tachypnoea continue, they may require IV inotropes and/or continuous positive airway pressure (CPAP) to improve LV contractility.

Cardiogenic shock can occur when there is sustained hypotension and poor organ perfusion despite adequate blood volume (Figure 17.5). This life-threatening condition may require the insertion of an intra-aortic balloon pump.

18 Advanced life support (ALS)

Figure 18.1 Chain of survival

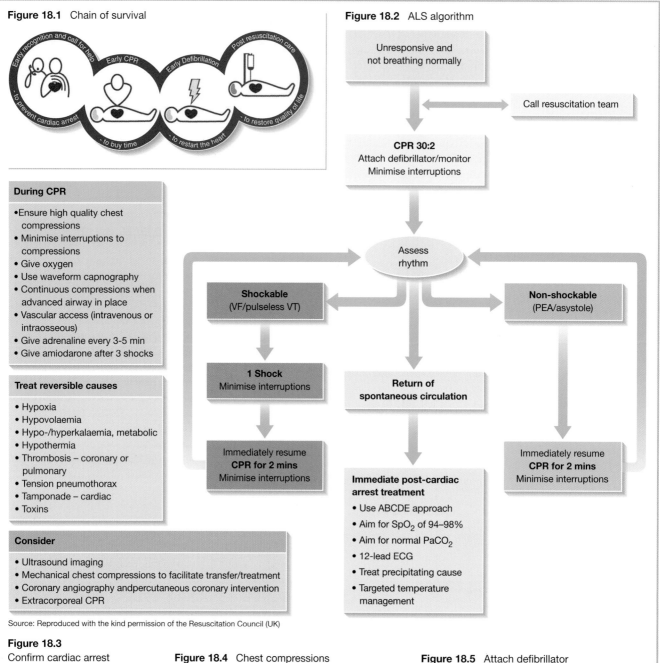

Figure 18.2 ALS algorithm

Unresponsive and not breathing normally

Call resuscitation team

CPR 30:2
Attach defibrillator/monitor
Minimise interruptions

Assess rhythm

Shockable
(VF/pulseless VT)

Non-shockable
(PEA/asystole)

1 Shock
Minimise interruptions

Return of spontaneous circulation

Immediately resume **CPR for 2 mins**
Minimise interruptions

Immediately resume **CPR for 2 mins**
Minimise interruptions

Immediate post-cardiac arrest treatment
• Use ABCDE approach
• Aim for SpO_2 of 94–98%
• Aim for normal $PaCO_2$
• 12-lead ECG
• Treat precipitating cause
• Targeted temperature management

During CPR
• Ensure high quality chest compressions
• Minimise interruptions to compressions
• Give oxygen
• Use waveform capnography
• Continuous compressions when advanced airway in place
• Vascular access (intravenous or intraosseous)
• Give adrenaline every 3-5 min
• Give amiodarone after 3 shocks

Treat reversible causes
• Hypoxia
• Hypovolaemia
• Hypo-/hyperkalaemia, metabolic
• Hypothermia
• Thrombosis – coronary or pulmonary
• Tension pneumothorax
• Tamponade – cardiac
• Toxins

Consider
• Ultrasound imaging
• Mechanical chest compressions to facilitate transfer/treatment
• Coronary angiography andpercutaneous coronary intervention
• Extracorporeal CPR

Source: Reproduced with the kind permission of the Resuscitation Council (UK)

Figure 18.3
Confirm cardiac arrest

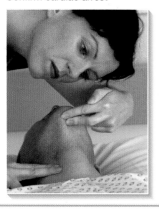

Figure 18.4 Chest compressions

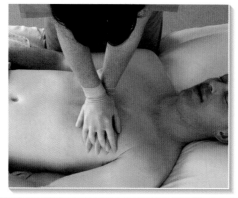

Figure 18.5 Attach defibrillator

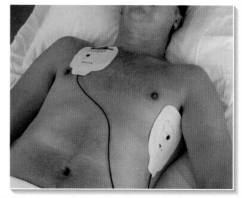

Emergency Nursing at a Glance, First Edition. Natalie Holbery and Paul Newcombe.
© 2016 John Wiley & Sons, Ltd. Published 2016 by John Wiley & Sons, Ltd. Companion website: www.ataglanceseries.com/nursing/emergencynursing

Cardiac arrest is a common scenario in an emergency department (ED). Some arrests occur in the department, but many patients are brought in by ambulance following an out-of-hospital cardiopulmonary arrest (OHCA) with resuscitation under way. Survival rates are bleak – less than 10% for OHCA and slightly higher for in-hospital cardiac arrests.

Chain of survival

There are four stages that contribute to successful outcome following cardiac arrest (Figure 18.1).

Early recognition and call for help

Because survival from cardiac arrest is often unlikely, the emphasis is on early identification and prevention in the deteriorating patient (Chapter 4). However, if cardiac arrest has occurred, early recognition and calling for the resuscitation team is essential.

Early cardiopulmonary resuscitation (CPR)

Early, good-quality CPR has been found to improve chances of survival. It increases the success of delayed defibrillation, but it should not delay defibrillation when available.

Early defibrillation

The most likely cause of OHCA is myocardial infarction (MI). The most likely initial arrhythmia in MI is ventricular fibrillation (VF) or pulseless ventricular tachycardia (VT). Where the presenting rhythm is VF/VT, defibrillation should be administered as soon as possible.

Post-resuscitation care

Return of spontaneous circulation (ROSC) is only the next step in the resuscitation continuum. The quality of post-resuscitation care will significantly influence patient outcome.

ALS algorithm (Figure 18.2)

Ensure personal safety

Safety of the area should be confirmed and universal precautions followed. Planning is key for an expected cardiac arrest arriving via the ambulance service.

Check response

If a patient is found apparently unconscious, the shoulders are gently shaken while asking loudly, 'Are you all right?' In a pre-hospital cardiac arrest with CPR in progress on arrival at the ED, this is not usually necessary.

Call for help

If alone with an unresponsive patient, help should be called by using the emergency buzzer.

Confirm cardiac arrest

The airway is opened using a head-tilt chin-lift manoeuvre (Chapter 7) while looking, listening and feeling for normal breathing and signs for life for no more than 10 seconds. If trained to do so, a carotid pulse is checked at the same time (Figure 18.3). Agonal breathing (occasional gasps) is common following cardiac arrest and should not be confused with normal breathing. In a pre-hospital cardiac arrest with CPR in progress on arrival at the ED, cardiac arrest should be reconfirmed before continuing.

Call resuscitation team

Depending on the context, the resuscitation team should be called and resuscitation equipment ('crash trolley') collected.

Start CPR

CPR is started as soon as cardiac arrest is confirmed. The heel of one hand is placed in the centre of the chest with the other hand on top (Figure 18.4). High-quality chest compressions are delivered to a depth of 5–6 cm and at a rate of 100–120 per minute. Ideally, a bag-valve-mask device connected to supplemental oxygen and an airway adjunct should be used to ventilate the patient initially (Chapter 7). Compressions and ventilations are delivered at a ratio of 30:2. Once the airway is secured, compressions are delivered continuously.

Attach defibrillator

As soon as it is available and while CPR is in progress (unless alone), a defibrillator should be attached to the patient's chest using self-adhesive electrodes (Figure 18.5).

Assess rhythm

If using an automated external defibrillator (AED), the machine's prompts are followed. Otherwise, CPR is briefly paused to assess the electrocardiogram (ECG) rhythm.

Treatment of shockable rhythms (VF/VT)

Once a shockable rhythm is confirmed, chest compressions are immediately resumed. Simultaneously, the defibrillator is charged to the appropriate energy level (depending on the type of defibrillator). All other personnel are instructed to stand back and remove supplementary oxygen. Once the defibrillator is charged, the person doing chest compressions stands clear and a shock is delivered. Without reassessing the rhythm or feeling for a pulse, CPR is restarted.

After 2 minutes, CPR is briefly paused and the rhythm reassessed. If VF/VT persists, further shocks are delivered following 2-minute cycles. After the third shock, 1 mg of adrenaline (epinephrine) and 300 mg of amiodarone are given intravenously. Further adrenaline 1 mg intravenous (IV) is given after alternate shocks along with one further dose of amiodarone 150 mg IV. If organised electrical activity compatible with a pulse is seen during rhythm reassessment, a central pulse is checked. If there is evidence of ROSC, post-resuscitation care is commenced. If there is no evidence of ROSC (or asystole), CPR is continued and the non-shockable algorithm followed.

Treatment of non-shockable rhythms (pulseless electrical activity [PEA]/asystole)

PEA is organised electrical activity without a pulse. Asystole is absent electrical activity and has a poor prognosis. CPR is delivered at 30:2 initially. Adrenaline 1mg IV is given as soon as possible. The rhythm is reassessed after 2 minutes and if organised electrical activity is seen, a pulse is checked. If there is evidence of ROSC, post-resuscitation care is commenced. If PEA or asystole persists, CPR is continued and adrenaline 1mg IV given every 3–5 minutes (alternate cycles). If VF/VT is seen at rhythm reassessment, the shockable algorithm is followed. Reversible causes (4 H's and 4 T's) should be identified and treated. The 4 H's and T's is a mnemonic used to remember the possible causes of cardiac arrest.

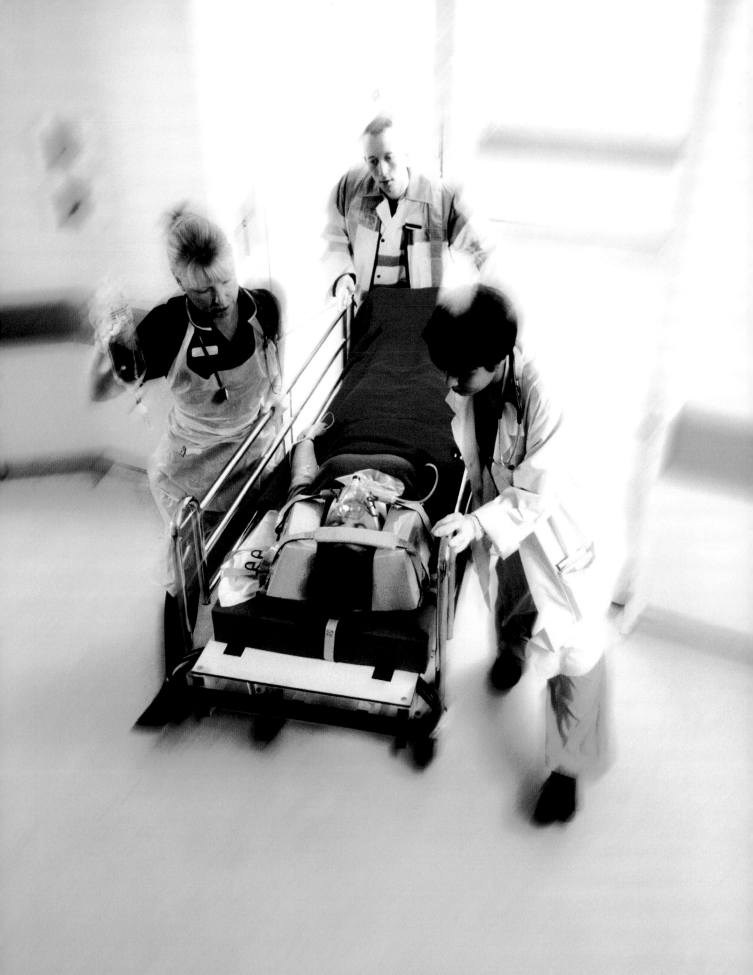

Disability

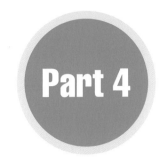

Part 4

19 Assessment of neurological function

Figure 19.1 AVPU

Patient:
- **A**lert   • Responds to **V**oice   • Responds to **P**ain   • **U**nresponsive

Figure 19.2 The GCS

Eyes open	
Spontaneously – eyes are open before the assessment starts	E4
To speech – eyes open on speaking or shouting to the patient	E3
To pain – eyes open on physical contact: shaking or trapezius pinch	E2
None – eyes do not open even to strong pain	E1

Verbal response	
Orientated – patient recalls own name, day, date and current location	V5
Sentences – patient uses coherent word combinations	V4
Words – single or unconnected words, random or meaningless	V3
Sounds – noises, but no discernible words	V2
None – patient makes no sound, even in response to pain	V1

Motor response

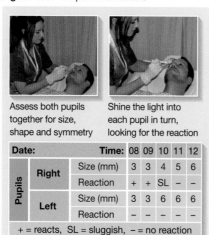

Obeys, **M6**   Localizes (trapezius), **M5**   Localizes (supra-orbital), **M5**

Normally flexes, **M4**   Abnormally flexes, **M3**   Extends, **M2**

None – no motor response, even to pain, **M1**

Figure 19.4 Central pain stimulus for assessment of consciousness

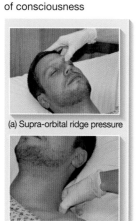

(a) Supra-orbital ridge pressure

(b) Trapezius pinch

Figure 19.5 Pupil observations

Assess both pupils together for size, shape and symmetry

Shine the light into each pupil in turn, looking for the reaction

Date:			Time:	08	09	10	11	12
Pupils	Right	Size (mm)		3	3	4	5	6
		Reaction		+	+	SL	–	–
	Left	Size (mm)		3	3	6	6	6
		Reaction		–	–	–	–	–

+ = reacts, SL = sluggish, – = no reaction

Figure 19.3 Recording and reporting the GCS

Date:			Time:	08	09	10	11	12	13	14	15
Eyes open	Spontaneously	E4		•	•	•					
	To speech	E3					•				
	To pain	E2						•	•		
	None	E1								•	•
Verbal response	Orientated	V5		•	•						
	Sentences	V4				•	•	•			
	Words	V3									
	Sounds	V2							•	•	
	None	V1									•
Motor response (record best arm)	Obeys commands	M6		•	•	•	•				
	Localises pain	M5						•	•	•	
	Normal flexion	M4									
	Abnormal flexion	M3									
	Extension	M2									
	None	M1									•

- The GCS does not distinguish left and right
- A patient's GCS must be reported in full
- On the chart above, the GCS at 1200 was E2 V4 M5

Figure 19.6 Limb assessment

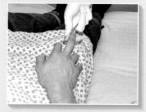

Where left and right are the same, mark with •

Peripheral pain may elicit spinal reflexes and does not demonstrate level of consciousness

Date:			Time:	08	09	10	11	12	13	14	15
Limb movement	Arms	Normal power		•	•	R	R				
		Mildly weak					L		R	R	
		Severely weak						L			
		Flexion							L	L	
		Extension									
		None								•	•
	Legs	Normal power		•	•	•	R				
		Mildly weak					L	R			
		Severely weak						L	R		
		Flexion									
		Extension								L	
		None								•	•

Emergency Nursing at a Glance, First Edition. Natalie Holbery and Paul Newcombe

Neurological function is a critical indicator of health and disease (Chapter 20). Assessing neurology provides a diagnostic baseline and ensures prompt detection of potentially catastrophic deterioration: this is a crucial role for emergency department (ED) nurses.

If the conscious level is impaired on initial assessment, observations should be done quarter-hourly to begin with, reducing to half-hourly then hourly only if the patient is stable. Any deterioration in conscious level (other than E4 to E3 [see later]), should trigger a full re-assessment on the ABCDE model (Chapter 4).

AVPU (Alert, Voice, Pain, Unresponsive)

AVPU (Figure 19.1) grades patients according to their immediate level of arousal. It provides little information and should only be used for initial triage. Patients assessed as 'P' (responding to pain) or 'U' (unresponsive) are at risk of airway compromise and should be moved to the resuscitation room. Patients assessed as 'V' (responding to voice) or 'A' (alert) are at less immediate risk but may deteriorate suddenly. All patients must be assessed promptly with the Glasgow Coma Scale (GCS).

GCS

The GCS (Figure 19.2) assesses consciousness: the brain's ability to engage with the world. It is not a numerical scale (the numbers are just a shorthand code) but a description of a patient's responses in three modalities: eye opening, verbal response and motor response.

Eye opening indicates **arousal**, the brain's receptivity to stimulus.
Spontaneously (E4): the eyes are already open before you start your assessment.
To speech (E3): the eyes open when you speak to the patient. Shout if necessary.
To pain (E2): the eyes open on physical contact. Start by shaking and shouting, proceeding to more concentrated pain stimulus (see later) if necessary.
None (E1): the patient's eyes do not open, even on strong painful stimulus.

Verbal response tests the brain's ability to use language to engage with its environment.
Orientated (V5): the patient tells you **all of**: their name, the day and date, and where they are (e.g. the name of the hospital).
Sentences (V4): the patient is not orientated but uses coherent combinations of words to express themself. Patients should be told the correct information (day, date and location).
Words (V3): single or unconnected words, apparently random or meaningless.
Sounds (V2): the patient makes sounds but no formed words are audible.
None (V1): the patient makes no sound, even in response to pain.

Motor response assesses the brain's ability to organise movement. If a patient does not obey, assess arm responses to centrally applied pain (e.g. trapezius pinch). If left and right differ, record the better arm.
Obeys commands (M6): the patient follows a simple motor command. 'Thumbs up' or 'Stick your tongue out' are ideal because patients are unlikely to do them spontaneously.
Localises (M5): the patient moves a hand to the source of a noxious stimulus. The limb may be too weak to reach the pain site but the movement is clearly intended to do so – it is the mental process that matters.

If you are using trapezius pinch, one hand must come above the nipple line.
Normal flexion (M4): the elbow bends and there is no rotation of the arm or unnatural posturing at the wrist. The movement is not clearly aimed at locating the pain source.
Abnormal flexion (M3): the elbow bends, but the arm rotates inwards and there may be posturing at the wrist; a clearly abnormal movement.
Extension (M2): the elbow straightens. There is often internal rotation of the arms and posturing at the wrist, and the whole body may stiffen.
None (M1): there is no movement, even on pain stimulus.

The GCS must be recorded in full (e.g. E2 V3 M5; Figure 19.3). The scale was not designed to be summed up, a practice that obscures much of the useful information obtained. The nature of the deficits matters.

Pain stimulus

Applying pain to patients is only justifiable if it produces clinically useful information.

Sternal rub does not clearly distinguish between localising and flexing and should **not** be used for assessment.

Supra-orbital ridge pressure (Figure 19.4) is effective in assessing motor responses but it often makes patients screw their eyes shut and so is less useful in testing eye opening. It is contra-indicated if a patient has skull fractures, and it requires skill to be done safely.

Trapezius pinch (Figure 19.4) allows both motor and eye-opening responses to be assessed together. A relatively safe procedure, it is ideal for repeated observations.

Nail-bed pressure can be used to assess limb function but **not** the motor response section of the GCS because it may elicit a spinal response.

Pupil assessment

Pupils should be symmetrical, circular and an appropriate size for the ambient light. They should constrict briskly to strong light. Examine both pupils together before passing the light from a pen-torch across each pupil in turn, assessing for constriction (Figure 19.5). Fixed, dilated pupils in the context of falling conscious levels signal a critical deterioration.

Limb assessment

This exam (unlike the GCS) is looking for left-right differences in limb power (Figure 19.6). If the patient is obeying commands, strength can be gauged by taking their hands and asking them to pull and push against you. Legs can be assessed by asking the patient to raise their knees as you push down on them. If the patient is moving spontaneously but not obeying, assess each limb by the strength needed to resist it.

Normal power: the patient can resist your strength.

Mildly weak: the patient's resistance is easily overcome.

Severely weak: the patient can move the limb, but not lift it off the bed.

When a patient does not move a limb spontaneously or to command, test the limb's response to **peripheral** pain.

Flexion: the limb pulls back towards the body.

Extension: the limb pushes away from the body.

No response: there is no response to peripheral pain.

20 The unconscious patient

Figure 20.1 Trauma

Source: Woodward S & Mestecky AM (eds) (2011) *Neuroscience Nursing*. Reproduced with permission of John Wiley & Sons, Ltd

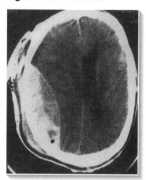

(a) A large extradural haematoma on CT with significant midline shift

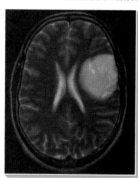

(b) A space-occupying lesion. A brain tumour on magnetic resonance imaging

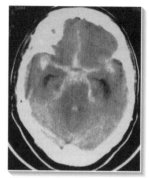

(c) Haemorrhage. White 'starfish' of blood in the basal cisterns typical in sub-arachnoid haemorrhage

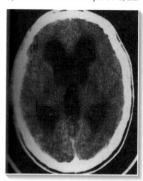

(d) Hydrocephalus. Dilated lateral and third ventricles on CT

Figure 20.2 Care of the unconscious patient

ED care of unconscious patients rightly focuses on resuscitation, diagnosis and referral. Nonetheless it is essential to assess and manage holistically the needs of vulnerable patients.		
Safety	• Poor awareness of self and surroundings	• Keep under constant supervision • Cot sides (beware trapping)
Observations	• Risk of deterioration • High risk to vital functions	• ¼-hourly neurological observation and vital signs • Reduce frequency to ½ hourly if stable for 1 hour • If any deterioration in neurology (not E4 to E3), re-assess ABCDE
Pain	• Patient may not be able to verbalise pain	• Observe for non-verbal signs: tachycardia, raised blood pressure, localising to pain sites, agitation, restlessness • Analgesia as required • Caution with opiates: possible neurological and respiratory depression
Nutrition/hydration	• Unable to eat and drink • Impaired/absent swallow • Risk of aspiration • Fluid and electrolyte status may affect conscious level	• Nil by mouth/tube • Blood sugar measurement. Treat abnormal results and re-assess • Insert naso/orogastric tube • Assess hydration: vital signs, urine output, condition of mouth, eyes and skin, blood results • Intravenous hydration • Mouth care
Elimination	• Impaired/absent bladder and bowel control	• If unable to use bottle/bedpan, catheterise • Measure urine output. Report if <0.5 ml/kg/hr • Record any bowel action
Hygiene	• Unable to maintain own hygiene • Risk of acquired infection, pressure damage, venous thromboembolism (VTE) • Loss of privacy and dignity	• Meet all hygiene needs promptly • Careful control of infection • Pressure-relieving mattress as soon as possible • VTE prophylaxis: anti-embolic stockings, pneumatic calf compression as indicated • Promote privacy and dignity
Psychological/social	• Possible confusion, agitation and fear • Possible language deficit • Family anxiety in uncertain and frightening situation	• Brief, clear explanations • Only one person talking at a time • Calm, re-assuring tone of voice • Use of touch to reassure • Keep family informed of situation and plans

Emergency Nursing at a Glance, First Edition. Natalie Holbery and Paul Newcombe

© 2016 John Wiley & Sons, Ltd. Published 2016 by John Wiley & Sons, Ltd. Companion website: www.ataglanceseries.com/nursing/emergencynursing

Consciousness

Many emergency department (ED) patients have lowered conscious levels. These people are unable to express or meet their own basic needs. Poor conscious levels reflect impaired brain functioning, a sign of serious illness, and pose an immediate threat to vital functions. ED nurses have a vital role in assessing, caring for and protecting such vulnerable patients.

Causes of lowered consciousness

Consciousness can be affected by diseases of the brain itself or by systemic diseases that disrupt the delicate homeostasis of the brain's environment.

Cerebral causes

- Head injury (Figure 20.1a)
- Tumours and abscesses (Figure 20.1b)
- Intracranial haemorrhage (Figure 20.1c)
- Hydrocephalus (Figure 20.1d)
- Stroke and transient ischaemic attack (Chapter 21)
- Infection
- Seizures (Chapter 22)
- Degenerative brain diseases: Parkinson's disease, multiple sclerosis, Alzheimer's, etc.

Systemic causes

- Hypoxia
- Circulatory failure: hypotension and cardiac arrest
- Acid-base imbalance
- High or low carbon dioxide
- Hyperglycaemia or hypoglycaemia
- Fluid and electrolyte imbalance
- Hypothermia or hyperpyrexia
- Liver or renal failure
- Alcohol or drug intoxication
- Anaesthesia and sedation.

Significance of lowered consciousness

Consciousness is a reflection of the brain's overall function. Impaired consciousness indicates either serious cerebral dysfunction or systemic disease so severe that the body has exhausted its ability to compensate and can no longer maintain the brain's essential homeostasis. A reduced conscious level means that all aspects of the brain's work may be impaired, with immediate threats to airway patency and respiratory function.

Assessment and management of patients with lowered conscious levels

Figure 20.2 sets out some of the most important aspects of nursing care for patients with lowered conscious levels. ED nurses should approach the assessment and emergency management of poorly conscious patients using the ABCDE model (Chapter 4). Nothing is gained by getting an early brain computed tomography (CT) scan if the brain in question is suffering ever more damage from hypoxia or poor perfusion while the scan is being done.

Airway

Poor consciousness can be the result of airway obstruction or the cause of it. Airway obstruction for any reason will rapidly lead to unconsciousness from hypoxia. Conversely, poor consciousness for any reason shows an impaired ability to self-maintain the airway and there is an imminent risk of obstruction.

Patients responding only to pain (Alert, Voice, Pain, Unresponsive [AVPU], Chapter 19) or with a summed Glasgow Coma Scale (GCS) of 8 or less are regarded as unable to protect their airways and should be assessed and managed accordingly (Chapter 7).

Breathing

The brain both manages the respiratory system and depends on it. Severe cerebral dysfunction can disrupt the brain's respiratory control. Equally, respiratory failure from any cause may lead to impaired consciousness, either from hypoxia or carbon dioxide retention. Poor conscious levels are often accompanied by altered breathing patterns.

Careful respiratory assessment is essential for patients with altered conscious levels (Chapter 8). While oxygen saturation monitoring is useful, there is no substitute for watching a patient's breathing to assess rate, depth and pattern. Respiratory observations should be recorded at the same frequency as neurological observations. Arterial blood gas analysis should be done to measure oxygen, carbon dioxide and carbon monoxide levels as well as acid-base balance.

Circulation

The brain is a small organ, making up about 2% of body mass, but it has such a high demand for oxygenated blood that it receives around 20% of cardiac output. Poor cerebral perfusion from profound hypotension or cardiac arrest quickly damages brain tissue, affecting consciousness. This damage soon becomes irreversible, leading to death or disability in survivors. The body's stress response mechanisms are designed to preserve brain perfusion as long as possible: impaired consciousness is a sign that circulatory failure has become critical.

Thorough cardiovascular assessment and resuscitation are essential for all patients admitted to an ED (Chapter 11). Patients with poor or fluctuating conscious levels should be continuously monitored and will need invasive blood pressure monitoring. Cardiovascular observations should be recorded at the same frequency as neurological observations.

Disability

Neurological observation is the subject of Chapter 19. The role of the nurse in assessing neurological function is critical to patient outcome: deterioration can be very rapid and early detection of change may make the difference between recovery and death or disability. Any change in neurological observations should trigger an immediate reassessment of ABCDE.

Exposure (and everything else)

Beyond immediate resuscitation, the priority in caring for unconscious patients is to establish the cause. This requires a careful evaluation of all the body's systems and as much information about the onset and history as can be obtained. Unconscious patients are unable to describe symptoms or relate their medical histories. Nurses in the ED must assess patients holistically and make no assumptions: the suspicion that a patient has been drinking, for instance, does not necessarily explain everything.

ED care is an essential stage in the patient journey. There is much emphasis nowadays on processing seriously ill patients through the ED as quickly as possible but however brief their stay, the care patients receive greatly affects the quality of their outcome. Nurses have the major role in preventing complications and promoting recovery at this early and critical stage.

21 **Stroke**

Figure 21.1 FAST

F Face	**A** Arms	**S** Speech	**T** Time
Has their **face** fallen on one side? Can they smile?	Can they raise both **arms** and keep them there?	Is their **speech** slurred?	**Time** to call **999** if you see any of these signs

Figure 21.3 Emergency care

Safety
- One-sided weakness and sensory loss. Possible aphasia and confusion
- High risk of falls, limb trapping in cot-sides, etc
  - Constant supervision

A
- High risk of compromise
  - Assess, support and monitor
  - Nil by mouth until swallow assessed: observe for dribbling, gurgling, 'wet' voice

B
- High risk of respiratory failure: altered pattern, aspiration pneumonia, pre-existing disease
  - Observe: rate, depth, pattern, SpO_2, arterial blood gas
  - Oxygen therapy
  - Chest X-ray may be indicated

C
- Pre-existing conditions
- Arrhythmias
- Risk of haemorrhage
- Hypertension is common after stroke
- Pyrexia worsens outcome
  - Cardiac and blood pressure (BP) monitoring, temperature, electrocardiogram
  - Aspirin 300 mg if not already given. Continue normal antihypertensives
  - If systolic BP >220 or diastolic >110, reduce gradually (intravenous labetalol)

D
- Neurological deficits may worsen
- Conscious level may deteriorate
  - Glasgow Coma Scale (GCS), pupil and limb observations; observe for facial weakness, eyelid droop
  - Capillary blood sugar
  - ROSIER
  - CT scan
  - **If GCS worsens (NOT E4 to E3), re-assess A, B, C**

E
- Holistic knowledge of patient essential to diagnosis and care
- Risk of complications
  - Previous and current medical history
  - Normal functional level: speech cognition, mobility, activities of daily living
  - Assess incontinence/retention
  - Assess skin condition: pressure-relieving mattress as soon as possible, frequent repositioning, venous thromboembolism assessment and prophylaxis
  - Gastric ulcer prophylaxis
  - Infection control

Figure 21.2 The ROSIER scale

Assessment:	Date .... / .... / .... Time ....
Onset of symptoms:	Date .... / .... / .... Time ....
GCS:	E = ... V = ... M = ... BP: .... / .... Blood sugar: .... mmol/L

If blood sugar <3.5 mmol/L, treat urgently and reassess when blood sugar is normal

Has there been loss of consciousness or syncope?	Yes ☐ (-1)	No ☐ (0)
Has there been seizure activity?	Yes ☐ (-1)	No ☐ (0)

Is there a **NEW ACUTE** onset (or on awakening from sleep)?

i.	Asymmetric facial weakness	Yes ☐ (+1)	No ☐ (0)
ii.	Asymmetric arm weakness	Yes ☐ (+1)	No ☐ (0)
iii.	Asymmetric leg weakness	Yes ☐ (+1)	No ☐ (0)
iv.	Speech disturbance	Yes ☐ (+1)	No ☐ (0)
v.	Visual field defect	Yes ☐ (+1)	No ☐ (0)

A ROSIER score of ONE or more suggests a stroke.
Scores of ZERO or less suggests stroke is unlikely but NOT definitely excluded.

Provisional diagnosis:

Stroke ☐

Non-stroke ☐ Specify ....

Source: Azlisham MN et al. *Lancet Neurology* 2005; 4 (11): 727–734. Reproduced with permission of Elsevier

Figure 21.4 Thrombolysis exclusions

- Time of onset >4.5 hours or not known
- Intracranial blood on CT scan
- Rapidly improving symptoms
- Seizure at onset
- Symptoms suggest subarachnoid haemorrhage: sudden headache, photophobia, neck stiffness
- Clotting disorders
- Blood sugar <2.7 or >22 mmol/L
- Pregnancy
- Recent lumbar puncture (1 week), major surgery or trauma (2 weeks), gastro-intestinal or urinary tract haemorrhage (3 weeks), or stroke or serious head injury (3 months)
- Previous intracranial haemorrhage
- Intracranial tumour, arterio-venous malformation or aneurysm

Every year in the UK, around 152,000 people suffer a stroke: roughly one every three and a half minutes. One in five die and fewer than half of survivors regain their former independence. There are approximately 1.1 million survivors in the UK. Good management reduces mortality by 25% and recurrence by 75%.

Incidence is age dependent with only 25% of patients under 65. Hypertension is the biggest risk factor, implicated in about half of all cases. Smoking doubles the risk regardless of other factors.

Aetiology

Ischaemic stroke is the loss of arterial blood flow to the brain, causing ischaemia and ultimately infarction (death) of tissue. There are four main causes:

1 **Thrombotic** (50%) – chronic damage to internal walls of arteries (atherosclerosis) prompts the build-up of a mass of platelets and fibrin. This thrombus may itself block the vessel, or lumps (thrombo-emboli) may break off and lodge in narrower branches. Hypertension, smoking and hyperlipidaemia are major risk factors.
2 **Cardio-embolic** (20%) – a damaged or arrhythmic heart may throw off small blood clots that block cerebral vessels. Atrial fibrillation, valve disease and previous myocardial infarction (MI) are the most common causes.
3 **Small vessel disease** (25%) – age-related thickening and loss of elasticity of small arteries deep in the brain.
4 **Other causes** (5%).

Onset and symptoms

The onset of stroke is sudden. Typically there is no headache and the patient may or may not lose consciousness. Specific symptoms depend on which areas of the brain have lost arterial supply. Common signs include:

- Weakness or paralysis (one-sided)
- Loss of sensation (one-sided)
- Facial weakness: drooping mouth/eyelid, lopsided smile
- Impaired use or understanding of language (aphasia)
- Impaired swallow (dysphagia)
- Confusion
- Reduced conscious level.

Diagnosis

Active treatment for stroke is only possible within a brief time frame. The FAST campaign (Figure 21.1) aims to improve public awareness of common stroke signs and the need for emergency medical attention.

The ROSIER scale (Figure 21.2) is used by emergency departments (EDs) for rapid identification of possible strokes. ROSIER scores key signs, with the aggregate score strengthening or weakening the suspicion of stroke. Patients must also be fully examined by a neurologist. The crucial investigation is computed tomography (CT) scanning, which distinguishes between ischaemic stroke and intracranial haemorrhage or other pathologies. Magnetic resonance imaging (MRI) scans give more information but may not be available in time.

Treatment

Assessment and resuscitation should be systematic, using the 'ABCDE' approach (Chapter 4; Figure 21.3). Prompt CT scanning is important but securing the patient's vital functions is essential.

Thrombolysis (clot breakdown) is the major active treatment for ischaemic stroke. Alteplase, a tissue plasminogen activator (tPA), must be given within 4½ hours of onset: this narrow window demands highly organised care but excludes the many patients whose time of onset is unknown. Patients at high risk of bleeding cannot receive the treatment (Figure 21.4). Giving thrombolysis to a patient with intracerebral or subarachnoid haemorrhage would have catastrophic consequences, so CT scanning is vital.

Thrombolysis is not a miracle cure: of every 1,000 patients who receive it, 80 will live more independently as a result.

Anti-platelet therapy is given when intracranial haemorrhage has been ruled out. An initial 300 mg of aspirin is followed by daily doses of aspirin or clopidogrel. Heparin is reserved for patients with venous sinus thrombosis or carotid artery dissection.

Intra-arterial treatments use angiographic techniques to extract the thrombus or inject alteplase directly onto it.

Blood pressure may be high but should not be actively reduced unless the systolic is above 220 mmHg or the diastolic above 110. If necessary, intravenous labetalol should be started cautiously and titrated to effect.

Conservative management and rehabilitation are crucial to recovery for all stroke patients: delaying rehabilitation worsens outcome. Emergency care focuses on resuscitation, diagnosis and referral, but preventing complications through good nursing care is always a priority. A sacral ulcer will prevent a patient from sitting out of bed, possibly for weeks or months.

Related conditions

Transient ischaemic attack (TIA) is an episode of stroke symptoms that resolve spontaneously within 24 hours. TIA has the same causes as stroke and patients have a high risk of going on to suffer a full stroke. All TIA patients should be referred to a stroke team for follow-up.

Intracerebral haematoma (ICH), or haemorrhagic stroke, is an arterial bleed into brain tissue. Onset is sudden, typically with severe headache, vomiting and poor consciousness. Focal signs such as one-sided weakness and speech deficit make it easy to confuse ICH with ischaemic stroke, hence the importance of early CT scanning.

Sub-arachnoid haemorrhage is an arterial bleed into the subarachnoid space around the brain, usually from an aneurysm. It presents as sudden severe headache, often with loss of consciousness. Photophobia and neck rigidity typically follow and focal signs (limb and speech deficits) are common.

Silent stroke is a cerebral infarct without immediately obvious symptoms, often identified when patients are investigated for problems with memory, cognitive function or mood change.

Carotid artery dissection is a tear in the lining of the artery creating a pocket in which blood pools and clots. Emboli break off, causing strokes. It may be spontaneous but is usually associated with previous head or neck trauma.

Venous sinus thrombosis is a blood clot blocking the sinuses draining venous blood from the brain. Venous congestion raises intracranial pressure, obstructs capillary flow and causes ischaemia, oedema and haemorrhage.

22 Seizures

Figure 22.1 Emergency management of seizures

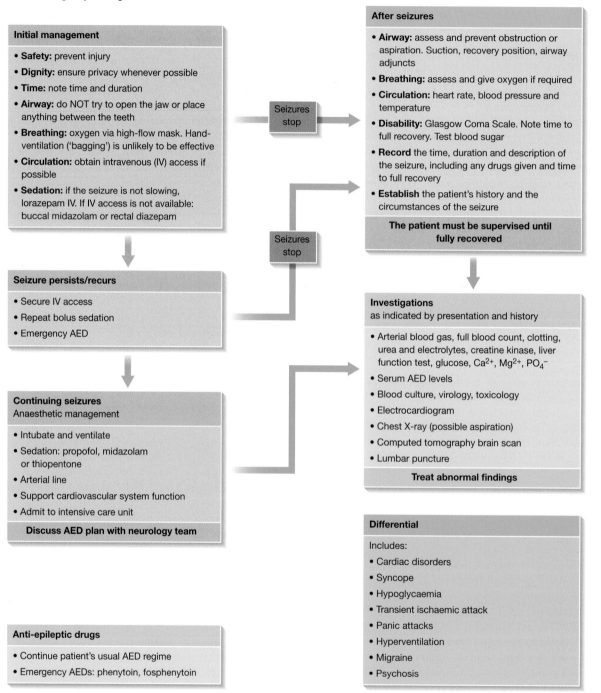

Initial management

- **Safety:** prevent injury
- **Dignity:** ensure privacy whenever possible
- **Time:** note time and duration
- **Airway:** do NOT try to open the jaw or place anything between the teeth
- **Breathing:** oxygen via high-flow mask. Hand-ventilation ('bagging') is unlikely to be effective
- **Circulation:** obtain intravenous (IV) access if possible
- **Sedation:** if the seizure is not slowing, lorazepam IV. If IV access is not available: buccal midazolam or rectal diazepam

Seizures stop

Seizure persists/recurs

- Secure IV access
- Repeat bolus sedation
- Emergency AED

Seizures stop

Continuing seizures
Anaesthetic management

- Intubate and ventilate
- Sedation: propofol, midazolam or thiopentone
- Arterial line
- Support cardiovascular system function
- Admit to intensive care unit

Discuss AED plan with neurology team

Anti-epileptic drugs

- Continue patient's usual AED regime
- Emergency AEDs: phenytoin, fosphenytoin

After seizures

- **Airway:** assess and prevent obstruction or aspiration. Suction, recovery position, airway adjuncts
- **Breathing:** assess and give oxygen if required
- **Circulation:** heart rate, blood pressure and temperature
- **Disability:** Glasgow Coma Scale. Note time to full recovery. Test blood sugar
- **Record** the time, duration and description of the seizure, including any drugs given and time to full recovery
- **Establish** the patient's history and the circumstances of the seizure

The patient must be supervised until fully recovered

Investigations
as indicated by presentation and history

- Arterial blood gas, full blood count, clotting, urea and electrolytes, creatine kinase, liver function test, glucose, Ca^{2+}, Mg^{2+}, PO_4^-
- Serum AED levels
- Blood culture, virology, toxicology
- Electrocardiogram
- Chest X-ray (possible aspiration)
- Computed tomography brain scan
- Lumbar puncture

Treat abnormal findings

Differential

Includes:

- Cardiac disorders
- Syncope
- Hypoglycaemia
- Transient ischaemic attack
- Panic attacks
- Hyperventilation
- Migraine
- Psychosis

Emergency Nursing at a Glance, First Edition. Natalie Holbery and Paul Newcombe
© 2016 John Wiley & Sons, Ltd. Published 2016 by John Wiley & Sons, Ltd. Companion website: www.ataglanceseries.com/nursing/emergencynursing

Seizures are a common reason for emergency hospital attendance and often occur while patients are in the emergency department (ED). ED nurses focus on maintaining patient safety and securing vital functions, but they should not overlook the need for careful holistic assessment.

Seizures and epilepsy

Any brain can suffer a seizure in extreme circumstances (e.g. severe hypoglycaemia, electrocution): in such cases, seizures do not usually recur once the precipitating factor is resolved. A diagnosis of **epilepsy** is made on the basis of a tendency to have recurrent seizures, not a single episode.

Around 600,000 people are estimated to be affected by epilepsy in the UK; two-thirds of sufferers have their condition adequately controlled with drugs.

Causes

Some seizures are **symptomatic**, a sign of underlying disease or damage. This can be the result of serious **systemic disease**: metabolic imbalance (hypoglycaemia, fluid and electrolyte imbalance, renal or liver failure), overdose or withdrawal of certain drugs (including antidepressants, antipsychotics, cocaine and alcohol), hypertension (e.g. eclampsia) or electrocution.

Seizures can be symptomatic of **acute brain disease**: intracranial haemorrhage, intracranial lesions (e.g. tumours) or infection (meningitis, encephalitis and abscesses).

Epilepsy, the tendency to have recurrent seizures, can also be symptomatic of **chronic brain injury**, either congenital or acquired (head injury, haemorrhage, stroke, meningitis, encephalitis, tumours or intracranial surgery).

Most epilepsy is **genetic** (or **idiopathic**). Here, a low seizure threshold is thought to have a genetic cause rather than being symptomatic of disease or damage. Genetic epilepsy typically presents first in childhood or adolescence.

People with epilepsy are more prone to seizures if their threshold is affected by factors including exhaustion, sleep, severe hunger, stress and changes in anti-epileptic medication or its absorption. Some people's seizures are triggered by specific stimuli such as flashing lights, music or performing mental arithmetic.

Symptoms

The outward signs of a seizure depend on which areas of the brain are affected.

In **focal seizures**, abnormal activity is confined to one hemisphere of the brain, often to a distinct focus. Patients do not lose consciousness but awareness may be impaired. There are various types: motor (jerking of the face, head or limbs on one side), sensory (abnormal sensations), psychic (abnormal thoughts, perception or emotions) and autonomic (abnormal respiratory and cardiovascular signs). Focal seizures with impaired awareness involve automatic behaviours, often repetitive and occasionally bizarre (e.g. fidgeting, walking or undressing). They are often referred to as **complex partial seizures** or **temporal lobe seizures**.

Focal seizures are usually symptomatic of brain disease, and are often the first sign of conditions such as brain tumours or encephalitis. Focal seizures of all types may progress to secondary generalised seizures, usually tonic–clonic.

In **generalised seizures**, both sides of the brain are affected and the patient loses consciousness. Generalised seizures are more common than focal.

The most common form of seizure is the **tonic–clonic**, a stiffening of the trunk and limbs followed by rhythmic jerking, usually followed by a **post-ictal** period of low consciousness. Tonic–clonic seizures can be symptomatic of systemic or brain disease, or the product of congenital epilepsy. Other types of generalised seizure are almost always congenital in origin. They include absence seizures (a brief loss of awareness often mistaken for daydreaming) and the relatively rare myoclonic, tonic or atonic forms.

Status epilepsy describes a seizure lasting more than 5 minutes, or seizures that recur without recovery in between. Convulsive status epilepsy is a medical emergency.

Drug therapy

Two classes of medication are used to manage seizures:

1 **Sedative drugs** stop seizures by suppressing brain activity generally but at the cost of worsening and prolonging poor consciousness post-ictally. Benzodiazepines such as lorazepam, midazolam and diazepam are used. Sedation may be necessary to establish control and manage airway and breathing if seizures are prolonged or frequent.
2 **Anti-epileptic drugs** (AEDs) are prescribed when there is a risk of recurrent seizures. Common AEDs include carbamazepine, clobazam, clonazepam, ethosuximide, gabapentin, lamotrigine, leviteracetam, phenobarbitone, phenytoin, sodium valproate and vigibatrin.

Most patients are managed with a single drug, some with combinations. Altering a patient's AED regime requires specialist advice.

Emergency nursing care

Assessment and management focuses first on stopping the seizures and then on assessing patients (the 'ABCDE' approach; Chapter 4) and establishing the cause (Figure 22.1). If a patient has never had seizures before, there is a high risk of serious systemic or cerebral disease. Diagnosing epilepsy (rather than managing acute seizures) is complex and has profound implications for patients: it is to be undertaken only by specialists.

Many patients brought to hospital with seizures have established epilepsy: a seizure can be part of their normal life. For these patients, it is important to establish whether the seizure is typical of their normal pattern and whether there have been any changes (e.g. medication or lifestyle) that might have triggered the seizure. ED staff should resist the urge to overinvestigate what for the patient may be an almost routine event.

Psychological and social considerations

Epilepsy has a profound impact on patients and those around them, potentially affecting employment, social and leisure activities, and personal relationships. There remains a stigma attached to the condition that has roots in traditional notions of spiritual possession.

Pseudo-epilepsy

It is an unfortunate fact that some people present to an ED with pseudo-seizures. Pseudo-epilepsy is often a manifestation of underlying psychological problems, and it requires specialist diagnosis and management.

23 Headache

Figure 23.1 Types of primary headache

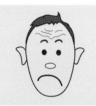

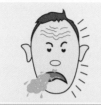

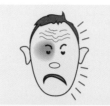

Tension-type headache

- 30 mins to continuous
- Mild to moderate
- Pressure/tightness
- Bilateral
- Not worse with activity

Migraine

- 4–72 hours
- Moderate to severe
- Throbbing/pulsating
- Unilateral
- Nausea and vomiting
- May have aura (15–20% of people)

Cluster headache

- 15 mins–3 hours
- Severe
- Pain behind one eye
- Unilateral
- Restless/agitated
- Unilateral tearing

Source for Figures 23.1 and 23.4: Hughes T & Cruickshank J (2011) *Emergency Medicine at a Glance*. Reproduced with permission of Thomas Hughes and Jaycen Cruickshank

Figure 23.2 History taking in headache

Assessment	History	Observations
• Location • Type of pain • Severity/intensity of pain • Time of onset • Duration • Frequency • Context/influencing factors • Exacerbates/relieves pain • Associated neurological signs and symptoms	• History of headaches, including family history • ? Recent (3 months) head trauma • Medication • Allergies • Diet • Alcohol intake • Smoking behaviour	• Signs of distress • Temperature, pulse and respirations • Blood pressure (BP) • Glasgow Coma Scale • Photophobia • Neck stiffness

Figure 23.3 Analgesia approach for headache

Step one	Step two	Step three
Simple oral analgesia – aspirin 600–900 mg or Ibuprofen 400–600 mg	**Rectal analgesia** – diclofenac suppositories 100 mg	**Specific anti-migraine drugs** – triptans
Anti-emetic – prochlorperazine 3–6 mg/metoclopramide 10 mg	**Anti-emetic** – domperidone suppositories 30–60 mg	**Anti-emetic** – domperidone 10 mg/metoclopramide 10 mg

Figure 23.4 Headache red flags

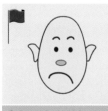

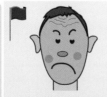

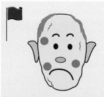

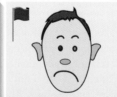

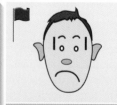

Subarachnoid bleed

- Severe sudden onset
- ↑BP
- Family history
- Warning bleed
  – symptoms may settle

Meningitis

- Non-blanching rash
- Neck stiffness
- Fever

Subdural haematoma

- Elderly, falls
- Anticoagulant
- Alcoholic

Glaucoma

- ↑Intraocular pressure
- Red eye
- Unilateral
- Cloudy cornea
- Blurred vision

Giant cell arteritis

- ↑Eyrthrocyte sedimentation rate
- Tender arteries
- Loss of vision

Emergency Nursing at a Glance, First Edition. Natalie Holbery and Paul Newcombe
© 2016 John Wiley & Sons, Ltd. Published 2016 by John Wiley & Sons, Ltd. Companion website: www.ataglanceseries.com/nursing/emergencynursing

Headache is a commonly reported complaint among adults. It can be a debilitating condition that has an impact on work and home life. It accounts for about 1–3% of emergency department (ED) attendance.

Headaches are classified as primary or secondary. Primary headaches are not caused by an underlying disease and usually first occur before 50 years of age. Examples include migraine, tension-type headache and cluster headache. Figure 23.1 compares the three main primary headaches.

Secondary headaches are symptoms of a disease process, medical condition or trauma. Some secondary headaches are life threatening. ED nurses must be aware of red flags associated with these conditions and their immediate management. Types of primary headaches and causes of secondary headaches are now discussed.

Migraine

Migraine is a debilitating condition that predominantly affects adults but can also affect children (usually from 12 years of age). It is characterised by unilateral or bilateral pulsating or throbbing pain lasting 4–72 hours and moderate or severe in nature. Migraine in children tends to last 1–72 hours. Nausea, photophobia (sensitivity to light) and phonophobia (sensitivity to noise) are common. An aura is present in 15–20% of patients with migraine and is characterised by flickering lights, partial loss of vision, numbness, pins and needles or speech disturbance. Treatment involves oral analgesics such as non-steroidal anti-inflammatory drugs (NSAIDs) and paracetamol. Opioids should be avoided. Triptans are commonly used. Because nausea is common, an anti-emetic should be offered. Patients who complain of photophobia or phonophobia will be more comfortable in a quiet, darkened environment. They do not need to be admitted and should seek ongoing care from their general practitioner. A headache diary may be suggested to determine triggers if these are not already known to the patient.

Tension-type headache

Tension-type headache is the most common primary headache. It is characterised by bilateral constricting or tightness pain lasting minutes to days. The pain is mild to moderate. Nausea, vomiting and photophobia are not usually present. Treatment involves oral analgesia such as NSAIDs and paracetamol. Patients do not need to be admitted. They should receive advice about which analgesia to use and seek ongoing advice from their general practitioner. They may also benefit from maintaining a headache diary to determine triggers.

Cluster headache

Cluster headaches predominantly affect men and there may be a family history of the condition. Alcohol is often a precipitating factor and many patients complain of their headache waking them. Cluster headaches are characterised by unilateral pain, usually near the eye and severe in nature. Tearing, nasal congestion, eyelid oedema or facial sweating are also defining features. As the name suggests, pain is clustered over short periods of time. It lasts from 15 minutes to 3 hours and can occur up to 8 times per day. The patient will then have weeks or months without pain. In the ED, cluster headaches are treated with high-flow oxygen (at least 12 litres) via a non-rebreathing mask. Subcutaneous or nasal triptans are also recommended. Patients do not need to be admitted. They should be advised to avoid alcohol during cluster headache bouts because it is thought to exacerbate the condition. They should seek ongoing care from their general practitioner and explore prophylactic treatment.

Primary headache management

The main goal of primary headache management is to identify the type of headache and provide analgesia. Good history taking is essential. Figure 23.2 outlines some key facets of the history.

Analgesia should be provided in a timely fashion and according to local guidelines. It is good practice for analgesia to commence at triage and in a step-wise approach as outlined in Figure 23.3. Anti-emetics should also be offered. Opioids should be avoided because they can be a contributing factor in medication overuse headache.

Secondary headache

Secondary headaches can be caused by a number of disease processes or medical conditions. It is important to take a full history to determine the cause and rule out life-threatening causes. Such causes include infection, aneurysm, trauma, medication overuse, dehydration and tumours. The ED management of secondary headache will be determined by the cause.

Investigations may include blood tests, computed tomography (CT), lumbar puncture or a combination of these. All patients should be offered analgesia in a timely manner and attempts should be made to address the cause. For example, if a patient is dehydrated, intravenous (IV) fluids should be commenced. If infection is suspected, antibiotics should be commenced as soon as possible. If a subarachnoid haemorrhage (SAH) is suspected a CT should be performed in the ED.

Medication overuse is the most common cause of secondary headache and is most often found in patients taking medication for primary headache. Those taking regular aspirin, paracetamol and NSAIDs (alone or in combination) for ongoing pain of any origin are also at risk of medication overuse headache. These patients should be advised to abruptly stop taking the medication for at least 1 month. It should be explained to them that symptoms will get worse before they improve.

Red flags

Approximately 3–5% of patients presenting to an ED with headache will have a life-threatening cause. Figure 23.4 lists these causes and their significant concerning features (red flags). Nurses must be familiar with these red flags in order to expedite treatment and reduce the risk of morbidity and mortality.

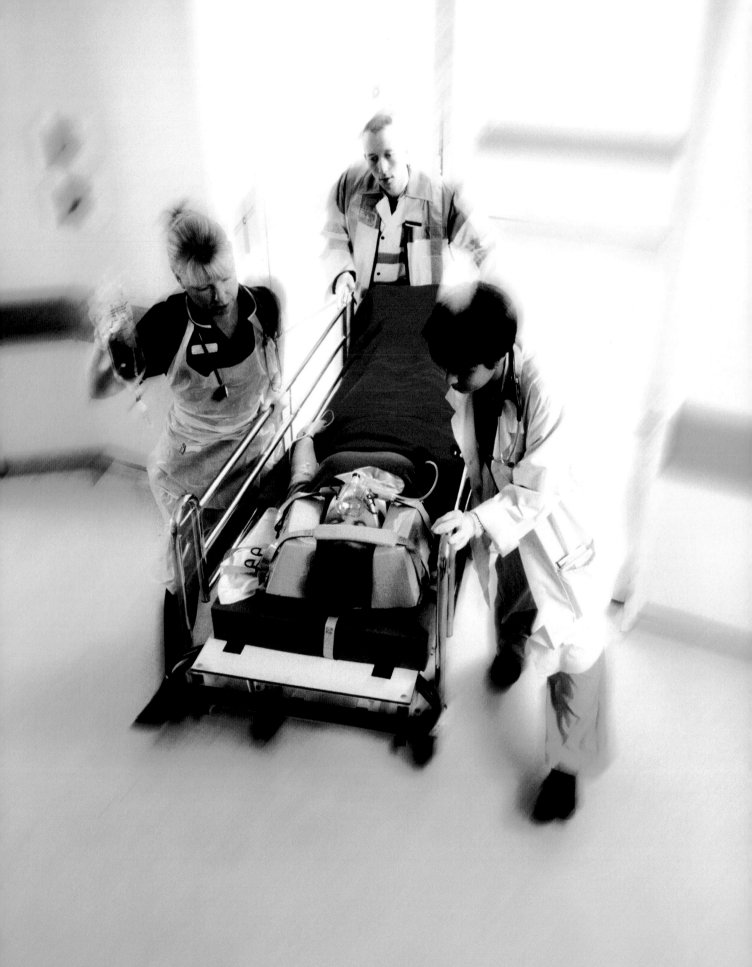

Emergency presentations and conditions

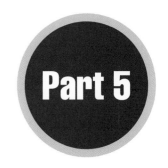

Part 5

Chapters

24 Abdominal pain

Figure 24.1 Causes of acute abdominal pain

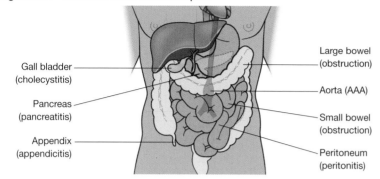

Gall bladder (cholecystitis)

Pancreas (pancreatitis)

Appendix (appendicitis)

Large bowel (obstruction)

Aorta (AAA)

Small bowel (obstruction)

Peritoneum (peritonitis)

Figure 24.2 General management

- Oxygen – if hypoxic or critically ill
- Intravenous (IV) access and blood tests
- Ongoing monitoring
- Consider IV fluids
- Analgesics
- Anti-emetics
- Consider nil by mouth
- Consider NG tube
- Pre-operative preparation?

Figure 24.3 Abdominal pain assessment

P	**Precipitating factors** Did anything trigger the pain?
Q	**Quality** What does the pain feel like?
R	**Region and radiation** Where is the pain?
S	**Severity and associated symptoms** How bad is the pain? What other symptoms do you have?
T	**Timing and treatment** When did the pain start? Does it come and go? Have you taken anything? Did it help?

Associated symptoms?
- Nausea/vomiting
- Anorexia
- Weight loss
- Indigestion
- Dysphagia
- Constipation
- Diarrhoea
- Wind
- Distension
- Urinary
- Fever
- Malaise

Figure 24.4 Types of abdominal pain

Visceral	• Stretching/inflammation of hollow viscus/organ • Dull ache, cramping or colic • Difficult to localise • Not aggravated by movement • Accompanied by anorexia, nausea and malaise
Parietal (somatic)	• Irritation or inflammation of parietal peritoneum • Sharp, stabbing or burning • Easily localised • Aggravated by movement • Confirmed by guarding and rebound tenderness
Referred (radiating)	• Shared nerve pathway with affected organ • Pain experienced away from the source • Common patterns • Shoulder tip pain in acute abdomen

Figure 24.5 Abdominal examination

Inspection	• Does the patient look well? • Distension, scars, hernias?
Auscultation	• Bowel sounds present?
Palpation	• Gently elicit tenderness • Masses, organomegaly? • Guarding, rebound tenderness?
Percussion	• Dull – fluid or solid mass • Tympanic – excess gas • Masses, organomegaly?
Rectal exam	• Haemorrhoids, skin tags? • Enlarged prostate? • Impacted stool, blood?

Abdominal quadrants

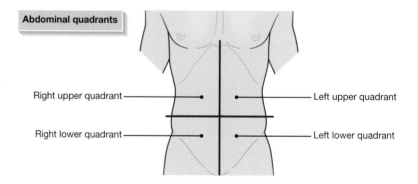

Right upper quadrant

Left upper quadrant

Right lower quadrant

Left lower quadrant

Figure 24.6 Types of bowel obstruction

	Small bowel	**Large bowel**
Age	Younger	Older
Cause	Adhesions	Malignancy
Onset	Rapid	Insipid
Pain	More severe	Less severe
Vomiting	Early, profuse	Late, faeculent
Distension	Late	Early
Constipation	Late	Early

Abdominal segments

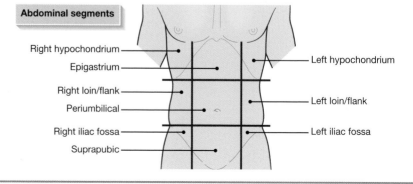

Right hypochondrium

Epigastrium

Right loin/flank

Periumbilical

Right iliac fossa

Suprapubic

Left hypochondrium

Left loin/flank

Left iliac fossa

Emergency Nursing at a Glance, First Edition. Natalie Holbery and Paul Newcombe.

A bdominal pain is a common presentation to the emergency department (ED). Underlying pathology can range from mild and self-limiting to severe and life threatening – the acute abdomen (Figure 24.1). Careful assessment is paramount. The focus of management is supportive care and rapid referral to the surgical team (Figure 24.2).

Assessment

A structured approach to history taking is advocated (Figure 24.3). The type of abdominal pain present can indicate the nature of the underlying disease (Figure 24.4). The patient's past medical history (PMH) may also be relevant, particularly any previous surgical history but also cardiovascular disease, diabetes and other long-term conditions. There may be medications taken that have an effect on the gastro-intestinal (GI) system (e.g. opiates [constipation], antibiotics [diarrhoea]). Social history may also be relevant (e.g. diet, smoking, alcohol, illicit drug use, foreign travel). Family history might reveal genetically linked diseases such as cancer or inflammatory bowel disease. Vital signs might show an inflammatory response, fever or shock. The doctor or nurse practitioner will perform a physical examination (Figure 24.5). Further investigations might include:

- Electrocardiogram (ECG) to rule out cardiac cause
- Urinalysis
- Blood tests
- X-rays
- Computed tomography (CT)
- Ultrasound scan (USS).

Appendicitis

Appendicitis is the most common cause of an acute abdomen and subsequent abdominal surgery. It occurs most frequently in children and young adults. Diagnosis is challenging because many patients present with atypical symptoms. Obstetric or gynaecological causes should be considered in women. As the appendix becomes blocked and inflamed, diffuse visceral pain is experienced in the lower abdomen. This may be accompanied by nausea, anorexia, diarrhoea, fever or general malaise. Pain then migrates to the right iliac fossa and becomes more severe. Physical examination demonstrates guarding and rebound tenderness. If the appendix has ruptured, symptoms of peritonitis are seen. Blood tests usually show raised inflammatory markers. CT may be used to confirm diagnosis. Open or laparoscopic appendicectomy is usually performed, although serial evaluation may be carried out first.

Cholecystitis

Cholecystitis is another common surgical emergency. It occurs more frequently in women, people with high cholesterol and increased age. It is characterised by gall bladder inflammation caused by blockage with gallstones. Rupture can lead to abscess formation or peritonitis. Dull pain may begin centrally, but then become more severe and localise to the right upper quadrant. Pain may be exacerbated by eating and deep breathing. Anorexia, fever, nausea and vomiting are often present. Jaundice may be seen in severe cases. Physical examination elicits guarding and rebound tenderness. Liver function tests may be raised. USS is the investigation of choice. Intravenous (IV) antibiotics may be given as an adjunct to general supportive care. Cholecystectomy is usually performed laparoscopically.

Pancreatitis

Acute pancreatitis occurs as a result of a range of different causes, but most commonly gallstones and alcohol. Chronic pancreatitis is usually caused by alcoholism. Autodigestion of pancreatic tissue by prematurely activated digestive enzymes is the main pathophysiological process, resulting in inflammation and oedema. Necrosis can lead to haemorrhage, abscess formation and peritonitis. Fluid shifts occur as pancreatic enzymes join the systemic circulation, eventually causing multi-organ failure. Pain tends to be severe, burning, localised to the epigastrium and relieved by sitting forwards. Fever, anorexia, nausea and vomiting are common. Abdominal examination reveals tenderness in the epigastrium. In severe pancreatitis the patient may be shocked. Amylase and lipase are raised. CT scanning may be used to confirm diagnosis. Treatment of hypovolaemic shock is the priority. Surgery is not usually indicated. In severe cases the patient is transferred to the intensive care unit (ICU).

Bowel obstruction

Both small and large bowel obstruction are common causes of abdominal pain (Figure 24.6). Paralytic ileus and pseudo-obstruction also occur and have similar symptoms. Above the obstruction, fluid and gas accumulate and the intestinal lumen dilates, becomes oedematous and causes fluid and electrolyte shifts. Strangulation occurs as the blood supply is compromised. Finally, necrosis and perforation result in leakage of bowel contents and peritonitis. Auscultation shows reduced or absent bowel sounds. An erect chest X-ray is taken to determine perforation from air under the right diaphragm. Patients require analgesics, anti-emetics, a nasogastric (NG) tube and IV fluids. Surgery is indicated for evidence of strangulation or perforation.

Peritonitis

Peritonitis is a secondary process related to the conditions detailed earlier, but also as a result of insults such as abdominal trauma. Inflammation of the peritoneum results in hypovolaemic shock due to the large surface area. Pain is sharp and localised initially, but becomes severe and diffuse as it progresses. The patient will have shallow breathing and be reluctant to move. The abdomen has board-like rigidity. The patient will need resuscitation with fluids, broad-spectrum IV antibiotics and preparation for urgent laparotomy.

Abdominal aortic aneurysm (AAA)

A dissecting or ruptured AAA may cause older patients to present with abdominal, chest or back pain, or collapse. Patients may look well initially and then rapidly deteriorate. Abdominal pain is classically described as tearing and radiates to the back. There may be a difference in left and right blood pressure. Femoral pulses may be weak or absent with mottled skin. A pulsatile mass may be visible and/or palpable. Chest X-ray, USS and CT may be used to confirm the diagnosis. IV fluid should be withheld or limited and the patient should be rapidly transferred to theatre. Mortality is 60–80%.

25 Gastrointestinal bleed

Figure 25.1 Causes of GI bleed

- Peptic ulcer disease
  - gastric ulcer
  - duodenal ulcer
- Oesophageal varices
- Oesophagitis
- Vomiting (Mallory–Weiss tear)
- Haemorrhoids
- Inflammatory bowel disease
- Crohn's disease
- Cancer

Figure 25.2 Types of GI bleed

- Haematemesis
  - vomiting blood
  - bright red blood = recent bleeding
  - brown 'coffee grounds' = old blood
  - associated with upper GI bleed
- Malaena
  - black, tarry stool
  - results from digested blood
  - usually associated with upper GI bleed
- Haematochezia
  - fresh blood passed per rectum
  - usually associated with lower GI bleed

Figure 25.3 Relevant history in GI bleed

- Previous GI bleed
- Dyspepsia (heartburn)
- Alcohol consumption
- Liver disease
- Clotting disorders
- Medication
  - anticoagulants
  - steroids
  - NSAIDs

Figure 25.4 Endoscopic image of a deep gastric ulcer

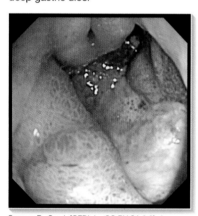

Source: By Samir [GFDL by CC BY-SA 3.0] via Wikimedia Commons

Figure 25.5 Oesophageal varices

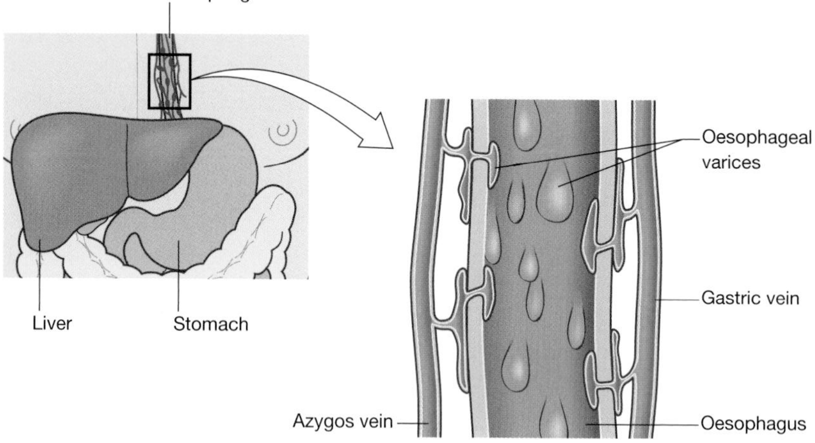

Oesophagus

Liver

Stomach

Oesophageal varices

Gastric vein

Azygos vein

Oesophagus

Figure 25.6 Sengstaken–Blakemore tube

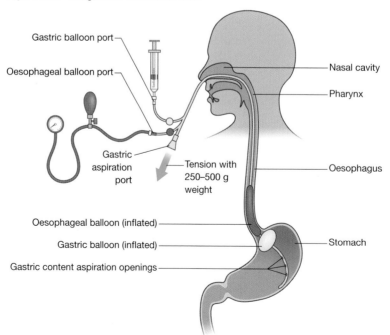

Gastric balloon port

Oesophageal balloon port

Gastric aspiration port

Tension with 250–500 g weight

Nasal cavity

Pharynx

Oesophagus

Oesophageal balloon (inflated)

Gastric balloon (inflated)

Gastric content aspiration openings

Stomach

Gastrointestinal (GI) bleeding is a common presentation to the emergency department (ED). While a standardised approach to initial assessment and management should be undertaken, identification of the cause is vital because underlying pathology ranges from minor to life threatening (Figure 25.1).

Assessment

Depending on the condition of the patient, an 'ABCDE' approach (Chapter 4) may need to be taken. Patients with a history of, or ongoing, significant haematemesis or per rectum bleeding, those with known oesophageal varices and those with evidence of shock and/or a reduced level of consciousness should be managed in the resuscitation room.

An accurate history from the patient, a carer or pre-hospital personnel should ascertain the type of GI bleeding (Figure 25.2) and relevant risk factors (Figure 25.3). It is important to distinguish haematemesis from haemoptysis, which is expectorated blood from the lungs. It is essential to determine the duration of symptoms and an estimate of the amount of blood lost. Along with presenting vital signs, this should guide the fluid replacement regimen.

Management

Airway

The combination of copious vomiting and reduced level of consciousness threatens airway patency. Airway equipment should be prepared, particularly suctioning. Lateral positioning might be useful. An anaesthetist should be called and intubation equipment prepared if necessary.

Breathing

The shocked patient should receive high-concentration oxygen via a non-rebreathe mask. Monitor respiratory rate and oxygen saturation levels.

Circulation

Ongoing haemodynamic monitoring is essential including heart rate, blood pressure and cardiac monitoring. More invasive monitoring may be necessary, via urinary, central venous and arterial catheters. Large-bore intravenous (IV) access should be gained in both antecubital fossae. Bloods should be sent for full blood count (FBC), urea and electrolytes (U&E), liver function tests (LFTs), clotting, glucose and crossmatch. Evidence of shock should be treated with fluid challenges; otherwise, fluid replacement may be prescribed. Saline should be avoided in known alcoholic liver disease (ALD) because of altered sodium levels. Blood products may be prescribed depending on blood loss, haemoglobin or clotting levels. Activation of a massive haemorrhage protocol may be necessary, if available (Chapter 61). Accurate fluid balance is essential. Significant GI bleeding can lead to cardiac arrest. Resuscitation equipment should be prepared.

Disability

Ongoing monitoring of level of consciousness and blood sugar is important.

Exposure

Management of vomiting and per rectum bleeding is the focus of care. Blood is an irritant to the GI tract and vomiting is inevitable in upper-GI bleeding; however, anti-emetics can be given. The patient will also need mouth care and may well be nil by mouth (NBM). Pain may also be present and analgesics should be administered

guided by accurate pain assessment. Repeated episodes of malaena can be difficult to manage in the context of the critically ill patient. It is important that the patient's skin and dignity are protected. Patients may also require significant reassurance.

The identification of upper- or lower-GI bleeding may determine referral: medics – upper; surgeons – lower. However, gastroenterology and liver specialists may also be available. Once stable, the patient may need endoscopy.

Peptic ulcer disease (PUD)

PUD is the most common cause of GI bleeding. Peptic ulcers occur in the stomach (Figure 25.4), but more frequently in the duodenum. Gastric ulcers (GUs) form when acid and pepsin erode the lining of the stomach where the protective mucosa is already damaged (due to non-steroidal anti-inflammatory drugs [NSAIDs], for example). Duodenal ulcers (DUs) occur due to abnormally high levels of acid and pepsinogen in chyme leaving the stomach. If damage is severe enough or involves a blood vessel, GI bleeding occurs. Helicobacter pylori (H pylori) is the main cause of PUD. This is a bacteria commonly found in the human stomach, although most people are asymptomatic. H pylori colonisation causes inflammation and damage to the mucosa and also increases acid production.

On endoscopy, if an ulcer is found and still bleeding or at high risk of re-bleeding, then endoscopic therapy can be administered. This may include:

- Injection with epinephrine (adrenaline)
- Thermal haemostasis
- Mechanical clips.

In the minority of cases where one or more of these therapies are unsuccessful, surgical repair is indicated. Drug therapy for PUD includes:

- Antacids and alginates
- Antisecretory drugs
  - Histamine H2 receptor antagonists
    - ranitdine, cimetidine.
  - Proton pump inhibitors (PPI)
    - lansoprazole, omeprazole.
- H pylori eradication ('triple') therapy
  - PPI
  - 2 antibiotics.

Oesophageal varices

ALD results in cirrhosis in about 10% of heavy drinkers. Irreversible fibrosis (scarring) and the development of nodules severely affects liver function and causes portal hypertension. Resistance to blood flow due to scarring results in the development of collateral circulation where blood supply bypasses the liver and is shunted mainly to veins of the lower oesophagus and stomach (Figure 25.5). Because these veins are not intended to carry such large volumes of blood, they dilate and become fragile. These vessels are prone to rupturing with catastrophic consequences and a 50% mortality.

The patient presents with copious haematemesis (which may be projectile) and malaena. Bleeding is further promoted by altered clotting, which often accompanies severe ALD. Endoscopic variceal band ligation is the first treatment choice, followed by sclerotherapy. If endoscopy is unavailable or bleeding is uncontrolled, vasoconstrictors such as glypressin should be given. A Sengstaken-Blakemore tube (Figure 25.6) may be inserted (with adequate provision for airway protection) while more definitive therapy is arranged, such as surgery.

26 Genitourinary conditions

Figure 26.1 Symptoms of a UTI

- Dysuria (pain or burning sensation on micturition)
- Lower abdominal pain
- Urinary frequency
- Urinary urgency
- Passing small volumes
- Malodorous urine
- Cloudy urine
- Haematuria
- Urinalysis (if positive, send for microscopy, culture and sensitivity [MC&S]):
  - blood
  - protein
  - leucocytes
  - nitrites

Figure 26.2 Symptoms of pyelonephritis

- Signs of UTI (Figure 26.1)
- General malaise
- Fever/rigors
- Loin/back pain
- Nausea/vomiting
- Anorexia
- Diarrhoea

Figure 26.3 Bladder distension in urinary retention

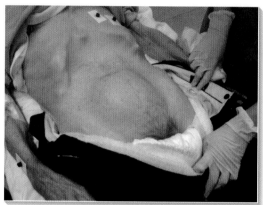

Source: By Frivadossi [GFDL by CC BY-SA 3.0] via Wikimedia Commons

Figure 26.4 Testicular torsion

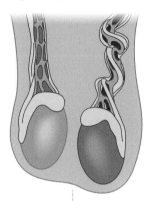

Normal testicle | Testicular torsion

Figure 26.5 Paraphimosis

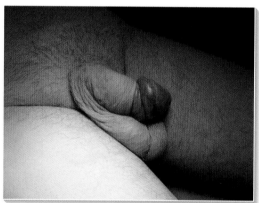

Source: [GFDL by CC BY-SA 3.0] via Wikimedia Commons

Emergency Nursing at a Glance, First Edition. Natalie Holbery and Paul Newcombe © 2016 John Wiley & Sons, Ltd. Published 2016 by John Wiley & Sons, Ltd.
Companion website: www.ataglanceseries.com/nursing/emergencynursing

Urinary tract infection (UTI)

Patients with UTI frequently present to an emergency department (ED). Owing to anatomical differences UTI is very common in women, but uncommon in men and usually reflects underlying pathology, such as benign prostatic hypertrophy (BPH). Women who are sexually active are more at risk, as are individuals who have an indwelling urinary catheter or comorbidities.

Most patients are well, but UTI can cause sepsis so careful assessment is important. Assessment includes history, vital signs and urinalysis. Symptoms of a UTI are listed in Figure 26.1.

UTI usually resolves on its own within 4–5 days. Antibiotics (e.g. Trimethoprim) can reduce recovery time and are often prescribed, particularly for recurrent UTIs. Patients should also be encouraged to increase oral fluid intake.

Pyelonephritis

A potential sequel to UTI is infection of the kidney(s) – pyelonephritis. A patient usually presents feeling unwell. Differential diagnoses include appendicitis and renal colic. Symptoms of pyelonephritis are listed in Figure 26.2.

The patient may be treated at home with oral antibiotics and analgesics – avoid non-steroidal anti-inflammatory drugs (NSAIDs). If they are unwell, they may require admission for intravenous (IV) antibiotics and IV fluids. Careful monitoring for sepsis and renal failure is important.

Acute urinary retention

Urinary retention tends to occur in older men as a result of BPH, particularly when large volumes of fluid are consumed or voiding is delayed. It may also be caused by constipation, UTI, anaesthetic agents, strictures, neurological disorders or blood clots caused by bladder cancer.

In BPH, the patient may report a history of urgency, frequency, nocturia, hesitancy, dribbling or poor flow. They usually present with severe lower abdominal pain, a distended abdomen (Figure 26.3) and an inability to pass urine. With a background of chronic retention, the patient may be pain-free and pass small volumes of urine (overflow). Backflow of urine to the kidneys may cause hydronephrosis (distension) and renal impairment.

Once the patient has presented to the ED, passing a urinary catheter is usually the only option and will swiftly relieve symptoms. If there are blood clots, a large-bore or three-way irrigation catheter may be needed. If it is not possible to pass a catheter via the urethra, expert help is required and a suprapubic catheter may be considered. Bloods should be taken to check renal function. Post-drainage diuresis may occur, so vital signs, accurate fluid balance and the provision of oral or IV fluids may be required. Specialist referral is needed to identify the cause and for planning definitive management. The patient being discharged home will require education regarding catheter care and community follow-up.

Renal colic

Renal or ureteral colic is a frequent cause of acute abdominal pain. It is more prevalent in men and recurrence is common. Renal calculi or kidney stones cause obstruction in the ureters. Pressure in the lumen causes dilation, smooth muscle contraction and spasms. The obstruction is often partial so renal failure is unlikely.

Renal colic is one of the most intense forms of pain. Pain is in the flank or loin, comes in waves and may radiate to the back, groin or genitals – loin to groin pain. The patient is often pale, sweaty, tachycardic, agitated and vomiting. Blood is found on urinalysis. CT scanning aids diagnosis. Differential diagnosis includes appendicitis.

Early pain relief is the main priority. The pain responds well to NSAIDs because they reduce inflammation and inhibit ureteric smooth muscle contraction. They can be given rectally if the patient is vomiting. Caution should be taken in patients with existing renal disease and a history of gastrointestinal (GI) bleeding. Opiates are the second-line analgesics in renal colic. Anti-emetics can be given if the patient is vomiting or nauseous. Routine bloods should be taken to check renal function. Patients are encouraged to increase fluid intake (oral or IV) to flush the stones out. Stones that don't pass spontaneously may be removed by lithotripsy, ureterorenoscopy or surgery.

Testicular torsion

Testicular torsion is a surgical emergency occurring in adolescents and young males. Reduced blood supply through the spermatic cord occurs due to the testicle twisting inside the scrotum (Figure 26.4). Damage to the testicle is determined by the number of rotations and the time elapsed before surgery.

There may be a history of sport preceding the torsion, but not normally trauma. Testicular pain may be severe, radiating to the abdomen and accompanied by vomiting. The testicle may be red, hot and swollen. Differential diagnoses include epididymitis, orchitis, testicular cancer and renal colic.

The priority is for referral to a surgical team so that urgent surgery can be arranged. In the meantime, symptomatic relief (analgesics, anti-emetics) can be provided. In an incomplete torsion, the testicle can be untwisted and blood flow restored. Both testicles will be anchored with sutures to prevent recurrence. In a complete torsion, necrosis may have occurred and the testicle will be removed. The patient will require counselling before surgery to prepare them for this possibility.

Paraphimosis

This occurs when a tight foreskin is retracted and the glans of the penis swells (Figure 26.5). This is a urological emergency because necrosis can occur. Paraphimosis may result from failing to pull the foreskin forward to its natural position after cleaning or catheterisation. Other causes include scarring, vigorous sexual activity, infection and piercing. Pain usually accompanies the swelling.

Careful attempts at manual compression of the glans and retraction of the foreskin are often successful. Ice packs may also be useful. If simple methods fail, then urgent referral to urology is required.

27 Acute kidney injury (AKI)

Figure 27.1 Classification of AKI

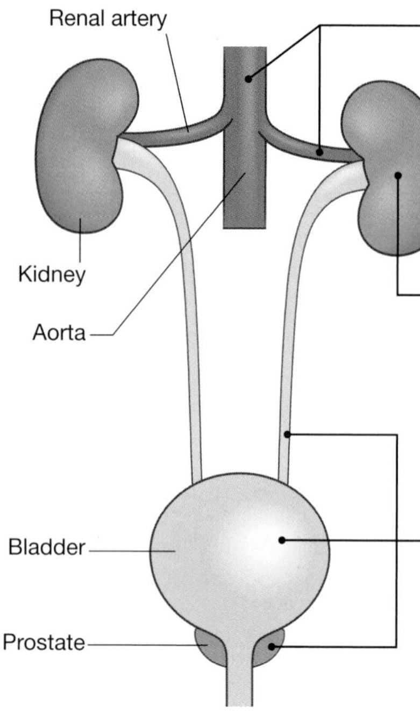

Renal artery
Kidney
Aorta
Bladder
Prostate

Pre-kidney injury
- Common in emergency department
- Results from decreased renal perfusion
- Caused by hypovolaemia or reduced cardiac output
- Leads to reduced glomerular filtration rate
- Usually reversible once underlying cause is corrected
- Can lead to intrinsic renal failure if cause not reversed

Intrinsic kidney injury
- Results from damage to the nephron itself
- May be irreversible
- Acute tubular necrosis most common
- Causes include inflammation, toxins, drugs and infection

Post-kidney injury
- Obstruction to flow in the urine-collecting system
- Can be above or below the bladder
- Causes include enlarged prostate and renal colic

Figure 27.2 Patients at greatest risk of AKI

- 65 years or over
- Previous AKI
- Long-term conditions
  - chronic kidney disease
  - heart failure
  - liver disease
  - diabetes
- Confusion or dependence on carer for hydration
- Dehydration
- Hypovolaemia
- Oliguria
- Sepsis
- Deteriorating early warning scores
- Nephrotoxic drugs
  - Non-steroidal anti-inflammatory drugs
  - some antibiotics (aminoglycosides)
  - angiotensin-converting enzyme inhibitors
  - angiotensin II receptor antagonists
  - diuretics
  - iodinated contrast agents
- Urological obstruction

Figure 27.3 Patient assessment

Airway A
- Intact unless ↓LOC
- Halitosis

Breathing B
- ↑Respiratory rate?
- ↓SpO₂?
- Kussmaul breathing
- Dyspnoea/shortness of breath
- Pulmonary oedema

Exposure E
- Anorexia
- Nausea/vomiting
- Dry, itchy skin
- Infection
- Oedema
- Urinalysis
  - blood
  - protein
  - leucocytes
  - nitrites
  - glucose

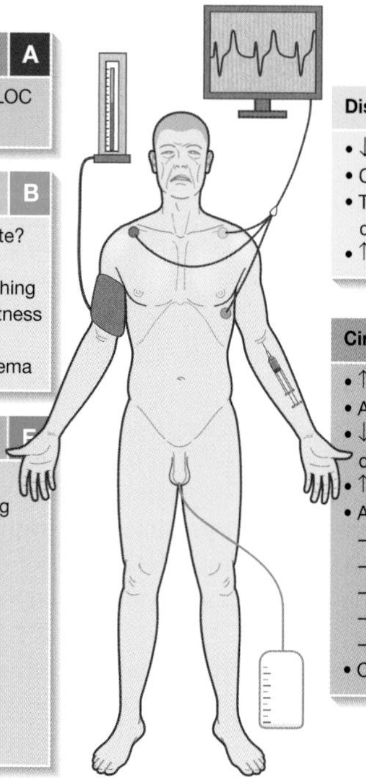

Disability D
- ↓LOC
- Confusion/irritability
- Tremors, twitching, convulsions
- ↑BG

Circulation C
- ↑HR?
- Arrhythmias
- ↓BP if shock or dehydration
- ↑BP if fluid retention
- Altered blood results:
  - ↑urea
  - ↑creatinine
  - ↑K⁺
  - anaemia
  - metabolic acidosis
- Oliguria or anuria

Figure 27.4 Management

Airway A
- Monitor and secure if necessary

Breathing B
- O₂ to maintain SpO₂ >94%
- CPAP for pulmonary oedema
- Ventilate if necessary
- Chest X-ray

Exposure E
- Infection control measures
- Personal care
- Nutritional support
- Anti-emetics

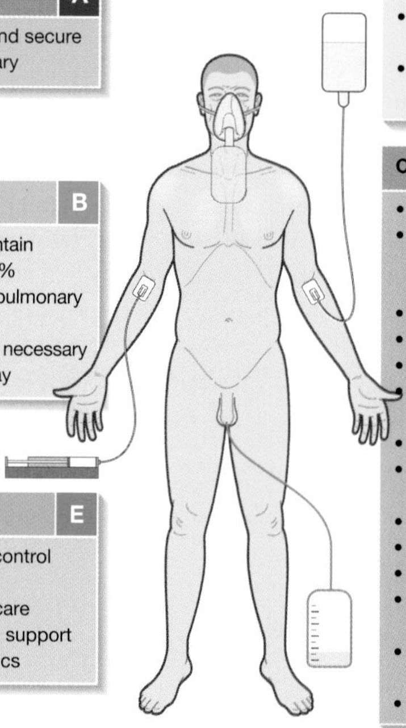

Disability D
- Monitor Glasgow Coma Scale (GCS)
- Monitor blood glucose level

Circulation C
- IV access
- Consider central venous catheter and arterial line
- CVP monitoring
- IV fluids
- Consider inotropes
- Maintain MAP >75 mmHg
- NEWS
- Hourly urine measurements
- Fluid balance
- Record weight
- ECG and monitoring
- Calcium resonium for ↑K⁺
- IV Insulin and glucose for ↑K⁺
- Consider RRT

Emergency Nursing at a Glance, First Edition. Natalie Holbery and Paul Newcombe.

Acute kidney injury (AKI) is common in unwell patients presenting to the emergency department (ED). It is seen in 13–18% of all people admitted to hospital and inpatient mortality rates are 25–30%. Previously known as acute renal failure, AKI covers a wide variety of conditions that affect the kidney and is often a complication of other illnesses. As renal function deteriorates over hours or days, injury becomes permanent. Waste products build up in the body, which can be fatal.

Classification of AKI is determined by the anatomical location of the cause (Figure 27.1). Pre-kidney injury is the most common cause due to reduced renal perfusion as a result of dehydration or shock. Those at highest risk of AKI are identified in Figure 27.2.

Assessment

Assessing for AKI is based on having heightened clinical suspicion in high-risk patients (Figure 27.3). An 'ABCDE approach' (Chapter 4) should be taken and vital signs recorded using a National Early Warning Score (NEWS) chart (Chapter 5).

Airway

A patient may well have an intact airway unless there is a reduced level of consciousness (LOC). Vomiting may present a risk.

Breathing

Again, breathing may be normal if the patient is not acutely unwell. If AKI is established, they may be tachypnoeic and hypoxic. If metabolic acidosis is present due to poor renal function, then Kussmaul breathing is likely. These are deep, sighing breaths to blow off carbon dioxide in compensation. If the patient has hypertension and fluid retention, pulmonary oedema may be identified by crackles on chest auscultation and pink, frothy sputum.

Circulation

Heart rate (HR) may be normal, but it may be raised due to compensation for low blood pressure (BP). Conversely, blood pressure may be raised due to existing hypertension. Arrhythmias may be present due to hyperkalaemia. Peaked T waves are a common sign, but more serious arrhythmias can develop. Blood should be urgently tested for full blood count (FBC), urea and electrolytes (U&E) and glucose, and an arterial blood gas (ABG) considered. Urine output should be accurately measured, preferably via a urinary catheter. Hourly fluid balance should be carefully recorded. When a patient has an arteriovenous fistula for dialysis, the other arm should be used for blood pressure and blood tests.

Disability

If not unwell, a patient may be alert with intact cognition. However, rising urea and other toxins cause a range of neurological symptoms, including drowsiness, confusion and irritability. Raised blood glucose (BG) may also be seen, even in the absence of diabetes.

Exposure

Again, raised urea and other toxins affect a number of body systems such as the gut and skin. Oedema may be present in the lower legs. A full infection screen should be carried out. Urinalysis is likely to reflect damage to the kidneys with blood and protein most common. Urinary obstruction may also be evident and can be confirmed by ultrasound scan (USS).

Diagnosis

AKI is diagnosed by:

- Rise in creatinine >26 μmol/L within 48 hours, or
- Rise in creatinine >50% within 7 days, or
- Fall in urine output <0.5 ml/kg/hour for 6 hours.

Management (Figure 27.4)

Airway

Monitor and secure as required.

Breathing

Provide supplemental oxygen to maintain oxygen saturation above 94%. Chest X-ray can help detect infection and pulmonary oedema. Pulmonary oedema can be managed pharmacologically and with continuous positive airway pressure (CPAP).

Circulation

Intravenous (IV) access should be established, taking care to avoid arms with a fistula if present. If the patient is hypotensive with signs of shock, fluid resuscitation or replacement is commenced. Careful cardiovascular monitoring and fluid balance should be undertaken to monitor for response and tolerance. Patients with existing cardiovascular disease may not tolerate rapid fluid administration. Central venous pressure (CVP) monitoring will help guide fluid management. Inotropic drugs may be considered if fluids alone are insufficient to maintain mean arterial pressure (MAP) >75 mmHg. Hyperkalaemia is treated with calcium resonium for cardiac protection and then potassium is forced into the cells with an insulin and glucose infusion. Salbutamol nebulisers can also be used. Regular monitoring of potassium levels and electrocardiogram (ECG) testing are essential.

Disability

Continue neurological observations and hourly BG. Offer reassurance to the patient and carers.

Exposure

Uremic patients are particularly susceptible to infection so scrupulous infection control measures should be followed. Personal care and nutrition should be addressed when appropriate. Anti-emetics are given to treat nausea and vomiting.

Renal replacement therapy (RRT)

Patients should be referred immediately to the renal or critical care team for RRT if any of the following are not responding to medical management:

- Hyperkalaemia
- Metabolic acidosis
- Symptoms or complications of uraemia
- Fluid overload
- Pulmonary oedema.

RRT for AKI is usually provided in an intensive care unit (ICU) setting. It consists of passing the patient's blood through a circuit via a machine to a semipermeable membrane that acts as a filter. Waste products and water (the ultrafiltrate) are removed by convection or diffusion. Replacement fluid is added and the blood is returned to the patient. RRT methods include:

- Haemodialysis
- Haemofiltration
- Haemodiafiltration.

28 Diabetic emergencies

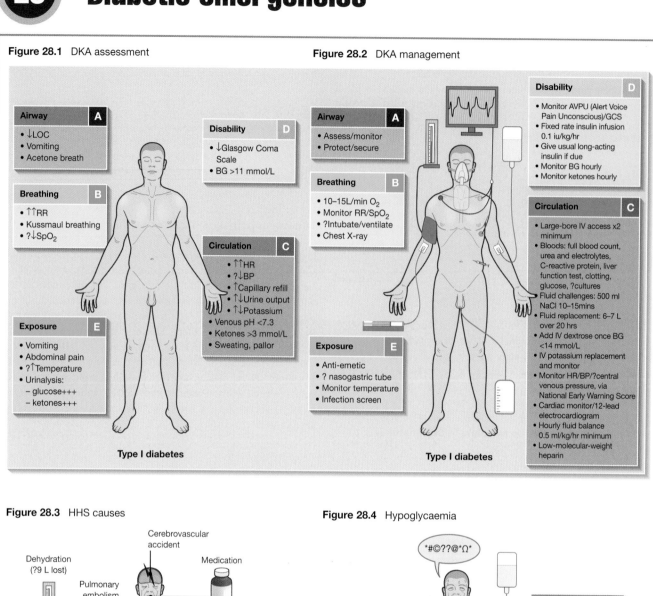

Figure 28.1 DKA assessment

Airway A
- ↓LOC
- Vomiting
- Acetone breath

Breathing B
- ↑↑RR
- Kussmaul breathing
- ?↓SpO₂

Disability D
- ↓Glasgow Coma Scale
- BG >11 mmol/L

Circulation C
- ↑↑HR
- ?↓BP
- ↑Capillary refill
- ↑↓Urine output
- ↑↓Potassium
- Venous pH <7.3
- Ketones >3 mmol/L
- Sweating, pallor

Exposure E
- Vomiting
- Abdominal pain
- ?↑Temperature
- Urinalysis:
  – glucose+++
  – ketones+++

Type I diabetes

Figure 28.2 DKA management

Airway A
- Assess/monitor
- Protect/secure

Breathing B
- 10–15L/min O₂
- Monitor RR/SpO₂
- ?Intubate/ventilate
- Chest X-ray

Disability D
- Monitor AVPU (Alert Voice Pain Unconscious)/GCS
- Fixed rate insulin infusion 0.1 iu/kg/hr
- Give usual long-acting insulin if due
- Monitor BG hourly
- Monitor ketones hourly

Circulation C
- Large-bore IV access x2 minimum
- Bloods: full blood count, urea and electrolytes, C-reactive protein, liver function test, clotting, glucose, ?cultures
- Fluid challenges: 500 ml NaCl 10–15mins
- Fluid replacement: 6–7 L over 20 hrs
- Add IV dextrose once BG <14 mmol/L
- IV potassium replacement and monitor
- Monitor HR/BP/?central venous pressure, via National Early Warning Score
- Cardiac monitor/12-lead electrocardiogram
- Hourly fluid balance 0.5 ml/kg/hr minimum
- Low-molecular-weight heparin

Exposure E
- Anti-emetic
- ? nasogastric tube
- Monitor temperature
- Infection screen

Type I diabetes

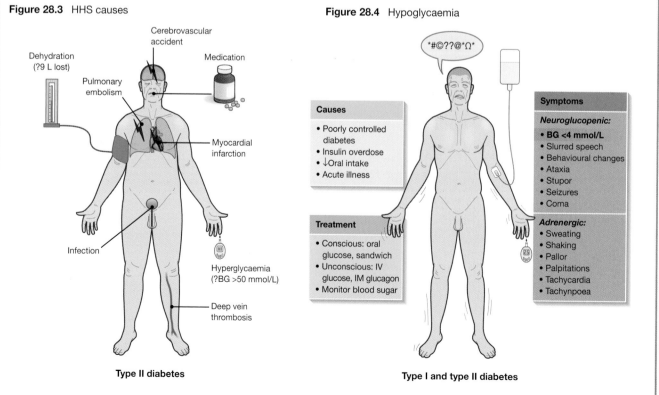

Figure 28.3 HHS causes

- Dehydration (?9 L lost)
- Cerebrovascular accident
- Medication
- Pulmonary embolism
- Myocardial infarction
- Infection
- Hyperglycaemia (?BG >50 mmol/L)
- Deep vein thrombosis

Type II diabetes

Figure 28.4 Hypoglycaemia

*#©??@*Ω*

Causes
- Poorly controlled diabetes
- Insulin overdose
- ↓Oral intake
- Acute illness

Treatment
- Conscious: oral glucose, sandwich
- Unconscious: IV glucose, IM glucagon
- Monitor blood sugar

Symptoms

Neuroglucopenic:
- **BG <4 mmol/L**
- Slurred speech
- Behavioural changes
- Ataxia
- Stupor
- Seizures
- Coma

Adrenergic:
- Sweating
- Shaking
- Pallor
- Palpitations
- Tachycardia
- Tachynpoea

Type I and type II diabetes

Emergency Nursing at a Glance, First Edition. Natalie Holbery and Paul Newcombe.

Diabetes mellitus is an increasingly common long-term condition that causes a large number of chronic health problems and often presents as a comorbidity. However, there are a number of circumstances that result in the presentation of potentially life-threatening diabetic emergencies to an emergency department (ED), namely:

- Diabetic ketoacidosis (DKA)
- Hyperosmolar hyperglycaemic state (HSS)
- Hypoglycaemia.

Diabetic ketoacidosis (DKA)

Patients with type I diabetes have limited or absent production of insulin from the pancreas. This is often the result of an autoimmune process. Type I diabetes usually manifests in children, adolescents or young adults. There are a range of circumstances that are known to precipitate DKA in patients with type I diabetes, but about 25% of presentations occur in undiagnosed diabetics. Causes include:

- Stress
- Infection
- Acute illness
- Drugs/alcohol
- Accidental/intentional insulin omission
- Unstable diabetes.

Pathophysiology of DKA

DKA is characterised by:

- Raised blood glucose ([BG]; hyperglycaemia)
- Raised blood ketones (ketonaemia)
- Acidosis
- Hypovolaemic shock (Figure 28.1).

A combination of little or no insulin production and the release of counter-regulatory hormones (glucagon, cortisol, growth hormone, epinephrine) due to a stress response, causes severe hyperglycaemia (BG >11 mmol/L). Insulin resistance also occurs. Because cells are unable to use available glucose, lipolysis occurs to generate an alternative energy source. The liberated free fatty acids are metabolised by the liver into ketones. These are excreted in the urine and by the lungs, but because ketones are acidic they lower the pH, hence ketoacidosis. The body responds by increasing the rate and depth of respiration (Kussmaul breathing) to 'blow off' carbon dioxide in an attempt to correct the acid-base imbalance. Raised ketones also contribute to a reduced level of consciousness (LOC), abdominal pain, nausea and vomiting.

Fluid losses of 7L occur in DKA and are responsible for the high mortality rate. Hypovolaemic shock occurs as a result of hyperglycaemia-induced osmotic diuresis, vomiting, reduced oral intake and increased insensible losses, including sweating and raised respiratory rate (RR). As blood sugar rises, the threshold for reabsorption of glucose from the renal tubules is exceeded. This causes increased urinary excretion and subsequent increased urine output due to osmotic diuresis. Electrolytes, namely potassium, are also lost. Potassium shifts out of the cells due to the lack of insulin. Because of the resulting fluid volume deficit, the body's compensatory mechanisms are activated causing increased heart rate (HR) and contractility, increased peripheral vascular resistance and eventually reduced urine output. Blood pressure (BP) and organ perfusion drops once compensatory mechanisms are exceeded. Before the production of insulin in the 1920s, DKA had a 100% mortality.

Management of DKA

DKA should be considered in all acutely ill patients with diabetes and also in any patient presenting with acute illness of unknown cause, particularly children and young adults and especially those in a coma. Patients are often brought in by ambulance as a priority call but they may also self-present.

The goals of management in DKA are

- Early identification
- Swift 'ABCDE' approach (Chapter 4)
- Restoration of circulating volume
- Clearance of ketones/suppression of ketogenesis
- Correction of electrolyte imbalance (potassium)
- Reduction of BG
- Identification and treatment of underlying cause (Figure 28.2).

Specialist input may be required and the patient should be transferred to the intensive care unit (ICU).

Hyperosmolar hyperglycaemic state (HSS)

Formerly known as hyperosmolar non-ketotic syndrome (HONK), HHS is ten times less common than DKA, but has a similar mortality rate. Because HHS occurs in people with type II diabetes, patients tend to be older. Likely causes reflect this (Figure 28.3).

The key pathophysiological differences are that insulin resistance and a usually insipid onset cause significant hyperglycaemia (sometimes >50 mmol/L), whereas insulin production is just sufficient to prevent ketosis. Dehydration is often even more significant in HHS (>9L lost). Some patients with type II diabetes present with features of both HHS and DKA.

Management is essentially the same as for DK, but because of the age of the patient, comorbidities and polypharmacy, caution needs to be exercised. Fluid, potassium and insulin administration should all be monitored carefully. Identification and treatment of the underlying cause are essential.

Hypoglycaemia

Hypoglycaemia or 'hypo' is a common occurrence in patients with both type I and type II diabetes (Figure 28.4). Hypoglycaemia is defined as <4 mmol/L. There are a number of causes that may result from poorly controlled or poorly managed diabetes, insulin overdose or acute illness.

Patients may present with bizarre behaviour or appear drunk, or they may be brought in by ambulance in a coma. Symptoms are characterised as neuroglucopenic (due to low glucose in brain cells) or adrenergic (due to the stress response). Hypoglycaemia is life threatening and needs to be identified swiftly via a thorough ABCDE approach. Early measurement of BG level is key. Accompanying family and friends may be useful in establishing usual patterns.

Treatment depends upon a patient's ability to consume oral carbohydrates. Sugary drinks, gels or tablets should be given if possible, followed by long-acting carbohydrates such as a sandwich, when appropriate. If the patient is unconscious or unable to take anything orally, intravenous (IV) access should be gained and IV glucose given urgently. Intramuscular (IM) glucagon can also be given if IV access is difficult. Ongoing monitoring of BG is essential. Patient education and referral to a diabetes specialist nurse on discharge may be necessary.

(29) Obstetrics and gynaecology

Figure 29.1 Changes in pregnancy

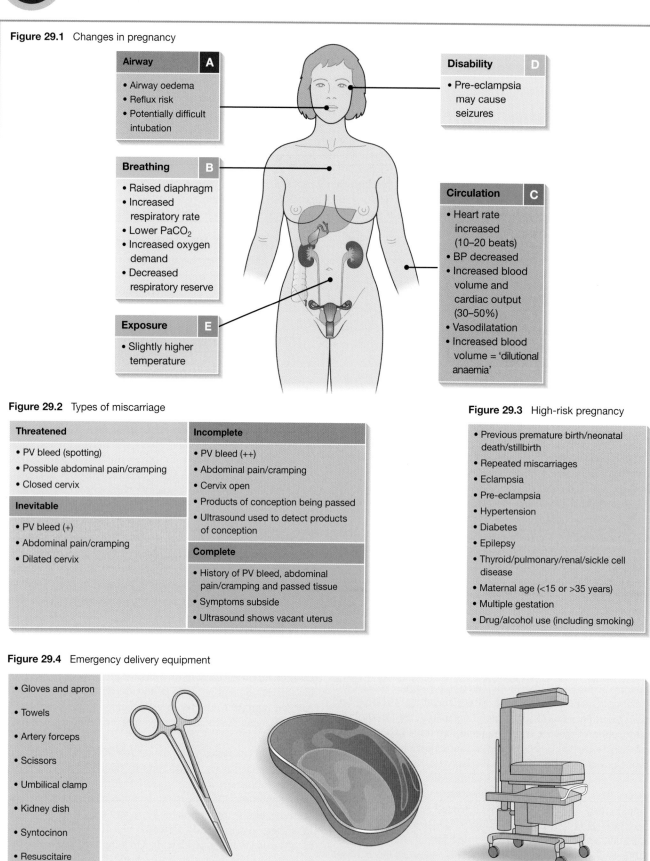

Airway	A
• Airway oedema
• Reflux risk
• Potentially difficult intubation

Disability	D
• Pre-eclampsia may cause seizures

Breathing	B
• Raised diaphragm
• Increased respiratory rate
• Lower $PaCO_2$
• Increased oxygen demand
• Decreased respiratory reserve

Circulation	C
• Heart rate increased (10–20 beats)
• BP decreased
• Increased blood volume and cardiac output (30–50%)
• Vasodilatation
• Increased blood volume = 'dilutional anaemia'

Exposure	E
• Slightly higher temperature

Figure 29.2 Types of miscarriage

Threatened
- PV bleed (spotting)
- Possible abdominal pain/cramping
- Closed cervix

Inevitable
- PV bleed (+)
- Abdominal pain/cramping
- Dilated cervix

Incomplete
- PV bleed (++)
- Abdominal pain/cramping
- Cervix open
- Products of conception being passed
- Ultrasound used to detect products of conception

Complete
- History of PV bleed, abdominal pain/cramping and passed tissue
- Symptoms subside
- Ultrasound shows vacant uterus

Figure 29.3 High-risk pregnancy

- Previous premature birth/neonatal death/stillbirth
- Repeated miscarriages
- Eclampsia
- Pre-eclampsia
- Hypertension
- Diabetes
- Epilepsy
- Thyroid/pulmonary/renal/sickle cell disease
- Maternal age (<15 or >35 years)
- Multiple gestation
- Drug/alcohol use (including smoking)

Figure 29.4 Emergency delivery equipment

- Gloves and apron
- Towels
- Artery forceps
- Scissors
- Umbilical clamp
- Kidney dish
- Syntocinon
- Resuscitaire

Emergency Nursing at a Glance, First Edition. Natalie Holbery and Paul Newcombe
© 2016 John Wiley & Sons, Ltd. Published 2016 by John Wiley & Sons, Ltd. Companion website: www.ataglanceseries.com/nursing/emergencynursing

Obstetric problems

Pregnant women may present to an emergency department (ED) with pregnancy or non-pregnancy related conditions. ED nurses need to be familiar with anatomical and physiological changes in pregnancy (Figure 29.1) to aid assessment and decision making. Regardless of the nature of their presentation, pregnant patients may feel anxious presenting to the ED. Nurses should offer reassurance to the patient and her partner, and be familiar with local resources and referral pathways. General care principles and the most common pregnancy related conditions are presented below.

General principles

Any woman of child-bearing age who presents with abdominal pain or vaginal bleeding should be asked about the potential for pregnancy. A pregnancy test should be performed with informed consent. Results of the pregnancy test should be shared with the patient and documented in the notes.

Domestic abuse is known to commence or escalate during pregnancy. ED nurses should be alert to signs and symptoms of domestic abuse (Chapter 37) and sensitively approach the patient if concerned.

Most pregnant patients will carry hand-held maternity notes. Whenever possible, assessment and discharge information should be recorded in these as well as ED notes.

Ectopic pregnancy

Usually occurring at 6–10 weeks gestation, ectopic pregnancy is the most common life-threatening condition in early pregnancy. The embryo develops in the fallopian tube rather than the uterus, sometimes causing fallopian tube rupture and haemorrhage. Some patients may not know they are pregnant. The classic signs are abdominal pain, amenorrhoea, new vaginal bleeding and syncope. However, other signs such as diarrhoea, vomiting, dizziness, back pain and shoulder tip pain may also be present. These latter signs often indicate tubal rupture. If ectopic pregnancy is suspected, a urine pregnancy test should be performed. If this is negative and pregnancy is still suspected, a blood test can be done. An ultrasound, ideally transvaginal, should be performed to confirm diagnosis. Ectopic pregnancies may spontaneously resolve (tubal abortion) or require surgery, usually a laparoscopy. ED nurses should monitor pain, provide analgesia and fluids as required, and give psychosocial support.

Miscarriage

Miscarriage, also known as spontaneous abortion, is thought to occur in up to 20% of known pregnancies. There are four types of miscarriage and each will require different management (Figure 29.2). Women who present to an ED are often distressed and require psychosocial support. Most women do not present as haemodynamically unstable and should be cared for in a private room in majors whenever possible. If haemodynamic instability is present (usually due to haemorrhage), a woman should be cared for in the resuscitation area. Management of haemorrhage in miscarriage is similar to any major haemorrhage and is outlined in Chapter 61.

Hyperemesis

Hyperemesis is uncontrolled vomiting during pregnancy that results in dehydration, electrolyte imbalance and weight loss. Hospitalisation is usually required. Symptoms usually commence from 8–9 weeks and continue up to 20 weeks of pregnancy. Management in the ED includes intravenous (IV) fluids, administration of electrolytes (e.g. potassium) and dietary and lifestyle advice. Eating smaller meals more frequently may help, and ginger has been shown to reduce nausea in some cases. Fatigue is known to exacerbate nausea and vomiting, and women should therefore be encouraged to increase their rest.

Pre-eclampsia

Pregnant women are usually screened for pre-eclampsia in antenatal clinics and it is therefore a relatively uncommon ED presentation. However, pre-eclampsia is considered an obstetric emergency, so ED nurses should be familiar with its presentation and management. Symptoms include headache and epigastric pain. Severe pre-eclampsia may be associated with visual disturbance, altered mental state, oedema or shortness of breath. The patient's blood pressure (BP) should be checked, along with other vital signs, urine tested for the presence of protein (proteinuria) and bloods taken (full blood count [FBC], urea and electrolytes [U&E], liver function tests [LFTs], clotting screen). Pre-eclampsia should be suspected if BP is elevated or there is proteinuria. A referral to the obstetric team should be made. ED nurses should commence a fluid balance chart and administer antihypertensive medication as prescribed. The goal is to achieve a BP of less than 160 mmHg systolic. A decision may be made to take the patient to theatre for urgent delivery. ED nurses should communicate the plan and provide psychosocial support.

Thromboembolism

Thromboembolism, the collective term for deep vein thrombosis (DVT) and pulmonary embolism (PE), is a potentially life-threatening condition. Pregnant women are at increased risk of thromboembolism due to hypercoagulability. The condition can occur at any stage during pregnancy. Signs of thromboembolism in a pregnant patient are the same as in non-pregnant patients; pain and swelling of the affected leg, shortness of breath and tachycardia. Any one of these signs in a pregnant patient should be treated as possible DVT or PE. A clinical diagnosis is often made but a blood test (d-dimer) and scan will confirm diagnosis. ED nurses should administer anticoagulant medication as soon as possible and provide analgesia, fluids and psychosocial support as required.

Emergency delivery and labour

On occasions women, and sometimes children, present to an ED in labour. In most cases the pregnancy is known, while in others the pregnancy is undisclosed. The latter is more common in children and young women. Unless delivery is imminent, the ED nurse should notify the maternity unit and arrange for immediate transfer to the labour ward.

Unless high risk (Figure 29.3), delivery in the ED can occur in a cubicle in majors; however, local guidelines should be followed. A midwife should be notified and equipment prepared (Figure 29.4). It may also be appropriate to notify the neonatal team. A doctor and ED nurse should stay with the patient until delivery. If the baby is crying, they should initially be placed on the mother's chest. If not crying, the baby should be wrapped in towels and rubbed to stimulate a response. If the baby does not respond, neonatal life support should be initiated. The neonatal team should be notified urgently.

Artery forceps and scissors are used to clamp and cut the cord when appropriate. Syntocinon is administered intramuscularly after delivery to facilitate placental delivery. The mother and baby should then be transferred to the maternity unit.

Early pregnancy assessment units (EPAUs)

Many hospitals have dedicated units that provide urgent assessment and support during the early stages of pregnancy. They generally do not require a referral, allowing women to attend as they need to. Patients presenting to an ED with non-life threatening early pregnancy related conditions can be sent straight to the EPAU, although local policy should be followed. The majority of EPAUs do not operate out of hours; ED nurses therefore need to be familiar with pregnancy related conditions and their management.

Gynaecological problems

Most women with gynaecological problems who present to an ED complain of per vaginal (PV) bleeding or pelvic pain. Some hospitals have emergency gynaecological units where patients may self-present or be redirected from triage.

Vaginal bleeding

Vaginal bleeding in non-pregnant women may be caused by structural or traumatic causes from the vagina, uterus or cervix. A doctor or nurse practitioner will perform a pelvic examination to establish the cause and determine the need for further investigations. Assessment of PV bleeding should include the following:
- Duration of bleeding
- Colour of blood (red/brown)
- Amount of bleeding
- Number of pads used since bleeding started
- Last menstrual period
- Consideration of abuse (domestic/sexual/child).

If bleeding is severe and the patient is haemodynamically unstable, she should be cared for in the resuscitation area and have two cannulas inserted followed by administration of blood products. In this situation, the massive transfusion protocol may need to be activated.

Fortunately, most women with PV bleeding who present to an ED are not considered emergencies and are usually discharged home for ongoing care from their general practitioner or gynaecological team.

Pelvic pain

Pelvic pain may be associated with menstrual related problems such as dysmenorrhea, endometriosis or ovulation pain. Non-menstrual related pain may include pelvic inflammatory disease (PID), ovarian torsion or pelvic tumours (e.g. fibroids). Although pelvic pain is usually associated with gynaecological problems, other causes, such as urinary tract infection, appendicitis and inflammatory bowel disease, must be ruled out. Assessment should include the following;
- severity and nature of pain
- presence of vaginal discharge
- PV bleeding
- date of last menstrual period
- bowel habits
- urinary habits
- consideration of abuse (domestic/sexual/child).

A pregnancy test should be performed (with informed consent) in women of child-bearing age. Blood tests and an abdominal/pelvic ultrasound are likely investigations. If a sexually transmitted infection is suspected, the assessment should occur in a private area. Chapter 36 outlines the assessment and care of patients with sexually transmitted infections.

Pain should be managed in a timely manner and commenced at triage. Referral to the gynaecological team may be required and admission will be determined by the diagnosis and severity of illness.

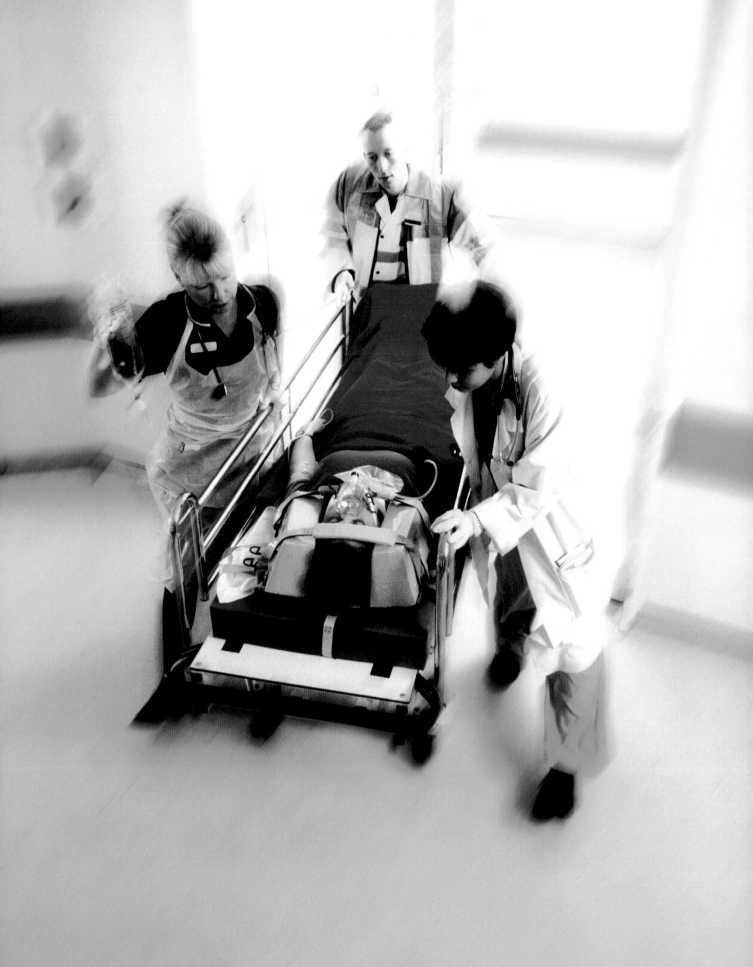

Poisoning and overdose

Part 6

Chapters

30 Poisoning: Assessment and management

Figure 30.1 Common toxins with antidotes

Toxin	Antidote/treatment
Digoxin	Digibind®/Digifab®
Acute dystonic reaction (e.g. metoclopramide, prochlorperazine)	Procyclidine
Cyanide	Cyanokit® (Hydroxocobalamin)/dicobalt edetate/sodium nitrite
Benzodiazepines	Flumazenil (Anexate®)
Ethylene glycol/methanol (anti-freeze)	Fomipezole®/ethanol
Paracetamol	N-Acetylcysteine (Parvolex®)
Warfarin	Vitamin K (Konakion®)/Prothrombin complex concentrate (e.g. Beriplex®)
Opioids	Naloxone
Iron	Desferrioxamine
Beta-blockers	Atropine, glucagon, intotropes, and pacing
Calcium channel blockers	Calcium, atropine, glucagon, intotropes and pacing
Organophosphates	Atropine/Pralidoxime®
Carbon monoxide	Oxygen

Figure 30.2 Assessment

Assessment

- Are there any signs and symptoms?
- What drug/substance has been taken?
- What type of preparation is it? (e.g. enteric coated, modified release)
- What dosage was taken?
- What is the patient's weight?
- What time was it taken?
- Single or staggered dose?
- How was it taken (intravenous (IV), intramuscular, inhaled, oral, absorbed, per rectum, per vagina)?
- Was anything taken with it? (consider above questions for each co-ingestant)
- Is there any significant past medical history? (e.g. renal/liver problems)

Figure 30.3 Common effects of toxic substances on body

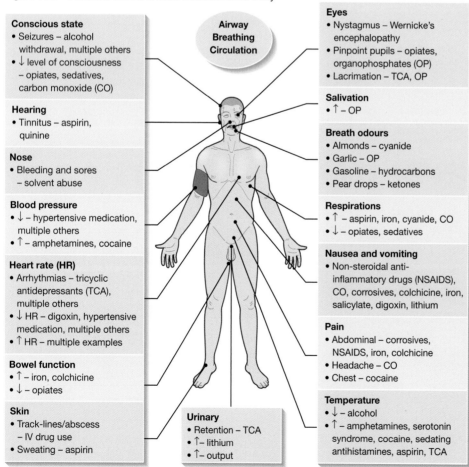

Conscious state
- Seizures – alcohol withdrawal, multiple others
- ↓ level of consciousness – opiates, sedatives, carbon monoxide (CO)

Hearing
- Tinnitus – aspirin, quinine

Nose
- Bleeding and sores – solvent abuse

Blood pressure
- ↓ – hypertensive medication, multiple others
- ↑ – amphetamines, cocaine

Heart rate (HR)
- Arrhythmias – tricyclic antidepressants (TCA), multiple others
- ↓ HR – digoxin, hypertensive medication, multiple others
- ↑ HR – multiple examples

Bowel function
- ↑ – iron, colchicine
- ↓ – opiates

Skin
- Track-lines/abscess – IV drug use
- Sweating – aspirin

Airway
Breathing
Circulation

Eyes
- Nystagmus – Wernicke's encephalopathy
- Pinpoint pupils – opiates, organophosphates (OP)
- Lacrimation – TCA, OP

Salivation
- ↑ – OP

Breath odours
- Almonds – cyanide
- Garlic – OP
- Gasoline – hydrocarbons
- Pear drops – ketones

Respirations
- ↑ – aspirin, iron, cyanide, CO
- ↓ – opiates, sedatives

Nausea and vomiting
- Non-steroidal anti-inflammatory drugs (NSAIDS), CO, corrosives, colchicine, iron, salicylate, digoxin, lithium

Pain
- Abdominal – corrosives, NSAIDS, iron, colchicine
- Headache – CO
- Chest – cocaine

Temperature
- ↓ – alcohol
- ↑ – amphetamines, serotonin syndrome, cocaine, sedating antihistamines, aspirin, TCA

Urinary
- Retention – TCA
- ↑ – lithium
- ↑ – output

Figure 30.4 Activated charcoal

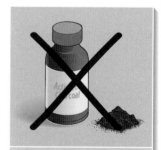

Activated charcoal is not effective in the ingestion of:
- Cyanide
- Ethanol
- Ethylene glycol
- Iron
- Lithium
- Malathion
- Methanol
- Petroleum distillates
- Strong acids and alkalis

Emergency Nursing at a Glance, First Edition. Natalie Holbery and Paul Newcombe.

Overdose, poisoning and acute alcohol intoxication are common presentations to an emergency department (ED) and the assessment and management of this group of patients presents a number of challenges for nursing and medical teams. While a number of antidotes and methods of decontamination and elimination are available for certain types of poisoning (Figure 30.1), management of the poisoned and intoxicated patient is generally supportive (e.g. monitoring for 6 hours post-ingestion; treating symptoms if/when they arise). The National Poisons Information Service (NPIS) and its online database, Toxbase, provide comprehensive sources of information relating to toxicology, and all ED staff should have access to, and consult these resources when caring for patients who have been poisoned.

Assessment

Effective treatment of a poisoned patient is expedited when those treating the patient have clear information relating to the overdose or poisoning episode. However, and particularly when dealing with an unknown substance, the need for an accurate subjective history should not distract a nurse from initiating an 'ABCDE' assessment of all patients (Chapter 4). This ensures that any life-threatening complications are managed as a priority.

The questions in Figure 30.2 could be used to elicit pertinent information from patients who have deliberately or accidentally overdosed. However, this can be problematic: patients may present with a reduced level of consciousness rendering direct questioning impossible, or they may be unreliable historians. Consider, for example, the patient with suicidal ideation who is reluctant to be helped, or the curious toddler and confused, visually impaired, older patient who are unable to provide an accurate history.

In situations where this information is unreliable or unavailable, a nurse should consider what other sources of information are available to them. For example, can a family member corroborate or offer information? If there are empty packets of medication, what date were the drugs dispensed? Are there any old patient notes? In addition, observing the patient for signs and symptoms of overdose, such as those highlighted in Figure 30.3, can often provide clues as to the type of substance that has been taken.

Decontamination and elimination

The process of decontamination attempts to reduce absorption of toxins into the systemic circulation. In contrast, methods of elimination (e.g. haemodialysis) aim to maximise toxin removal from the system.

Activated charcoal (AC)

The large surface area of the granules in AC makes it particularly adept at binding to toxins and preventing the absorption of toxic substances by the gastrointestinal tract. AC is only indicated for use in substances that have been ingested within the past hour (or 2 hours in the case of medicines that delay gastric emptying (e.g. tricyclic antidepressants (TCAs), aspirin, enteric-coated and modified-release preparations). Reconstituted with water to achieve the desired concentration, AC is administered as a single dose or, occasionally, in multiple doses. Its unpalatable taste can induce vomiting, which in turn will reduce efficacy of the treatment. As such, consider anti-emetic medication and mixing the solution with a non-caffeinated drink. Nurses need to consider the following in order to avoid airway management complications:

- Is the patient cooperative and alert?
- Does the airway need to be secured before proceeding?

It should be noted that decontamination with AC is not universally indicated and Figure 30.4 outlines the substances for which AC is generally regarded as ineffective.

Whole bowel irrigation (WBI)

WBI with polyethylene glycol is generally used to expedite the passage of drugs that have been swallowed by 'body stuffers' involved in drug smuggling. It is administered in large volumes as an oral solution, by mouth or nasogastric tube.

Gastric lavage (GL)

'Stomach pumping' is now rarely used in practice. Its efficacy has been questioned and there are very few poisoning scenarios in which toxicology experts recommend gastric irrigation – namely, large life-threatening overdoses of substances taken within an hour, which cannot be removed by other means. The passage of a large orogastric tube into the patient's stomach facilitates removal of toxic substances through an irrigation/aspiration technique. The main risk factor from GL is aspiration, and therefore nursing care is primarily concerned with maintaining a safe airway.

Other methods

Haemodialysis is not routinely carried out in an ED but it is the gold standard treatment for large lithium and toxic alcohol overdoses. Patients undergoing this treatment will require admission to the intensive care unit (ICU).

Urine alkalinisation is a process by which increasing the pH (alkalinity) of urine by administering sodium bicarbonate enhances the excretion of weak acid toxins, such as moderate levels of salicylate (aspirin). It is an adjunct in treating methotrexate poisoning.

Referral and follow-up

A number of variables will dictate the referral and follow-up protocols for these patients. Admission for observation and further treatment may be required and, in some cases, specialist input (e.g. liver, renal, cardiology) may be sought. Intentional overdose may require the involvement of psychiatric services once the patient is suitable for medical discharge. Finally, nurses should always have a low threshold for initiating safeguarding children and vulnerable adult protocols in situations where poisoning incidents have occurred.

Poisoning: Prescription and non-prescription drugs

Figure 31.1 Tricyclic antidepressant overdose: Assessment and management

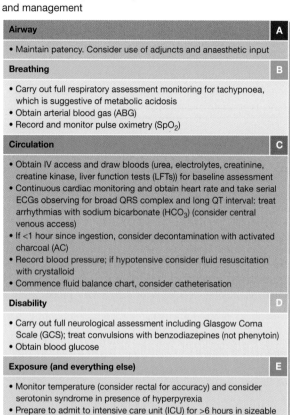

Airway **A**
- Maintain patency. Consider use of adjuncts and anaesthetic input

Breathing **B**
- Carry out full respiratory assessment monitoring for tachypnoea, which is suggestive of metabolic acidosis
- Obtain arterial blood gas (ABG)
- Record and monitor pulse oximetry (SpO_2)

Circulation **C**
- Obtain IV access and draw bloods (urea, electrolytes, creatinine, creatine kinase, liver function tests (LFTs)) for baseline assessment
- Continuous cardiac monitoring and obtain heart rate and take serial ECGs observing for broad QRS complex and long QT interval: treat arrhythmias with sodium bicarbonate (HCO_3) (consider central venous access)
- If <1 hour since ingestion, consider decontamination with activated charcoal (AC)
- Record blood pressure; if hypotensive consider fluid resuscitation with crystalloid
- Commence fluid balance chart, consider catheterisation

Disability **D**
- Carry out full neurological assessment including Glasgow Coma Scale (GCS); treat convulsions with benzodiazepines (not phenytoin)
- Obtain blood glucose

Exposure (and everything else) **E**
- Monitor temperature (consider rectal for accuracy) and consider serotonin syndrome in presence of hyperpyrexia
- Prepare to admit to intensive care unit (ICU) for >6 hours in sizeable overdose

Figure 31.3 Paracetamol treatment nomograph

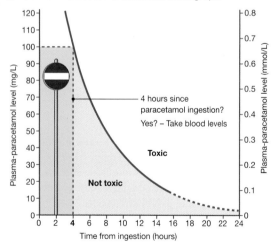

- 4 hours since paracetamol ingestion? Yes? – Take blood levels
- Toxic
- Not toxic

Time from ingestion (hours)

Figure 31.4 Treatment with Parvolex (NAC)

- <1 hour consider AC
- >1 hour but <4 hour: commence NAC immediately in significant or staggered overdose; otherwise wait for 4 hours for blood levels
- >4 hours: await bloods and treat if over the treatment line (in toxic 'zone')
- Refer to TOXBASE guidance

N.B. NAC is most effective if commenced within 8 hours of ingestion

Figure 31.2 Signs and symptoms of paracetamol overdose

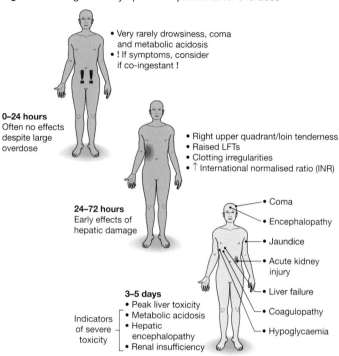

- Very rarely drowsiness, coma and metabolic acidosis
- ! If symptoms, consider if co-ingestant !

0–24 hours
Often no effects despite large overdose

- Right upper quadrant/loin tenderness
- Raised LFTs
- Clotting irregularities
- ↑ International normalised ratio (INR)

24–72 hours
Early effects of hepatic damage

- Coma
- Encephalopathy
- Jaundice
- Acute kidney injury
- Liver failure
- Coagulopathy
- Hypoglycaemia

3–5 days
- Peak liver toxicity
- Metabolic acidosis

Indicators of severe toxicity
- Hepatic encephalopathy
- Renal insufficiency

Figure 31.5 Opioid overdose: Assessment and management

Airway **A**
- Maintain patency. Airway at risk secondary to central nervous system depression
- Consider risk of withdrawal-related vomiting in opioid-dependent patients whose symptoms are 'reversed' with naloxone
- Consider use of adjuncts and anaesthetic input

Breathing **B**
- Carry out full respiratory assessment monitoring for bradypnoea secondary to respiratory depression
- Consider lowest dose of naloxone/naloxone infusion sufficient to raise respiratory rate to adequate level (particularly in opioid-dependent patients)
- Record and monitor SpO_2. Give O_2 if hypoxic
- Obtain ABG if bradypnoeic and/or ↓level of consciousness

Circulation **C**
- Obtain IV access and draw bloods for baseline assessment
- Consider intraosseus access if venous access difficult
- If <1 hour since ingestion, consider decontamination with AC
- Record BP and HR
- Record 12-lead ECG and connect to cardiac monitor
- Serial ECGs in **methadone** overdose

Disability **D**
- Carry out full neurological assessment including GCS; treat convulsions with benzodiazepines (not phenytoin)
- Observe for opioid withdrawal in patients receiving naloxone
- Obtain blood glucose

Exposure (and everything else) **E**
- Record temperature
- Inspect body for injection sites/abscess in IV drug users
- Inspect body for opioid patches
- Prepare to admit to ICU for >6 hours in sizeable overdose
- Monitor for 6 hours post-naloxone and 12 hours in modified-release preparations
- Anticipate agitation and withdrawal in opioid-dependent patients

Emergency Nursing at a Glance, First Edition. Natalie Holbery and Paul Newcombe.
© 2016 John Wiley & Sons, Ltd. Published 2016 by John Wiley & Sons, Ltd. Companion website: www.ataglanceseries.com/nursing/emergencynursing

Overdose and poisoning from prescription and non-prescription drugs is commonly encountered in an emergency department (ED). The differentiation between prescribed and non-prescribed drugs in this context reflects the use and abuse of illicit recreational drugs and the harmful effects of prescribed medication taken in excessive quantities. Both scenarios can present as either accidental or intentional poisoning episodes.

Prescription drugs

There is a seemingly inexhaustible list of prescribed substances that could be ingested alone or in combination with other medications or substances. For this reason, consultation with the National Poisons Information Service (NPIS) and its online database, Toxbase, is of paramount importance in guiding the management and nursing care of these patients. With the exception of paracetamol and salicylate (aspirin) poisoning, blood toxicology is of limited use in the detection of substances that may have been ingested.

Tricyclic antidepressants (TCAs)

After illicit opiate use, TCA (e.g. amitriptyline and dosulepin) overdose represents the largest group of drugs responsible for patient deaths. TCA overdose is particularly dangerous because of the cardiovascular toxicity of large doses that cause significant electrocardiogram (ECG) changes. The presence of signs and symptoms can be rapid (within 30 minutes of drug ingestion) and deterioration can be precipitous. Patients present with a range of clinical signs and symptoms but the general picture, initially, is that of vasodilation. An 'ABCDE' approach (Chapter 4) to such patients should be adopted (Figure 31.1).

Other antidepressants

Other antidepressant medications such as selective serotonin re-uptake inhibitors (SSRIs) (e.g. fluoxetine, sertraline and citalopram), venlafaxine and mirtazapine are generally safer in overdose than their older TCA counterparts. However, an ED nurse should ensure that a thorough and systematic assessment and re-assessment of patients takes place, and refer to TOXBASE and the NPIS for guidance.

Lithium

Lithium is used to treat bipolar depression and, even at therapeutic levels, has notable side effects. It is characterised by having a narrow therapeutic index and, accordingly, chronic toxicity can readily occur. Lithium is **not** adsorbed by activated charcoal and severe lithium toxicity is therefore eliminated through haemodialysis.

Paracetamol

Paracetamol poisoning is common and represents half of all drug overdose related presentations in the UK. It is the leading cause of acute liver failure and subsequent transplantation. There are rarely any initial signs and symptoms of a toxic paracetamol overdose, a factor which can delay treatment, with devastating consequences. (Figure 31.2).

Prompt treatment (<8 hours) guided by a treatment normograph (Figure 31.3) with N-acetylcysteine (NAC/Parvolex®), is uniformly effective even in patients who have ingested a potentially fatal dose and/or who have pre-existing liver damage. Treatment of paracetamol poisoning is outlined in Figure 31.4. Increasingly, staggered overdoses are becoming common and can be difficult to treat.

Opioids

Opioids are widely used in both community and clinical settings to treat moderate to severe pain. Illicit use is dealt with separately. Opioids such as codeine are commonly available over the counter in a number of different preparations and strengths. Opioid overdose is reversed with the administration of naloxone, a drug that blocks opiate receptors but has a shorter half-life than the opioids it treats. To counter this, an infusion of naloxone is often given in significant overdoses. The ABCDE approach should be used to guide intervention and patient care (Figure 31.5).

Benzodiazepines

Benzodiazepines are commonly used in an ED for procedural techniques such as relocation of dislocated limbs. Like opioids, they are also drugs of dependency and complete reversal of overdose can precipitate withdrawal seizures in some patients. Large doses of benzodiazepines are associated with depression of the respiratory centre and, in attempts of deliberate self-harm, this effect is commonly exacerbated with concomitant use of alcohol. The reversal agent flumazenil, however, should only be used when medical staff can be certain that presenting signs and symptoms are directly attributed to benzodiazepine use (e.g. reversing the effect of midazolam post-procedure).

Salicylate

Ingestion of a large amount of aspirin (salicylate) can be dangerous because of difficulties in managing complex acid-base and electrolyte derangement. Depending on the dose, symptoms can vary from tinnitus, nausea, vomiting and abdominal pain to hyperventilation, seizure and coma. Owing to their size, children are at particular risk from salicylate poisoning. If timing allows, decontamination with activated charcoal (AC) is indicated, and haemodialysis may be required. Urine alkalinisation with sodium bicarbonate is also of value in salicylate elimination.

Non-prescription drugs

Patterns and trends in illicit drug use are influenced by many factors including age and gender. Although there is an overall downward trend in recreational drug use (RDU) in the UK, there has been a significant increase in the availability and abuse of newer novel psychoactive substances such as mephedrone or 'legal highs'.

Patient assessment follows the same ABCDE approach outlined earlier and treatment is largely supportive; it should be directed by specialist toxicology resources. Urine screening for RDU is occasionally used to identify unknown toxic ingestion, but it has limited utility because it is unable to differentiate between acute and chronic drug use.

Heroin and methadone

Treatment priorities for heroin and methadone overdose are addressed earlier in relation to opioid overdose. An ED nurse should be aware that methadone has a longer half-life than other opioids and that heroin can also be smoked and snorted.

Cocaine

A cocaine-induced myocardial infarction (MI) is precipitated by vasospasm as opposed to a thromboembolic event. As such, the treatment of choice is intravenous (IV) benzodiazepines and drugs such as glyceryl trinitrate (GTN).

32 Poisoning: Other substances

Figure 32.1 Sources of carbon monoxide

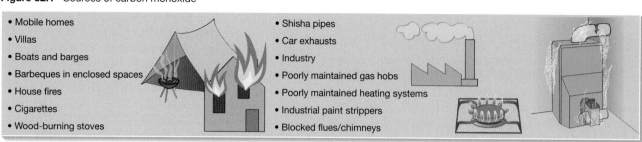

- Mobile homes
- Villas
- Boats and barges
- Barbeques in enclosed spaces
- House fires
- Cigarettes
- Wood-burning stoves

- Shisha pipes
- Car exhausts
- Industry
- Poorly maintained gas hobs
- Poorly maintained heating systems
- Industrial paint strippers
- Blocked flues/chimneys

Figure 32.2 Signs and symptoms of carbon monoxide poisoning

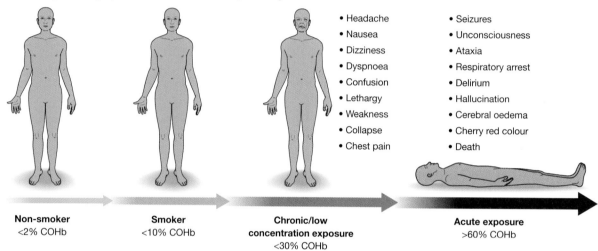

- Headache
- Nausea
- Dizziness
- Dyspnoea
- Confusion
- Lethargy
- Weakness
- Collapse
- Chest pain

- Seizures
- Unconsciousness
- Ataxia
- Respiratory arrest
- Delirium
- Hallucination
- Cerebral oedema
- Cherry red colour
- Death

Non-smoker
<2% COHb

Smoker
<10% COHb

Chronic/low concentration exposure
<30% COHb

Acute exposure
>60% COHb

Figure 32.3
Questions to ask

- Is more than one person in house affected?
- Do symptoms disappear when away from house?
- Are symptoms worse in winter/when cooking?
- Does smoke/condensation accumulate in rooms?
- Is it black/sooty on or around appliances?
- Is there a yellow/orange flame instead of blue from gas appliances?

Figure 32.4 Carbon monoxide poisoning: Assessment and management

Airway   A

- Maintain patency. Consider use of adjuncts and anaesthetic input

Breathing   B

- Venous/arterial COHb measurement
- Do not rely on pulse oximetry: peripheral measurement not able to distinguish between O_2Hb and COHb
- Commence 100% oxygen therapy via tight-fitting non-breathe mask (CO half-life reduced by administering high-flow O_2)
- Arterial blood gas to assess ventilation and presence of metabolic acidosis

Circulation   C

- Obtain intravenous access and draw bloods (U&E, FBC, CK, Troponin) for baseline assessment
- Continuous cardiac monitoring, obtain heart rate and take serial electrocardiograms observing for broad QRS complex and long QT interval. Treat arrhythmias and electrolyte imbalance
- Record blood pressure; if hypotensive, consider fluid resuscitation with crystalloid
- Assess colour of perfusion: skin can appear 'cherry-red'

Disability   D

- Carry out full neurological assessment including Glasgow Coma Scale; treat convulsions with benzodiazepines
- Consider possibility of ↑intracranial pressure and cerebral oedema
- Obtain blood glucose

Exposure (and everything else)   E

- Monitor temperature
- Consider cyanide poisoning if house fire
- Prevent re-exposure – multi-agency response may be required (e.g. social services input)
- Treat other personnel who may have been exposed
- Health promotion advice re: CO detectors
- Consider low threshold for further treatment in high-risk groups, e.g. pregnancy (i.e. HBOT)

Emergency Nursing at a Glance, First Edition. Natalie Holbery and Paul Newcombe
© 2016 John Wiley & Sons, Ltd. Published 2016 by John Wiley & Sons, Ltd. Companion website: www.ataglanceseries.com/nursing/emergencynursing

With the exception of carbon monoxide poisoning, accidental or intentional poisoning that originates from non-drug sources is an uncommon emergency department (ED) presentation. The National Poisons Information Service (NPIS) and its online database, Toxbase, are of particular use in ascertaining treatment priorities in this rarely seen poisoning scenario.

Environmental sources

Carbon monoxide (CO) poisoning

CO is a colourless, odourless and tasteless gas present in small quantities in the atmosphere. It is produced by the incomplete combustion of fossil fuels, and common sources are depicted in Figure 32.1. The most common presentation of CO poisoning to an ED occurs accidentally, either from smoke inhalation in a house fire or as a result of poorly ventilated or malfunctioning domestic gas appliances. Although increasingly less common, failed suicide attempts from intentional inhalation of CO (i.e. from motor vehicle exhaust fumes) occasionally present to an ED.

Pathophysiology

At high concentrations of oxygen, haemoglobin in red blood cells forms loose bonds with oxygen to form oxyhaemoglobin (HbO_2). In this way, oxygen is delivered to individual cells in the tissues of the human body, where the concentration of oxygen is low, and released. In the presence of CO however, oxygen is unable to compete with CO's greater affinity for Hb. CO binds tightly and more readily than oxygen to haemoglobin, thereby creating carboxyhaemoglobin (COHb). The resultant hypoxic insult is felt most keenly in those organs where oxygen demand is greatest: the heart and brain.

Signs and symptoms

Figure 32.2 illustrates how signs and symptoms of CO poisoning are dependent on the level of exposure. At lower levels, patients may be unaware of their, often chronic, exposure to CO. Consequently, they may present to triage with vague symptoms that are non-specific, mimicking other commonly seen presentations (such as flu). Nurses at triage should therefore have a low threshold of suspicion for CO poisoning in the patient presenting with dizziness, nausea and, in particular, a non-traumatic headache. Triage nurses should consider eliciting answers to the questions suggested in Figure 32.3. In contrast, high-concentration exposures (<60%) can be rapidly fatal with collapse and death occurring within minutes.

Treatment

Figure 32.4 outlines the management priorities for CO-poisoned patients. Treatment is largely directed at optimising oxygen delivery and reducing the half-life of CO from approximately 320 minutes (without oxygen) to 80 minutes (with oxygen). Use of hyperbaric oxygen therapy (HBOT) reduces this half-life further still to approximately 20 minutes.

Animal toxins

Snake bites

The adder is the only poisonous snake indigenous to the UK and fatalities from adder bites are extremely rare. Although a licence is required, exotic, venomous snakes can also be kept as pets.

Envenomation by any poisonous snake is likely to produce localised symptoms at the site of the snake bite (swelling, erythema and pain) that radiate distally from the affected limb. However, anaphylactoid-type reactions can occur and should be managed as for ana-phylaxis (Chapter 13). Systemic reactions are more likely in children, owing to their smaller size, and after envenomation by highly poisonous snakes (e.g. cobra, mamba). Treatment is largely supportive (pain control and limb immobilisation) although a number of antivenoms can be used in patients who develop systemic effects.

Household sources

A number of household substances are implicated in accidental overdose although most (particularly those ingested by children) turn out to be non-toxic. Toxbase provides a comprehensive list of common low-toxicity items.

Sodium hydroxide (caustic soda)

Ingestion of strongly alkaline substances found in products such as drain cleaner primarily cause oesophageal burns and gastrointestinal (GI) perforation. Patients are likely to require intubation, endoscopy, admission to intensive care and extensive treatment.

Sodium hypochlorite and hydrogen peroxide

Sodium hypochlorite of <10% strength is found in many household disinfectants (e.g. bleach) and small quantities (<100 ml for a child and <300 ml in adults) are unlikely to produce too many ill-effects. Hydrogen peroxide is found in a wide variety of products including chlorine-free bleach and hair dye. Large ingestions of hydrogen peroxide are likely to cause haemetemesis, oropharyngeal burns and GI perforation.

Toxic alcohols

Toxic alcohols such as methanol and ethylene glycol are chemical additives used in antifreeze products associated with automobile maintenance (e.g. engine coolant, screen wash and de-icer). Ingestion of large amounts can be extremely dangerous because initial inebriation gives way to metabolic acidosis and, if untreated, acute kidney injury. Effects are dose-related and may be blunted in chronic alcohol abusers. Nursing priorities for these patients involve, whenever possible, establishing an accurate history of ingestion and a systematic 'ABCDE' assessment (Chapter 4). Treatment priorities are similar to the management of the acutely intoxicated patient (Chapter 33). Fomepizole is the antidote of choice in the treatment of poisoning. Haemodialysis may be required.

Industrial sources

Cyanide

Cyanide poisoning should be considered in patients presenting to an ED with smoke inhalation and who display signs of hypoxia. Cyanide poisoning is rapidly fatal if untreated. All patients should receive high-flow oxygen and the appropriate antidote (Chapter 30). Owing to the potential for contamination, in the event of respiratory arrest, a facemask must be used to deliver rescue breathing.

Organophosphates (OPs)

Worldwide, organophosphate (OP) poisoning is a leading cause of death, mainly suicide, among agricultural workers. Signs, symptoms and onset of action are dependent on exposure levels, but vary from GI and neurological dysfunction to respiratory collapse. The antidote to OP poisoning is atropine. Risk of personal exposure to toxins can be minimised by the use of personal protective equipment.

33 Alcohol misuse

Figure 33.1 Acute alcohol intoxication: Assessment and management

Airway | A

- Alcohol is a central nervous system (CNS) depressant and reduces LOC; maintain patency
- Consider use of adjuncts (oropharyngeal airway, nasopharyngeal airway)
- Do not delay requesting anaesthetic input if Glasgow Coma Scale (GCS) score drops <8

Breathing | B

- Alcohol suppresses the respiratory centre: carry out full respiratory assessment monitoring for bradypnoea secondary to respiratory depression
- Record and monitor pulse oximetry (SpO$_2$). Give O$_2$ if hypoxic

Circulation | C

- Obtain IV access and draw bloods for baseline assessment
- Alcohol causes hypotension secondary to vasodilation and dehydration; consider fluid resuscitation
- The heart rate increases in an attempt to maintain blood pressure; obtain 12-lead electrocardiogram

Disability | D

- Alcohol can cause drop in blood glucose; check blood glucose levels and correct as necessary
  N.B. If correcting hypoglycaemia with IV dextrose, ensure IV Pabrinex is given, because carbohydrate loading exacerbates WE
- Perform full neurological assessment including GCS: have low threshold for considering head injury and WE
- Consider use of recreational drugs and unknown comorbidities
- Dependent drinkers who have recently ceased drinking may be at risk of acute alcohol withdrawal; observe for signs of alcohol withdrawal and seizure
- Nurse in lateral/recovery position if patient has reduced LOC

Exposure (and everything else) | E

- Alcohol reduces core temperature and patients are often found outside; monitor temperature and correct hypothermia with warming device
- Monitor regularly
- Deeply intoxicated patients are often incontinent of urine and faeces: maintain patient dignity
- Intoxicated patients often sustain other injuries: gain consent (if patient able to give it) and assess your patient fully for other injuries. Assess, clean and dress wounds, consider X-rays/referrals as appropriate
- Consider any safeguarding issues; is the patient with the alcohol problem responsible for any children?

Figure 33.2 Effects of excess alcohol on the body

- **Brain: short-term** – elation, slurred speech, malcoordination, agression; **long-term** – tiredness, neglect and reduced motivation, dependence, depression and anxiety, stroke and cerebral bleed, Wernicke's encephalopathy (WE) and Korsakoff's syndrome, dementia.
  Withdrawal – anxiety, fits, delirium tremens

- **Face**: jaundice, facial injury, rhinophyma, premature ageing

- **Throat**: mouth and larynx cancer

- **Eyes**: abnormal eye movements

- **Chest**: spider naevi, breast cancer, gynaecomastia reduced immunity – colds, pneumonia

- **Heart**: hypertension, cardiomyopathy, heart failure

- **Upper abdomen**: dyspepsia, gastritis, ulcer disease, oesphageal cancer, varices, pancreatitis, diabetes

- **Central abdomen**: central weight gain, ascites, malnutrition, caput medusa fatty liver, cirrhosis, hepatitis, cancer, portal hypertension, splenomegaly

- **Hands**: tremor, Dupuytren's contracture

- **Pelvis**: erectile dysfunction, infertility, low birth weight babies, fetal alcohol syndrome, testicular atrophy

- **Legs/bones**: myopathy, haematological dysfunction, thrombocytopenia, anaemia, traumatic fractures

- **Feet**: peripheral neuropathy

Figure 33.3 Alcohol units by drink

25 ml single spirit shot (40%) = 1 unit	Government advises alcohol consumption should not regularly exceed:
125 ml glass of wine (12.5%) = 1.5 units	
568 ml pint of beer (4%) = 2 units	
750 ml bottle of wine (12.5%) = 9 units	**Men:** 3–4 units daily
750 ml bottle of spirits (12.5%) = 30 units	**Women:** 2–3 units daily

Source: Office for National Statistics

Figure 33.4 Effect of excess alcohol

	Alcohol withdrawal syndrome	Delirium tremens/ withdrawal delirium
Symptoms of autonomic hyperactivity	Tremors, diaphoresis, nausea and vomiting, headache	Generalised seizures, hypertension, tachycardia, tachypnoea, tremors,
Neuropsychiatric signs and symptoms	Agitation, anxiety, auditory disturbance, clouding of sensorium, tactile disturbance, visual disturbance	Hallucination, confusion
Timing	6–24 hours. Peak in 24–36 hours and cease by 48 hours	1–4 days; persist up to 2 weeks

Figure 33.5 WE: Signs and symptoms

- Vision changes (movement of eye (nystagmus); double vision)
- Ataxia (balance, co-ordination and balance dysfunction)
- Acute confusion
- Hypotension with hypothermia

Emergency Nursing at a Glance, First Edition. Natalie Holbery and Paul Newcombe

© 2016 John Wiley & Sons, Ltd. Published 2016 by John Wiley & Sons, Ltd. Companion website: www.ataglanceseries.com/nursing/emergencynursing

Acute alcohol intoxication

Acute alcohol intoxication features heavily in the workload of emergency department (ED) staff, and presents significant challenges in effective management. However, in order to ensure that this vulnerable patient group receives optimal care, an emergency nurse needs to adopt excellent objective assessment management and health promotion skills.

As in all poisoning scenarios, a systematic 'ABCDE' approach (Chapter 4) to assessment should be adopted (Figure 33.1). In the presence of a reduced level of consciousness (LOC), unless the patient can give an appropriate and accurate history, the nurse must have a low threshold for considering other causes of a reduced LOC (e.g. head injury, drug use, hypoglycaemia). All patients with a threatened airway and a reduced LOC should be considered at risk of deterioration, and nursed in an appropriately resourced area.

Common complications

Head injury

The incidence of head injury in an acutely intoxicated patient has been estimated to be as high as 65%. In dependent drinkers, the risk factors for developing an intracranial bleed are even higher because of coagulopathy secondary to liver dysfunction. However, it can prove difficult establishing whether reduced LOC, vomiting, headache or amnesia are a result of inebriation or head injury. Performing a neurological assessment in an intoxicated patient can be very difficult, which often makes hospital admission and regular neurological observations the only safe clinical decision that can be made.

Chronic alcohol dependence

The long-term effects of drinking and alcohol dependency can have a detrimental effect on many of the body systems (Figure 33.2) and therefore, directly or indirectly, alcohol plays a role in many of the presentations seen in an ED.

Alcohol withdrawal syndrome

Although 'binge drinking' is generally said to occur when women drink more than 2–3 units in one sitting and men 3–4 units (Figure 33.3), the term can also apply to episodes of intense drinking (often a number of days) where the focus on becoming intoxicated becomes the primary objective. In this scenario, it is not uncommon for patients to attend an ED seeking medical help and/or to detoxify. However, abrupt cessation of alcohol consumption in the dependent drinker can cause a number of signs and symptoms that can vary in their severity (Figure 33.4). Nurses should observe for signs and symptoms of alcohol withdrawal syndrome (AWS) using a suitable assessment tool (e.g. the Clinical Institute Withdrawal Assessment of Alcohol Scale, Revised [CIWA-Ar]) in order to prevent progression of delirium tremens (DT), a medical emergency that can result in cardiovascular collapse.

Nursing care is focused on the identification of patients at risk from alcohol withdrawal and, when required, intervening with a symptom-triggered treatment regime administering medication such as chlordiazepoxide. Patients who demonstrate signs of AWS but choose to self-discharge must be advised to seek medical help while detoxifying from alcohol. 'Cold turkey' methods of abstinence from alcohol should **not** be encouraged.

Wernicke's encephalopathy (WE)

WE is a rapidly occurring and reversible acute neurological condition caused by thiamine deficiency. Dependent drinkers often have a poor dietary intake of thiamine and, although WE is relatively common and can be treated easily with parenteral thiamine (Pabrinex®), the signs and symptoms of WE are often indistinguishable from those of general intoxication (Figure 33.5). Untreated, WE can progress to an irreversible condition known as Korsakoff's psychosis (KP), which is characterised by short-term amnesia and confabulation. A large number of patients who progress to this stage require institutionalised care.

As such, treatment with Pabrinex is usually prophylactic. A nurse should also bear in mind that because carbohydrate loading can precipitate WE, intoxicated patients receiving intravenous (IV) glucose must be given Pabrinex to prevent this.

Challenges

Attitudes of staff

Frequent exposure to intoxicated patients can sometimes affect the objectivity of members of staff responsible for their care. Emergency nurses should not lose sight of the fact that these patients can become acutely unwell very quickly.

Mental health

Many patients with alcohol problems also have underlying mental health problems that may require intervention from a member of the psychiatric team. However, acutely intoxicated patients are unlikely to be able to fully participate in an assessment of their mental state and, as such, may require admission to 'sober up' first.

Referral complexities

Housing and financial problems, dysfunctional family relationships, concomitant drug abuse, requests for detoxification, mental health problems, self-neglect, etc. can make it very difficult for a nurse to know how to best help and direct individuals. Safeguarding children and vulnerable adult protocols must be considered and activated as necessary when caring for an acutely intoxicated patient.

Non-concordance, aggression and treatment necessity

Intoxicated patients are often non-concordant with assessment and treatment, and can be belligerent and aggressive. Their inability to maintain a safe environment, however, means nursing staff frequently have to encourage treatment and prevent, often unrealistic, attempts at self-discharge. This poses a number of difficult issues relating to consent, capacity, necessity of treatment and duty of care, which, in turn have to be balanced against zero-tolerance policies towards aggression. These issues are further exacerbated if staff-to-patient ratios are already sub-optimal (e.g. at night), and particularly if acuity of other patients remains high. The role played by effective communication skills, hospital security and the police cannot be understated.

Health promotion and screening tools

An ED nurse plays an important role in providing health promotion advice to patients attending with an alcohol-related illness or injury. The key to this is determining the best 'teachable moment' when the patient will be most receptive to advice on safe drinking limits. This can be facilitated by using screening tools – e.g. the Alcohol Use Disorders Identification Test (AUDIT), the Paddington Alcohol Test (PAT) and **CAGE:**

    C Have you ever felt you should cut down on your drinking?
    A Have people annoyed you by criticising your drinking?
    G Have you ever felt bad or guilty about your drinking?
    E Eye opener: Have you ever had a drink first thing in the morning to steady your nerves or to get rid of a hangover?

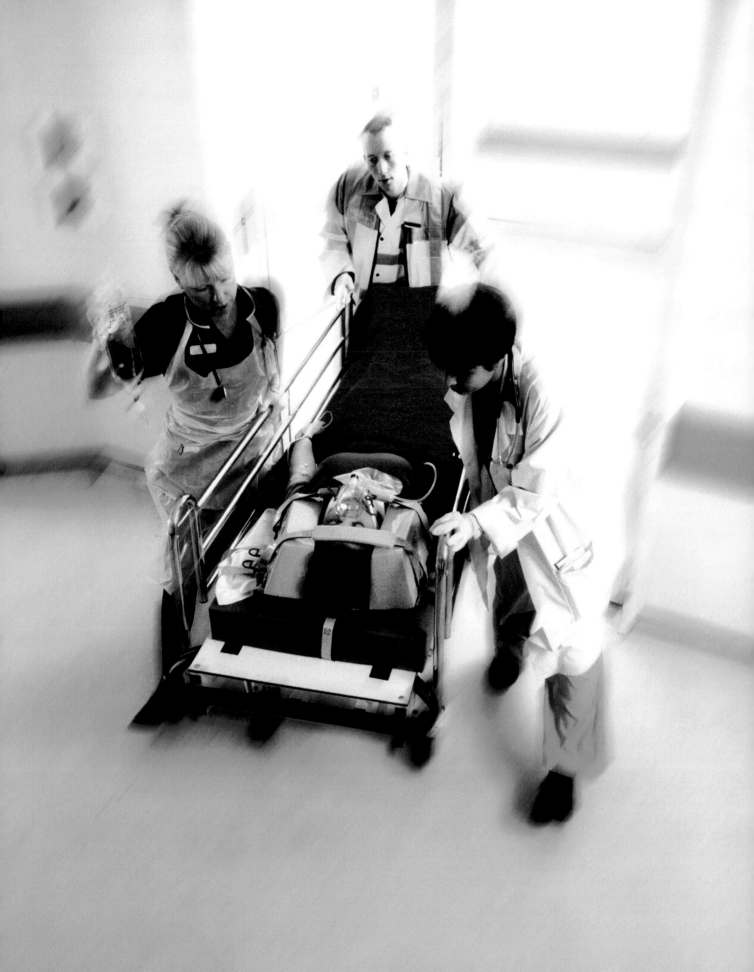

Infectious diseases

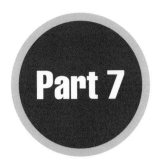

Chapters

34 Infectious diseases

Figure 34.1 Cellulitis

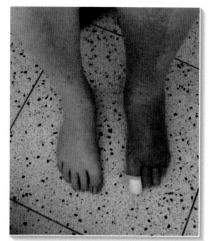

Source: By Colm Anderson [GFDL by CC BY-SA 3.0] via Wikimedia Commons

Figure 34.2 Impetigo

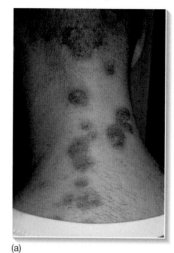 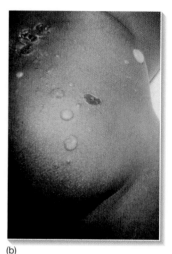

(a)   (b)

Source: By Åsa Thörn [GFDL by CC BY-SA 3.0] via Wikimedia Commons

Figure 34.3 Meningitis rash

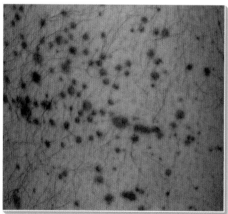

Source: Via Wikimedia Commons

Figure 34.4 Non-blanching rash and the tumbler test

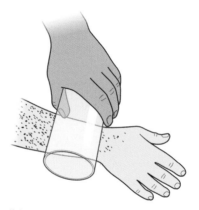 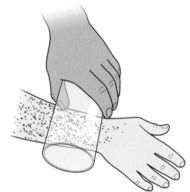

If the rash **does** fade under the tumbler's pressure, the person is unlikely to have meningitis. Repeat the test hourly because, although rarely, the rash can change.

Press the side of a glass tumbler against the rash; if it does NOT change colour, contact a doctor immediately.

Source: By Hektor [GFDL by CC BY-SA 3.0] via Wikimedia Commons

Emergency Nursing at a Glance, First Edition. Natalie Holbery and Paul Newcombe

The busy, fast-paced nature of emergency care, seeing hundreds of patients a day, necessitates strict adherence to infection control precautions. Attention to standard principles such as hand hygiene, correct use of personal protective equipment (PPE), and sharps and clinical waste disposal will reduce the risk to staff and patients. While most patients do not present with an infection, emergency department (ED) nurses must be familiar with the presentation, risks and management of a variety of infectious diseases. The most common seen in ED are outlined below here. Notifiable diseases are covered in Chapter 35.

Cellulitis

Cellulitis is an acute bacterial infection that affects the dermis and subcutaneous tissue (Figure 34.1). It is caused by a break in the skin, such as an insect bite or ulcer. The bacteria involved will depend on the cause. Patients present to an ED with a painful, red, swollen and hot limb (often a leg). They may report a history of a bite or be unaware of the cause. They are usually seen in minors or urgent care. They require oral or intravenous (IV) antibiotics and analgesia. Many EDs have ambulatory care pathways for cellulitis that allow a patient to be discharged, returning for IV antibiotics as required. Nurses should provide education about medication side effects, signs of deterioration, ongoing care and future prevention of infection. Staff should wear gloves and apron if there is contact with blood or other bodily fluid. Masks and visors are not required unless splash is likely.

Diarrhoea

Diarrhoea is a common presentation to an ED, often accompanied by abdominal pain or vomiting. It may be infectious or non-infectious. All cases of diarrhoea in the ED should initially be treated as infectious and the patient placed in a cubicle with a door whenever possible. Hand washing should not be replaced by alcohol gels because some diarrhoea-causing organisms are resistant to alcohol (e.g. *Clostridium difficile*). If a patient is dehydrated, fluids should be administered as prescribed. A stool sample may be required and it is good practice to commence a stool chart or document the type and frequency of diarrhoea in the patient's notes.

Human immunodeficiency virus (HIV)

HIV is a permanent, immunosuppressive blood-borne infection. The prevalence of HIV varies according to region, with London having the highest rate of infection in the UK. Risk factors for HIV include unprotected sexual activity, IV drug use and blood transfusion before 1985. Men who have sex with men remain the highest risk group. It is thought that up to 20% of people are unaware they are infected. Some EDs in high-risk areas have initiated routine HIV testing for adults to aid early diagnosis and treatment. Early diagnosis ensures faster access to treatment, improves health and quality of life, and reduces early mortality.

Patients may present to an ED with HIV-related symptoms or as a result of another condition. Symptoms of acute HIV infection include fever, fatigue, sore throat and, less commonly, rash and headache. ED nurses need to be aware of these symptoms because many can be incorrectly attributed to flu-like illness. Patients do not need to be isolated unless they are immunocompromised. Staff should wear gloves and apron if there is contact with blood or other high-risk bodily fluid. Masks and visors are not required unless splash is likely.

Impetigo

Impetigo is a bacterial skin infection most commonly seen in children (Figure 34.2). It is highly contagious and spread by close contact, including sharing towels and clothes. It is most commonly non-bullous (without blisters) but bullous in about 30% of cases. Non-bullous impetigo is characterised by red sores that eventually burst and form yellow crusts. It most commonly occurs on the face, usually nose and mouth. The sores are not painful but may be itchy. Bullous impetigo is similar except that the initial sores are fluid-filled blisters and more commonly occur on the trunk, arms and legs. Topical or oral antibiotics are generally prescribed. ED nurses should advise patients and/or carers to avoid close contact with others until the sores have stopped crusting, or for 48 hours after commencing treatment. Children should usually avoid school and nursery. If staff become infected, they should avoid contact with patients and see occupational health staff for advice. Patients with impetigo should be isolated if possible and staff should wear gloves and apron. Masks and visors are not required unless splash is likely.

Rash illness

There are a number of causes of rash illness seen in an ED. Examples include allergy, bites and stings, medication and infection. Some rashes are associated with mild conditions, while others are more serious. When a patient presents to an ED with a rash, the triage nurse should assess the rash distribution, progression, colour, texture and associated symptoms. ED nurses should be familiar with rashes that are associated with severe or life-threatening illness. Meningococcal rashes do not blanch or change colour when pressure is applied to the skin (Figures 34.3 and 34.4).

Treatment of a rash depends on the cause. If the patient is unwell, they may also need supportive therapy such as analgesia, fluid replacement and antipyretics. Isolation is recommended initially and staff should wear gloves and apron as a precaution. Masks and visors are not required unless splash is likely.

Respiratory syncytial virus (RSV)

Respiratory syncytial virus (RSV) is a common respiratory infection, usually seen in children. It is the most common cause of bronchiolitis in infants. Antiviral medication may be administered although treatment is mostly supportive. Fluid replacement and antipyretics should be administered as prescribed. Patients with RSV should be isolated if possible and staff should wear gloves and apron. Masks and visors are not required unless splash is likely.

35 Notifiable diseases

Figure 35.1 Notifiable diseases UK: Diseases notifiable to local authority proper officers under the Health Protection (Notification) Regulations 2010

- Acute encephalitis
- Acute infectious hepatitis
- Acute meningitis
- Acute poliomyelitis
- Anthrax
- Botulism
- Brucellosis
- Cholera
- Diphtheria
- Enteric fever (typhoid or paratyphoid fever)
- Food poisoning
- Haemolytic uraemic syndrome
- Infectious bloody diarrhoea
- Invasive group A streptococcal disease
- Legionnaires' disease
- Leprosy
- Malaria
- Measles
- Meningococcal septicaemia
- Mumps
- Plague
- Rabies
- Rubella
- Severe acute respiratorysyndrome
- Scarlet fever
- Smallpox
- Tetanus
- Tuberculosis
- Typhus
- Viral haemorrhagic fever
- Whooping cough
- Yellow fever

Figure 35.3 TB risk factors

- From India, Pakistan or Somalia
- Close contact with a person with active pulmonary TB
- Previous treatment for TB
- HIV, diabetes, kidney disease or solid organ transplant
- Taking corticosteroids or chemotherapy
- Homeless or living in overcrowded conditions
- Alcohol or drug misuse

Figure 35.4 VHF personal protective equipment

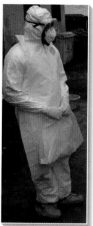

Source: By CDC global [GFDL by CC-BY-2.0] via Wikimedia Commons

Figure 35.2 Types of hepatitis

	Hepatitis A	Hepatitis B	Hepatitis C	Hepatitis D	Hepatitis E
Acute/chronic	• Acute	• Chronic • Can lead to cirrhosis and liver cancer	• Chronic • Can lead to liver disease	• Acute and chronic	• Acute
Spread	• Faecal–oral	• Blood borne	• Blood borne • Intravenous drug use	• Blood borne. Requires concurrent Hep B infection to replicate	• Faecal–oral
Prevalent area	• Africa • India • Pakistan	• South-east Asia • Tropical Africa • Parts of China	• Central and East Asia • North Africa	• Southern Italy, Middle East, North Africa and South America	
Symptoms	• Abnominal pain • Loss of appetite • Muscle/joint pain • Mild fever • Smokers lose taste for tobacco • Jaundice (later) • Itchy skin (later)	• Many patients are asymptomatic and unaware of diagnosis • Fatigue • Weight loss • Nausea • Abdominal pain • Flu-like symptoms • Jaundice (later)	• Many patients are asymptomatic and unaware of diagnosis • Fatigue • Weight loss • Nausea • Abdominal pain • Flu-like symptoms • Jaundice (later)	• Many patients are asymptomatic. Symptoms are similar to other types of hepatitis. Fever, abdominal pain, nausea and vomiting, fatigue, flu-like symptoms, weight loss, jaundice (later)	• Many patients are asymptomatic • Mild symptoms
Diagnostic tests	• Blood test	• Blood test	• Blood test	• Blood test	• Blood test
Treatment	• Self-limiting • No specific treatment; • Admission generally not required	• Antivirals depending on patient factors • Admit if unwell; may need supportive therapy	• Anti-virals although not always successful • Admit if unwell; may need supportive therapy	• No anti-viral treatment, admit if unwell, may need supportive therapy	• Self-limiting • No specific treatment • Admission generally not required unless HIV positive or pregnant
Ongoing care/ advice	• Full recovery usual • Hand hygiene • Reducing identified individual risks	• Education relating to identified individual risk factors	• Education relating to identified individual risk factors, especially safe needle use	• 6 month follow-up to determine if chronic condition	• Advise condition is self-limiting • Avoid alcohol until infection cleared

Emergency Nursing at a Glance, First Edition. Natalie Holbery and Paul Newcombe.
© 2016 John Wiley & Sons, Ltd. Published 2016 by John Wiley & Sons, Ltd. Companion website: www.ataglanceseries.com/nursing/emergencynursing

Public Health England mandates the reporting of certain infectious diseases in an attempt to swiftly detect possible outbreaks and epidemics. The responsibility for reporting lies with the doctor or nurse practitioner treating the patient. Notification needs to occur within 3 days of identification and within 24 hours if urgent.

New regulations allow for reporting suspected cases rather than waiting for laboratory results. Figure 35.1 lists the notifiable diseases in the UK at the time of publication. There follows a summary of the most common seen in an emergency department (ED).

Hepatitis

Hepatitis is a broad term to describe inflammation of the liver. There are many types of hepatitis virus (A–E), each with varying modes of transmission (Figure 35.2). Some patients with hepatitis B and C are asymptomatic. Symptoms common to all types of hepatitis are flu-like symptoms, abdominal pain, loss of appetite and nausea. Jaundice tends to be a later sign. Patients who are systemically well can usually return home with follow-up treatment, while others may require admission for supportive treatment such as fluids and analgesia.

Malaria

Malaria is a serious tropical disease contracted from mosquito bites. It cannot be transmitted from person to person. It is prevalent in Africa, Asia, Central and Southern America and parts of the Middle East where it is responsible for over 600,000 deaths. It is not found in the UK, although approximately 1,500 people are diagnosed each year after recent travel to those areas.

Patients will present generally unwell, with flu-like symptoms such as fever, sweats, headache, lethargy, vomiting, and occasionally diarrhoea and muscle aches. A history of recent travel (1–4 weeks) is significant, although some people have developed symptoms of malaria months after being bitten.

General infection control standards such as hand washing should be adhered to but because malaria is not transmitted person-to-person, there is no need for isolation or masks. Patients should have a blood test to determine the presence of the disease, and they may require supportive treatment such as analgesia and fluids if unwell. Treatment consists of a course of antimalarial medication. ED nurses should educate patients about antimalarial medication before future travel.

Meningococcal septicaemia

Meningococcal septicaemia is a systemic bacterial infection that is life threatening if not treated promptly. It is spread person-to-person by inhaling respiratory droplets or kissing. It can occur at any age but is most common in young children and adolescents.

Patients present with flu-like symptoms including fever, headache, painful joints and fatigue. Photophobia and vomiting may also be present. Infants may present as pale with fever, reduced or no feeding, restlessness, lethargy or inactivity. The distinctive rash is purpuric in nature; small pink or purple dots (petechia) form on the body (Chapter 34). The rash is non-blanching (i.e. it does not change colour when pressure is applied to it). Onset of symptoms is rapid. If meningococcal septicaemia is suspected, the patient should be moved to the resuscitation area and intravenous (IV) antibiotics administered as soon as possible. Management of septic shock is covered in Chapter 13. Parents and carers will often be anxious or distressed, and ED nurses should provide reassurance and support.

Tuberculosis

Tuberculosis (TB) is a bacterial disease that usually infects the respiratory system although it can infect other systems as well. It is less common than in the past, although parts of the UK such as London have seen a rise in recent times. TB is either active (infectious) or inactive (latent or non-infectious). Patients with inactive TB are not contagious, whereas those with active TB are. ED patients with suspected respiratory TB should be initially treated as having active TB until proven otherwise.

Patients present with a productive cough, fever, night sweats, weight loss and haemoptysis. Some patients complain of chest pain. The triage nurse should establish the presence of risk factors (Figure 35.3) and if TB is suspected the patient should be moved to a single cubicle. Current UK guidelines recommend masks and barrier nursing only for patients with multidrug-resistant TB. A sputum sample should be sent for testing. Patients should be encouraged to cough into tissues and dispose of them in clinical waste bins. Visitors should be restricted to those who have already had prolonged contact with the patient (usually family members).

Diagnosis in the ED is based on clinical symptoms and a chest X-ray. If the patient is unwell they may need to be admitted; otherwise they should be discharged home with ongoing treatment from their GP or the community respiratory care team.

Whooping cough

Whooping cough (pertussis) is a bacterial respiratory infection mostly seen in infants and children but which can occur at any age. It is highly contagious and spread through close direct contact. Infants are at highest risk of severe complications and death. It tends to be most prevalent in the summer months. Patients will present with a dry cough that is increasingly persistent. The cough resembles a 'whooping' sound. Treatment consists of antibiotics and, if well, the person will be discharged from the ED. Patients should be advised to stay away from school and work for 5 days to prevent infection spreading to others. Infants may be admitted to monitor breathing and prevent severe complications.

Viral haemorrhagic fever (VHF)

VHF is an umbrella term used to describe a number of infectious diseases such as the ebola virus. It is highly infectious. Signs and symptoms include fever and lethargy, in the early stages, followed by vomiting, bleeding (mucosal and gastrointestinal) and hypotension in the latter stage. Patients with suspected VHF should be isolated immediately and all clinicians should wear full personal protective equipment (Figure 35.4). Treatment is predominantly supportive and includes intravenous (IV) fluids, analgesia, antipyretics and, as relevant, antiviral medication.

36 Sexually transmitted infections

Figure 36.1 Herpes lesion

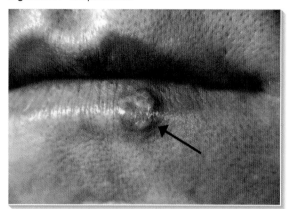

Source: Via Wikimedia Commons

Figure 36.2 Syphilis to genitalia

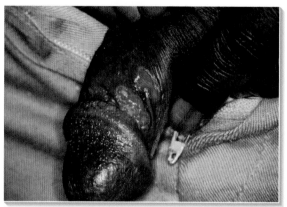

Source: CDC/M. Rein, VD via Wikimedia Commons

Figure 36.3 Syphilis rash to hands

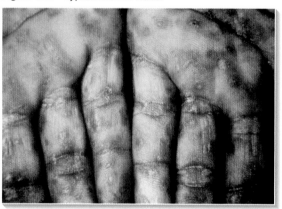

Source: CDC/Robert Sumpter via Wikimedia Commons

Emergency Nursing at a Glance, First Edition. Natalie Holbery trand Paul Newcombe
© 2016 John Wiley & Sons, Ltd. Published 2016 by John Wiley & Sons, Ltd. Companion website: www.ataglanceseries.com/nursing/emergencynursing

Sexually transmitted infections (STIs) are common in the UK. A number of sexual health and genitourinary medicine (GUM) clinics exist as drop-in centres for patients to access. However, some patients may also choose to attend an emergency department (ED), especially if out of hours. ED nurses therefore need to be familiar with common STIs and their management. STIs are most prevalent in young adults but can occur at any age, including in children. Local safeguarding procedures should be followed if children present with STIs.

Most patients self-present to an ED and may be anxious and embarrassed. A sensitive, non-judgmental approach is essential. Assessment in a private area is important to maintain confidentiality and increase the likelihood of an accurate assessment. A doctor or nurse practitioner will perform further assessments, including a genital examination. An ED nurse should act as a chaperone during this time and provide reassurance to the patient.

Testing for STIs usually involves a combination of tests including invasive (urethral/cervical), non-invasive (urine), self-taken (vulvo-vaginal), extra-genital (rectal/pharyngeal) or blood, depending on history and suspicion of infection. All procedures and tests should be explained to the patient, including how and when they will be informed of the results. This will depend on local services but should be within 14 days via their GP, local sexual health clinic or ED doctor or nurse practitioner. ED nurses should confirm current contact details to facilitate this process. They also need to advise patients about the importance of safe sex behaviours and encourage partner notification.

The most common STIs seen in the UK are outlined here. Human immunodeficiency virus (HIV) is covered in Chapter 34.

Chlamydia

Chlamydia is the most common bacterial STI in the UK. It is often asymptomatic and presentation to an ED may be due to signs related to untreated infection such as pelvic inflammatory disease (PID) or ectopic pregnancy. It also causes infertility if not treated. If symptomatic, women tend to experience vaginal discharge, bleeding between periods, dysuria and lower abdominal pain. Men experience penile discharge, dysuria, and burning or itching in the genital area.

If patients present with another STI, it is good practice to screen for chlamydia. It is often present with gonorrhoea infection. Testing female patients involves a urine sample or vaginal/cervical swabs. Male patients can produce a urine sample or have a urethral swab. If a patient has had receptive anal sex, a rectal swab is advised. Treatment is relatively simple with oral antibiotics, and retesting is recommended in 3 months.

Gonorrhoea

Gonorrhoea is another bacterial STI and similar to chlamydia in that women are often asymptomatic until the infection has caused PID or an ectopic pregnancy. It can also cause infertility in women. Men are more likely to be symptomatic, with penile discharge and dysuria present. Female patients may experience yellow or bloody vaginal discharge and dysuria. Testing female patients involves a urine sample or vaginal/cervical swabs. Male patients require a urethral swab. Treatment consists of a single-dose antibiotic, usually intramuscular (IM). Retesting is recommended in 3 months.

Genital herpes

Genital herpes is caused by the herpes simplex virus (HSV), usually HSV2. It is a lifelong viral infection that is characterised by intermittent painful vesicular lesions (Figure 36.1). Some patients do not present with lesions but may complain of nerve-like pain or dysuria, or be generally unwell. If vesicular lesions are present, they should be swabbed and sent for testing. If the patient presents with a first episode of infection, the recommended treatment is a 7-day course of antiviral (Acyclovir). This will not eradicate the infection but it will address initial signs and symptoms. Screening for other STIs is recommended.

Syphilis

Syphilis is a bacterial infection that is relatively uncommon in the UK, although numbers have increased over the past decade. Patients may present during the initial (primary) infection or during subsequent (secondary) infection. Primary infection is characterised by painless ulcers to the genital area (Figure 36.2). If left untreated, these resolve within approximately 6 weeks. Secondary infection follows non-treatment of the primary infection (6 weeks to 6 months) and patients may present complaining of feeling generally unwell and with a rash to their palms or feet (Figure 36.3). Syphilis in pregnancy is associated with miscarriage or stillbirth. Testing involves taking a swab of the ulcer or a blood test. Patients with syphilis should also be tested for HIV because they can develop neurological complications. Treatment of syphilis is with penicillin, usually IM in the first instance. ED nurses should advise patients that there is a risk of developing Jarisch-Herxheimer reaction, a condition found in penicillin treatment of syphilis. It is relatively short term (3–6 hours) and associated with fever, headache and myalgia. Antipyretics can be used to treat symptoms.

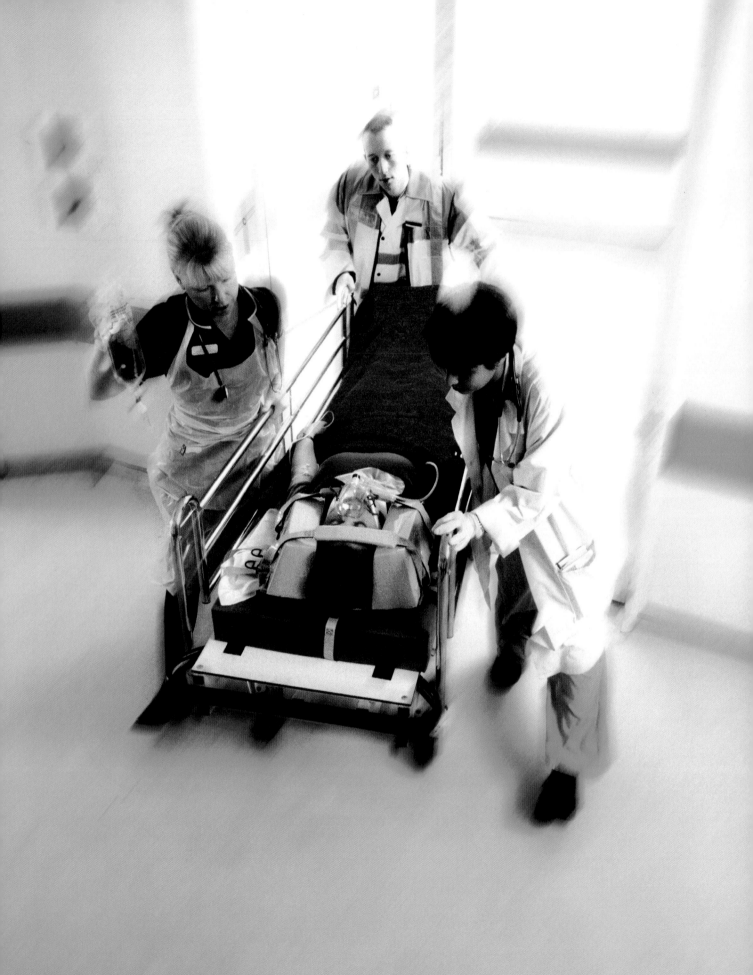

Vulnerable patient groups

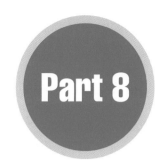

Part 8

Chapters

37 Domestic abuse

Figure 37.1 Protecting staff

- Do not approach or accuse suspected perpetrator
- Discuss concerns with patient in private
- Ensure documentation is secure
- Do not use family members as interpreters
- Report concerns to senior staff

Figure 37.2 Signs of domestic abuse

- Repeated attendance
- Unusual or change in behaviour when in presence of abuser
- Delay in seeking treatment
- Avoidance of eye contact
- Anxiety
- Physical
  - bruising
  - wounds
  - hand marks
  - human bite marks
  - cigarette burns
  - limb and facial injuries
  - unexplained injury
  - lethargy
  - abdominal injury (especially during pregnancy)
- Sexual
  - injury to genitalia and/or anus
  - bruising/wounds/bites to breasts
- Financial
  - limited/no access to funds
  - forcing changes to will
- Psychological
  - threatening behaviour
  - intimidation

Figure 37.3 British Medical Assocation: Recommended questions

- Do you ever feel afraid of your partner?
- Has your partner or ex-partner ever physically hurt or threatened you?
- Has your partner ever threatened or abused your children?

Emergency Nursing at a Glance, First Edition. Natalie Holbery and Paul Newcombe

Domestic abuse is defined in the UK as any violence, abuse or threatening behaviour between people over the age of 16 who are or have been in a relationship, regardless of gender or sexuality. This definition recognises that domestic abuse is increasing in young people, with females between the ages of 16 and 25 considered to be at greatest risk. The abuse may be physical, sexual, financial or psychological. Controlling and coercive behaviours are also indicative of domestic abuse.

One in four women and one in seven men experience at least one episode of domestic abuse in their lifetime. Thirty per cent of domestic abuse starts during pregnancy and existing abuse may worsen during this time. If children are involved, they are known to be in close proximity of abuse in up to 90% of episodes. Children are at increased risk of harm themselves if a parent or carer is experiencing domestic abuse.

People experiencing domestic abuse will often only contact the police after numerous abusive episodes. Nurses who work in emergency departments (EDs) are most likely to come into contact with victims of domestic abuse, and they may be the first to identify that abuse is occurring. It is therefore imperative to be aware of the signs of domestic abuse.

In an ED, the key principles of managing cases of suspected domestic abuse are treating injuries, safeguarding the patient, children (where relevant) and staff, documentation and reporting concerns. When children are involved, it is imperative that ED nurses follow local child protection guidelines. With violence and aggression towards healthcare workers on the rise, ED nurses need to ensure that they do not put themselves at risk of harm by following the principles outlined in Figure 37.1.

Signs of domestic abuse

People experiencing domestic abuse mostly present after an injury. Injuries may be minor or more severe, and they commonly include head, neck and facial injuries. Injuries to breasts and genitals may also occur. Other signs may be indicative but are not exclusively linked to domestic abuse (Figure 37.2).

The abuser often accompanies the patient and may hover or refuse to leave. They may stand over the patient and attempt to answer questions on the patient's behalf. In this situation, nurses should assess the patient on a one-to-one basis. This may be achieved by either asking the suspected abuser to leave, or by covertly carrying out the assessment in a private area.

Some patients may voluntarily disclose that they have been the victim of domestic abuse; however, most do not. Screening all patients in an ED for domestic abuse is not recommended. However, when it is suspected, ED nurses should feel confident enough to raise their concerns with the patient. Asking questions in a non-threatening, non-judgemental manner, and not in front of the suspected abuser, will increase the likelihood of a disclosure. This approach also avoids offending patients in cases where domestic abuse is not occurring. Figure 37.3 outlines the key questions recommended by the British Medical Association.

Management of domestic abuse

The first priority is to treat a patient's injuries or illness. Accurate and timely documentation is vital to ensure that injuries are properly recorded. Documenting in the patient's own words is also important. Documentation may be accessed at a later stage by a number of agencies including police, social workers, health visitors, GPs and legal professionals. In some EDs, photographs may be taken to further record injuries, and this should occur in line with local policy.

Patients are more likely to disclose that they have been the victim of domestic abuse if they are asked directly and believe that the person they inform will treat them with empathy, compassion and respect. Asking the patient without anyone else nearby, in a quiet room with closed doors (not curtained cubicles), creates a more secure and supportive environment.

There are numerous organisations that provide support and shelter for victims of domestic abuse. Providing contact details should be done carefully to avoid the perpetrator becoming aware and increasing the severity of abuse. ED nurses should not encourage the person to leave their abuser. Experienced case workers are available from professional organisations to ensure that actions are planned and safe.

Reporting domestic abuse

Confidentiality is a professional responsibility of all ED nurses. However, the Nursing and Midwifery Council (NMC) recognises that there are situations where breaching confidentiality is necessary – in particular, when it is believed that a person is at risk of harm. Reporting domestic abuse, as with other types of abuse, should not be done in isolation. Seeking advice and support from senior colleagues is recommended.

In such situations, the NMC recommends telling the person that information may be shared with other agencies. In relation to domestic abuse, this may be the police, social services or multi-agency groups such as the local Multi-Agency Risk Assessment Conference (MARAC). The NMC recommends that information sharing occurs with the patient's consent, although sharing information without patient consent is permitted to prevent abuse or serious harm to others. A multi-agency response is considered the best approach to address individual cases of domestic abuse. All ED nurses should be familiar with referral processes to the local MARAC and should work within local policies.

38 Sexual assault

Figure 38.1 Types of sexual assault

Rape
• Non-consensual, intentional penetration of vagina, anus or mouth with a penis
Assault by penetration
• Non-consensual, intentional penetration of vagina or anus with a body part or object
Sexual assault
• Non-consensual, intentional sexual touching

Figure 38.2 Potential injury in sexual assault

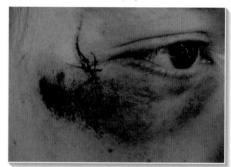

Source: By dbenzhuser [GFDL by CC BY-SA 3.0] via Wikimedia Commons

Figure 38.3 Principles of evidence preservation

Clothing
• Remove carefully into bags (ideally with patient standing over plastic sheet)
• Do not cut clothing (especially over/through damaged sections)
Wounds and skin
• Do not wash skin
• Take swabs from wounds
Mouth
• Avoid mouth care
Hair
• Comb pubic hair over clean sheet/paper and store in labelled evidence bag
Documentation
• Use body maps and/or photographs
• Document and securely store all evidence

Figure 38.4 Information sharing: Exceptional circumstances

• To protect the public
• To protect individuals
• To prevent a crime

The UK Sexual Offences Act 2003 presents three main definitions related to sexual assault (Figure 38.1). Commonalities of each include intentional sexually related acts without consent. Over 400,000 women are known to be sexually assaulted each year in the UK. Although sexual assault can occur in any age group, regardless of gender or sexuality, victims are most commonly women aged 16–24 years. In most cases the victim knows the perpetrator. Although the numbers of sexual abuse in the UK are significant, it is thought that fewer than half seek medical care.

Most victims of sexual assault do not report the crime to police. There are a number of reasons for this; fear of being blamed or not being believed are common reasons. It is important, therefore, that victims receive appropriate physical and psychosocial care and support if they attend an emergency department (ED).

Recognition

Patients who present after sexual assault may not disclose the assault. They may present with no obvious injuries and be seeking emergency contraception. Alternatively, they may present after domestic abuse. Sexual assault and rape are linked to domestic abuse and if a disclosure or signs of domestic abuse (Chapter 37) exist, nurses should consider the possibility of sexual assault. When there is suspicion of sexual assault, questions should be posed to the patient in a private area, away from family and visitors, in a non-judgmental and caring manner.

Patients may also present with injuries to the head, face, chest and genitalia, and these may include bruises, lacerations or bite marks (Figure 38.2). All EDs should have a clear process for managing patients after sexual assault.

Management

The ED care of a patient after sexual assault involves treating all injuries (including life threatening) first. If the patient has life-threatening injuries they will need to be cared for in the resuscitation area. If the injuries are not life threatening it is good practice to offer the patient a private cubicle, ideally with a door rather than a curtain.

Patients should be referred to a Sexual Assault Referral Centre (SARC) where further medical, forensic and psychological support can be offered. If a patient does not want to attend a SARC, their injuries should be assessed and a history of assault taken in the ED and clearly documented. Using the patient's own words when relevant is essential. Such records may be used at a later date for criminal proceedings.

Pelvic and genital examinations should be carried out by an experienced member of staff, usually a senior doctor. Some EDs have nurses who specialise in sexual assault examination and management, and who may also carry out these assessments.

Female patients who have been raped should be offered emergency contraception. Exposure to sexually transmitted infections, including human immunodeficiency virus (HIV), should also be considered. Screening for sexually transmitted infections (STIs) and HIV prophylaxis should be considered in the ED (Chapters 34 & 36). Some STIs will be undetected early on, so referral to a sexual health clinic for follow-up screening and counselling is recommended. A referral to other organisations such as victim support agencies and social services may be required. When children are involved (either as the patient or in the care of the patient), local safeguarding procedures should be followed.

Forensic considerations

Sexual assault is a crime and whenever possible evidence should be preserved. When evidence has been collected it should be correctly bagged, labelled and stored. The responsibility for collecting evidence and maintaining a chain of custody lies with the police or forensic medical officer/examiner. Treating injuries takes precedence, however. ED nurses should be aware of the procedures involved in preserving, collecting and handling evidence. Some common principles are outlined in Figure 38.3.

Support services

In the UK, SARCs exist to provide medical care, practical guidance and psychological support. SARCs are multi-agency organisations and offer healthcare, legal and practical advice, and psychological support. All ED nurses should be aware of local SARCs and other relevant services to support a victim beyond the ED. The patient may not wish to attend a SARC or contact the police, and ED nurses should respect this decision. ED staff can only share information with the police and social services in exceptional circumstances (Figure 38.4). Providing leaflets and/or contact details of local services is recommended.

39 The mental health patient in the emergency department (ED)

Figure 39.1 Issues to explore through questioning and observation

- Is the person currently aggressive and/or threatening?
- Do they pose a risk to self, you or others?
- Do they have any immediate plans (i.e. within the next few minutes or hours) to harm self, you or others?
- Might they abscond?
- Do they have a history of violence?
- Do they have a history of self-harm?
- Do they have a history of mental health problems?
- Do they appear to be experiencing any delusions or hallucinations?
- How collaborative are they?
- What is their level of social support and status (i.e. employment and housing status, partner/significant other, family members, friends)?

Figure 39.2 Assessment techniques

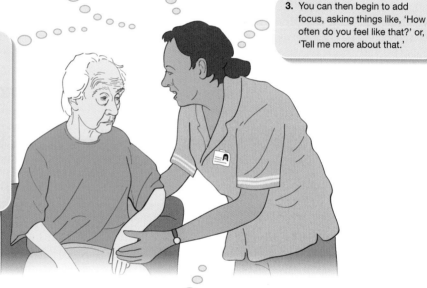

1. Active listening, an interest in the person's story, empathy, genuineness and looking for non-verbal cues will all help develop a rapport. Find out what the person wants, and why.

2. Open questions such as, 'What happened that led to you coming here today?' are a good starter. Other open questions might include, 'How do you feel?'

3. You can then begin to add focus, asking things like, 'How often do you feel like that?' or, 'Tell me more about that.'

4. As you explore important issues such as ideas about suicide, use more closed questions such as, 'Do you have a plan?' Then add further focus: 'What would you do?' 'What would happen for you to act on your ideas?'

5. Be explicit and name things. Ask specific questions, e.g. 'Do you want to kill yourself?' rather than being vague and missing opportunities to help the person talk about their real situation. 'Funnel in', with questions like 'Did you feel like killing yourself today?' 'Why was that?'

6. Allow short silences for the person – and sometimes yourself – to think:
   - Maintain good eye contact
   - Keep questions short and simple
   - Try and remain outwardly calm
   - Seek clarification when things aren't clear
   - Summarise periodically and at the end of the interview, including what has been agreed and any further interventions planned (e.g. referral to psychiatric services)

Emergency Nursing at a Glance, First Edition. Natalie Holbery and Paul Newcombe.

The key task for the ED nurse interviewing someone with mental health problems is to gain a rapid understanding of why the person has presented now and what immediate help they might need. The emphasis is on risk assessment and risk management. It is then a matter of knowing how to make a referral, what information to provide and to whom it should be given.

Rule out any physical cause for the person's presentation before considering mental health problems. If intoxicated from illicit drug use or alcohol, a full assessment must wait until the person can provide a coherent account and undertake a detailed interview.

If someone is known to mental health services, find out the person's care plan from their team and next appointments etc. Whenever possible, the clinician currently working with the patient should be involved in this assessment. Most hospitals will have a liaison psychiatry team and that is an obvious link, although there may also be home treatment teams to provide mental health assessments in the ED and arrange admission or community follow-up. The person – and/or carers/relatives – should be asked about what has changed to prompt this attendance at the ED.

Explore **current** risk within the context of the presenting problem, whether it is a mental disorder such as depression or an episode of self-harm or a suicide attempt. However, briefly exploring the risk history is a key part of this process.

Someone presenting for the first time obviously requires a fuller triage assessment before deciding about further assessment and/or a referral to specialist mental health services.

Factors to consider include precipitating events and any symptoms of mental disorder, how immediate the risk is, the frequency and severity of dangerous behaviours, the person's intent, their reasons for acting and the level of planning (Figure 39.1).

Interview techniques

State the purpose of the interview, that it will be brief and you will not be going into too much detail because it is likely that someone else will be asking similar questions later on. Outline possible outcomes. Focus on the relevant information as collaboratively and as conversationally as possible.

Active listening, an interest in the person's story, empathy, genuineness and looking for non-verbal cues will all help develop a rapport. Find out what the person wants, and why. For other interview techniques, see Figure 39.2.

Checking how congruent **what** the person says is with **how** they say it, their facial expressions and their body language are important parts of your assessment.

Explore what would make things better or worse, what might push the person into acting and what might stop them. It is useful to add what **you** think in terms of their risk.

Important skills are getting the relevant information without the person becoming emotionally overwhelmed and being able to 'close down' the interview, yet leaving the person knowing you have listened, validated their experience and understood. A simple statement can help, such as, 'This seems distressing for you so we won't go into that any further. I'll talk to my colleague who will see you later and she may pick it up then. But I'll make sure it doesn't get lost.'

Tell them what you will do next and help them remain safely in the department if you have concerns, while being specific about the risk of making a referral. Refer to the risk assessment matrix (Chapter 40) to help you summarise:

- What is the key problem?
- What is the level of risk – e.g. low, medium, high, very high?
- Is referral to the mental health liaison team or duty psychiatrist indicated?

Finally, a successful triage will determine **who** is at risk, **what** is the risk, **when** is the person at risk, **why** they are at risk, **where** they are at risk and **how** they are at risk.

The ED and the Mental Health Act 1983

If a police officer finds someone in a place to which the public have access, who appears to be suffering from mental disorder and in immediate need of care or control, they can detain the person under Section 136 of the Mental Health Act 1983 and take that person to a place of safety. The ED is **a** place of safety but mental health trusts should have a **designated** place of safety to which the person should be taken. Only if the police officer(s) suspect medical treatment is needed would it be appropriate to use the ED as the place of safety.

The person will be assessed by a registered medical practitioner and interviewed by an approved mental health professional (AMHP) to determine whether or not they should be further detained for ongoing assessment, and possibly treatment. The person can also be discharged from Section 136. This process **must** be completed within 72 hours from the time it is initiated, otherwise the person is automatically released from Section 136. The assessment can be undertaken in more than one place so if an examination reveals no medical treatment is required, the Mental Health Act assessment can be completed in the designated place of safety.

Section 4 may be used for someone suffering from a mental disorder warranting urgent detention in a hospital for assessment or for their own safety or the safety of others. It only requires the involvement of one approved doctor and an AMHP, and lasts for 72 hours.

There are other, specific legal requirements for the Act that need to be met regarding patients attending an ED but already detained in a psychiatric hospital, and the receipt and storage of section papers. Procedures need to be understood by staff and in place for out of hours as well as for when senior managers are available.

40 Risk assessment, self-harm and suicide

Figure 40.1 Mental health risk assessment matrix

Level of risk	Key risk factors	Pre-assessment action	Timescale for referral and assessment criteria
Low risk	• Minor mental health problems may be present but either no thoughts or plans regarding risk behaviours to self or others, or unlikely to act upon them • No evidence of immediate or short-term risk or vulnerability	• Treatment and follow-up arrangements managed by ED team • Possible referral to primary care services, e.g. GP or practice nurse • May benefit from mental health advice, e.g. safe alcohol consumption or non-statutory counselling services	• **Referral to liaison psychiatry team not necessary** • **Advice on further referral and/or management may be sought from liaison psychiatry service**
Medium risk	• Mental health problems present and/or has non-specific ideas or plans regarding risk behaviours to self or others • These either not dangerous or no immediate plans to act upon them • Potentially vulnerable in certain circumstances	• Should have specialist mental health assessment but no urgent action required if patient doesn't wish to engage • Should be advised to seek further help if necessary, e.g. from GP • Liaison team and GP to be informed as well as existing mental health services if already known	• **Non-urgent referral to liaison psychiatry team so person can be seen within 1.5 hours of arrival** • **Out of hours the person should be either seen by duty psychiatrist or referred to liaison team for next day follow-up**
High risk	• Serious mental health problems present, including possible psychotic features • Clear ideas or plans regarding risk behaviours to self or others • May have already self-harmed or carried out other risk behaviours • Mental state likely to deteriorate if left untreated and potentially vulnerable	• Urgent mental health assessment required and an action plan to be drawn up to address immediate and short-term risk factors • Key clinicians and others likely to be involved should be informed • Risk management plan to be agreed with patient before discharge can occur, or admission to psychiatric unit considered	• **Urgent referral to liaison psychiatry team to enable person to be seen within 1 hour of arrival** • **Attempts should be made to stop patient leaving department before mental health assessment completed** • **Police to be informed if patient absconds** • **Out of hours the patient should be fully assessed by duty psychiatrist**
Very high risk	• Serious mental health problems present, including possible psychotic features • Strong and immediate plans or ideas regarding risk behaviours to self or others • May have already self-harmed or carried out risk behaviours • Mental state very likely to deteriorate if left untreated • Is highly vulnerable	• Immediate mental health assessment needed by liaison psychiatry team or duty psychiatrist • Risk management plan to be instigated, addressing immediate and short-term risk factors, with ongoing treatment and care package, including considering possible admission to psychiatric unit • Key clinicians and others likely to be involved should be informed • If patient unwilling to engage, a Mental Health Act assessment should be arranged before they leave the department	• **Immediate referral to liaison psychiatry team, or duty psychiatrist out of hours, to enable the person to be seen at the earliest opportunity but no later than 1 hour of arrival** • **All possible attempts should be made to stop patient leaving department before mental health assessment** • **Police to be informed if patient absconds**

Emergency Nursing at a Glance, First Edition. Natalie Holbery and Paul Newcombe
© 2016 John Wiley & Sons, Ltd. Published 2016 by John Wiley & Sons, Ltd. Companion website: www.ataglanceseries.com/nursing/emergencynursing

Introduction

Always consider your own immediate safety and that of the patient. Is it safe to be in the room with this person? If the person tried to leave the emergency department (ED), would they be at immediate risk (Figure 40.1)?

Mental health patients rarely pose a threat to others. However, there may be a risk of violence because of the acuity and level of psychological and emotional disturbance experienced by those attending the ED, the stimulation of the environment and attitudes they may encounter from some staff. Clear policies need to be in place, including the role of security staff, restraint and what to do with patients who may abscond and would pose a risk to themselves or others. Nurses should be trained in effective de-escalation techniques.

Talking with someone about their ideas to self-harm or commit suicide can seem daunting, but it is easier if you understand some of the background, you develop a simple interview structure that suits you and you understand the limits of your role.

Self-harm

Self-harm is prompted by a range of factors and variety of complex motives (Box 40.1). It can be defined as any intentional act of self-poisoning or self-injury irrespective of the type of motivation or degree of suicidal intent. Of the numerous ways to self-harm, the most common are self-poisoning and cutting.

Some healthcare professionals view self-harm as 'attention seeking' or 'manipulative' but it is usually the only way the person can communicate their distress at that time. However, simple interventions can help (Box 40.2).

Suicide

Although a different phenomena, there is a direct relationship between self-harm and suicide. Between 7 and 10% of people who self-harm will kill themselves within a decade of self-harming. Over 400,000 people self-harm and more than 5,000 commit suicide each year.

Suicide is a common feature of many serious mental disorders, particularly depression. Most people who kill themselves have psychiatric disorders. Previous self-harm is a significant risk

---

> ## Box 40.1 Some motives for self-harm
>
> - A coping mechanism, often an unwanted response to unmanageable feelings
> - Relieving stress
> - Regulating unpleasant self-states
> - Increased sense of mastery and control

> ## Box 40.2 Helpful interventions for people who self-harm
>
> - A psychosocial assessment and brief follow-up treatment can help a person understand their behaviour, find safer alternatives and, most importantly, prevent further episodes
> - Listening, supporting and not judging
> - Helping the person think about skills and information that give them greater choices and control
> - Providing reasonable hope for recovery from their distress

---

factor, as is substance misuse, because it decreases inhibitions and increases impulsivity. Suicide is also a response to chronic physical illness, especially when associated with longstanding, poorly controlled pain. Although more women than men self-harm, three times as many men kill themselves.

There is evidence that neurobiological changes contribute to an increase in both suicidal ideation and suicidal acts. Indications of these changes should raise a nurse's concerns. They include the following:

- The person may misinterpret relatively neutral events, such as the expression on others' faces or chance comments, or view minor issues such as making simple mistakes as complete failure or humiliation
- The loss of problem-solving skills, particularly in interpersonal relationships
- An overwhelming feeling of needing to escape the situation but a sense of being unable to do so
- Thinking this state of affairs will continue forever and nothing will change to improve their future
- Behaviour based on emotions and drives not being well modulated, leading to the person doing things they would not have done previously, i.e. trying to kill themselves.

Risk assessment

Suicidal ideation commonly manifests in the person expressing feelings of hopelessness, that things will never get better and there is no way out other than to die, thinking this will bring relief from their suffering. Simple questions can be used to check this out, such as, 'How do you see your future?', 'What might change the way things are now?' and 'What might you do about how you're feeling?'

However, most people remain ambivalent about killing themselves despite their hopelessness, engaged in a see-saw battle between the wish to live and wish to die. This explains why, for example, someone can take a large overdose of medication and subsequently seek help. Tapping into this ambivalence and exploring other ways to escape unbearable feelings can help clinicians to negotiate safer alternatives.

If someone has attempted suicide, exploring the intent is crucial. For example, someone might take an overdose of relatively harmless antidepressant believing they will die, while someone else takes 30 paracetamol tablets believing it will not do any long-term harm. Also, having survived, might they try again?

A combination of factors contributes to a potentially suicidal act. In an ED, focus on what is susceptible to immediate change (i.e. the person's current situation). What might they do next? How vulnerable are they? Are they safe to go home? Do they require hospitalisation? Who needs to be informed? What can improve their situation? (See the risk assessment matrix in Figure 40.1.)

Suicide often seems to be an impulsive phenomenon, with the impulse to act being transient. If support is provided at the moment of impulse, the crisis may be defused. This is important when thinking about what to do with someone who presents in an ED. However, while the actual act may be impulsive, the person has usually already thought about what they might do and, if assessed sensitively, may reveal their thinking and possible plans.

41 Common mental health problems

Figure 41.1 Key features of psychosis

- **Hallucinations** are false sensory perceptions or perceptual phenomena arising without any external stimuli, such as hearing voices
- **Delusions** are false, firmly held beliefs it is difficult to dissuade the person from, despite contradictory evidence and other members of the same culture not believing them. They are not based on the person's cultural, religious, educational or social experience. Types of delusions include those of a paranoid or grandiose nature
- People may also describe receiving messages from songs, TV, the radio etc. and seeing significance in apparently unrelated things
- Another symptom of psychosis is thought disorder, which results in the type of incomprehensible speech sometimes seen when people are acutely disturbed

Key nursing issues

- As soon as it is clear someone is psychotic in the ED, consider where they will be safest while waiting to be seen
- If paranoid, they may feel more comfortable where they can see what is happening. If they are overstimulated, a quiet cubicle is probably best
- Explore how they feel about you and whether or not you are incorporated in their psychotic experience
- Think about how you would know if things were getting worse or better for the person, as a result of changes in their psychotic phenomena, rather than what is happening in the here and now

Figure 41.2 Key features of bipolar disorder

- Alternating episodes of mania (or hypomania) and depression
- Frequency and duration of episodes and asymptomatic periods are variable
- Remissions tend to get shorter over time
- Some individuals experience an episode of mania that quickly switches into depression, often as an indirect result of treatment used to manage the acute manic condition

The manic phase is diagnosed by the concurrent presence of at least three of the following symptoms:

- Grandiosity/inflated self-esteem
- Decreased need for sleep
- Pressure of speech
- Flight of ideas (rapidly racing thoughts and ideas flitting from one to another)
- Marked distractibility and irritability
- Increased goal-directed activity/psychomotor agitation
- Excessive involvement in pleasurable activities without regard for negative consequences (for example, buying sprees, sexual indiscretions, foolish business ventures)

In severe cases there may be psychotic symptoms (see Figure 41.1)

Key nursing issues

- Addressing physical problems, e.g. dehydration, exhaustion and lack of self-care
- Reducing external stimuli is essential, keeping the person in a cubicle or away from the main part of the ED
- Providing a nurse or security personnel will help prevent them becoming too disruptive
- Medication should also be considered if they are creating serious difficulties for other patients or becoming too distressed or irritable because of the constraints placed upon them

Figure 41.3 Key features of depression

A diagnosis of depression involves identifying depressed mood for at least two weeks, plus five other symptoms from the list below:

- Significant weight changes
- Sleep disturbance
- Feelings of worthlessness
- Diminished concentration
- Fatigue
- Hopelessness
- Guilt
- Marked diminished interest or pleasure in all or most activities
- Psychomotor retardation
- Poor memory
- Tearfulness
- Recurrent thoughts of death, suicidal ideation

Key nursing issues

- Because of the person's mental state, building a rapport will potentially be more difficult because they may be withdrawn, feeling unworthy of help, or unresponsive. More patience and time are likely to be needed
- Every person presenting with depression should be asked explicitly about whether or not they have any suicidal thoughts and/or plans because 15–20% of such people commit suicide

When interviewing the depressed person in the ED, consider:

- What do they mean by 'depression'?
- What is this experience like for the them?
- How does it affect their everyday functioning?
- What do they understand to be the cause(s)?
- What help do they want?

Figure 41.4 Key issues of borderline personality disorder

- Frantic efforts to avoid real or imagined abandonment
- Unstable and intense interpersonal relationships – alternating between idealisation and devaluation
- Identity disturbance – unstable sense of self
- Impulsivity
- Recurrent suicidal behaviour, threats, gestures or self-harming
- Unstable mood, including high levels of anxiety
- Feelings of emptiness, worthlessness
- Inappropriate anger
- Transient, stress-related paranoid ideation or severe dissociative symptoms

Key nursing issues

- Long-term, specialised therapy is needed to treat BPD. However, for nurses in the ED, remembering that the behaviour – no matter how difficult it seems – is neither really directed at you nor deliberate. You can help in responding calmly, consistently and clearly. This helps establish the clear boundaries that are essential
- However, boundaries need to be married to a compassionate response to the person's profound level of emotional disturbance, lack of coping and appropriate communication skills
- This is the time to be non-judgmental in your responses, to try and listen carefully and understand the person's situation but also to 'contain' their emotional intensity and disturbance by sticking with the 'here and now', not probing into difficult areas for the person, e.g. abuse, and giving them clear, unambiguous information about what will be happening
- If the person frequently attends the ED, it is worth having a care plan in place, ideally agreed with the relevant mental health team and/or liaison psychiatry team to ensure consistency

Emergency Nursing at a Glance, First Edition. Natalie Holbery and Paul Newcombe.
© 2016 John Wiley & Sons, Ltd. Published 2016 by John Wiley & Sons, Ltd. Companion website: www.ataglanceseries.com/nursing/emergencynursing

Acute psychosis

Acute psychosis is characterised by a loss of contact with reality, affecting a person's perception, thoughts, emotions and behaviour, with commonly seen acute symptoms including hallucinations and delusions (Figure 41.1). Psychosis has different causes, such as schizophrenia or bipolar disorder, but episodes can occur due to severe stress or severe cases of depression, various medical conditions (e.g. brain tumours, lupus and HIV/AIDS) and substance misuse. Effects from the disorder can be pervasive and cause significant, long-term impairment, but they can also be transient, intermittent or short term.

Asking questions of someone whose experience seems so different, even alien to our own, can seem very difficult. However, 'entering into the person's world', following their story and trying to understand **their** logic, by asking simple questions is key. Examples might be:

- 'When did you first notice this happening?'
- 'How did you know these people were thinking this?'
- 'What happened next?'
- 'Do you know why they might want to hurt you?'
- 'How did you find out you were special?'
- 'How does it affect you?'
- 'Do you feel safe?'

This neither denies the person's experience nor colludes with it. Most importantly, it will probably yield vital information for making a referral to the mental health team (e.g. to be able to report that the person is experiencing paranoid delusions, auditory hallucinations and receiving messages from the radio that leave them feeling very unsafe). This is far more effective than saying, 'He's behaving strangely' or 'We can't understand what he's saying.'

Also, while it may seem hard to comprehend what it is like to believe you are the victim, for example, of an 'alien conspiracy', the person is probably **feeling** terrified and a healthcare professional empathising with that feeling can be highly validating. Stress and anxiety are almost always at the root of acute psychotic episodes and both empathising with the feelings and trying to reduce that acute anxiety, either behaviourally or with the use of medication if necessary, can be very helpful.

Bipolar disorder

Bipolar disorder is a condition that causes extreme mood swings. Episodes of bipolar disorder can last for several weeks or longer (Figure 41.2). The person often experiences the manic phase as very creative and positive, and they may be reluctant to take any medication that blunts the heightened mood associated with mania.

Between episodes, people with bipolar disorder may re-establish their earlier lifestyle but it can often have profound adverse consequences on their quality of life, including their personal relationships and social functioning. Estimates of the lifetime risk of suicide range from 15 to 19%. An estimated third of individuals with bipolar disorder make a suicide attempt and this is most likely during a depressive episode.

Depression

Depression is a common and disabling psychiatric disorder and the largest single cause of disability in the world. It is far more than feeling 'down', miserable' or very sad (Figure 41.3).

The origins of depression can be genetic predisposition, medical conditions, social factors, relationship strain and life experiences, and psychological and neurobiological factors, although some people regard it as a natural part of the life cycle.

Depression has a symbiotic relationship with physical illness. Chronic illness, particularly when it is associated with severe pain, carries a significant risk of depression. If left untreated, depressive disorders will slow down rehabilitation from disabling physical illness, diminish pain tolerance and affect the individual's ability to seek help and treatment for physical disorders as well as their depression.

Borderline personality disorder (BPD)

People with BPD are likely to be a relatively common presentation in an emergency department (ED). BPD is a disorder of mood and interpersonal function, characterised by emotional instability, disturbed patterns of thinking or perception, impulsive behaviour and intense but unstable relationships with others (Figure 41.4).

ED attendance will often result from self-harm, suicide attempts or impulsive, dangerous behaviour such as binge drinking and substance misuse. In the ED a person's behaviour can often be challenging but it is important to understand the underlying vulnerability and anxieties that lead to this. Their early experience will often have been one of neglect, a traumatic childhood involving separation, trauma, and possible sexual, physical or emotional abuse.

The result is that they are left with a highly vulnerable temperament and unable to develop the emotional resilience, psychological coping strategies or simple trust in others – particularly carers – to enable them to function as others would.

Their relationships are often turbulent, with frequent arguments, repeated breakups, and a reliance on a series of maladaptive strategies that can both anger and frighten others – paradoxically driving them away – such as extreme or unpredictable behavioural and emotional responses. A profound fear of abandonment can result in frantic efforts to fend off loneliness and, as bad as they describe their experiences of being in the ED, ironically lead to repeat attendances.

Their damaging experiences are often re-enacted with staff in the ED. What is sometimes disparagingly described as attention seeking or manipulative behaviour is exactly that – attempts to get people to understand how distressed they are feeling or to do things for them, but without the simple social and communications skills that most people would use.

The terrible fear of abandonment described earlier, with each episode dredging up memories of past losses, can also explain the apparent incongruity of someone taking an overdose after having been left by a partner of only a few weeks.

It needs to be remembered that this is a highly vulnerable group of people. Between 60% and 70% of people with BPD will attempt suicide and 10% will complete the act.

42 The patient with dementia

Figure 42.1 The patient with dementia

ABCDE

- Systematic approach
- Assess and treat clinical needs
- Assess pain
- Provide pain relief

Environment

- Well lit
- Lighting to represent day and night
- Clear signage with text and icons
- Quiet room
- Space for family or carers
- Remove unnecessary equipment
- Adjacent to bathroom facilities whenever possible

Communication

- Take time for assessment and to determine patient's needs
- Face to face, make eye contact
- Clear, slow speech
- Involve family and carers
- Explain processes and plan in simple language

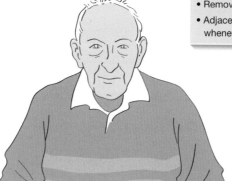

Screening

- Screen for dementia in ED
- Use a validated tool
- Involve family and carers in process

Nutrition

- Provide nutritious food and drink
- Determine what patient likes to eat and drink and provide this whenever possible
- If patient wears dentures ensure they are clean and *in situ*

Consent

- Assess for capacity using the Mental Capacity Act 2005
- Do not assume a patient with dementia has no capacity
- Involve family and independent mental capacity advocate (IMCA) to help make decisions

Figure 42.2 A dementia-friendly environment

Good lighting
- Natural light whenever possible
- In keeping with day and night

Clear signage
- Eye level
- Well-lit signs
- Sign placed on object, not adjacent to it
- Toilets and exits signposted

Colours
- Contrasting colours to identify walls, doors and handles

Noise
- Keep to minimum
- Consider doors and/or single cubicles

Flooring
- Non-slip
- Matt (non-shine)
- Plain colours
- Avoid patterns

Emergency Nursing at a Glance, First Edition. Natalie Holbery and Paul Newcombe

Background

'Dementia' is a generic term characterised by a loss of intellectual function. Memory, activities of daily living and social behaviour are often affected. Alzheimer's disease and vascular dementia are two types. It is estimated that around 800,000 people have dementia in the UK: a figure set to increase as the population ages. Dementia has received much media and government attention in an attempt to improve treatment and address gaps in health and social care.

The busy and noisy nature of emergency departments (EDs) can be unsettling for patients with dementia and other cognitive impairments. Emergency nurses need to ensure that patients with dementia are assessed and cared for as appropriate to their needs. Working closely with the patient, their carers and the multidisciplinary team is key to this.

The patient with dementia often presents with a condition or complaint unrelated to dementia. Assessment following the 'ABCDE' model (Chapter 4) remains the standard approach. However, particular attention to the environment and communication strategies is also necessary to ensure appropriate assessment and care (Figure 42.1). Capacity to consent to treatment should be assessed in line with the Mental Capacity Act 2005. It is incorrect to assume that all patients with dementia have no capacity to consent to treatment.

More time will be required to assess and communicate with a patient with dementia and at times they may need to be nursed one-to-one. This can be demanding in a time-pressured ED and will require a team approach to ensure that resources, including nursing time, are distributed appropriately. Attention to the patient's nutrition, hydration and pain relief (Chapter 6) will improve their experience and reduce distress and anxiety.

Communication

Patients with dementia often find it difficult to communicate their current concerns, including pain, as well as their medical history, medications and social circumstances. Involving carers or family members is crucial to gather this information. Contacting the patient's GP or carer by phone or requesting previous records may be required if the patient presents alone. Carers or family can also communicate what is normal behaviour for the patient.

A carer or family member should be encouraged to remain with the patient as a familiar face to reduce potential distress and confusion. Whenever possible, a carer or family member should also be present to provide reassurance during invasive procedures such as venepuncture and cannula insertion.

When communicating with a patient with dementia staff should, whenever possible, approach them from the front to gain their attention. It is recommended to address them formally at first. You can then clarify with the patient, carer or family member how the patient wishes to be addressed. Maintaining eye contact and positioning yourself at the same level as the patient is recommended to avoid intimidation and distress. Communicate using clear, slow speech and avoid the use of jargon. Short sentences are recommended and should relay only one message at a time. Tone of voice should be positive and friendly. Patients with dementia may struggle to find the right words to communicate their message. Listen carefully to them and try to observe their body language. Hurrying the person will worsen their confusion and distress. Remaining calm and asking them to explain in a different way may help.

Environment

EDs tend not to be dementia friendly although awareness of the need to address this is increasing among emergency nurses. Key features of a dementia-friendly environment are listed in Figure 42.2. In addition, there are measures that you can take on each shift to ensure that the environment is safe and appropriate for patients with dementia.

Whenever possible, placing the patient in a quiet room away from the noisiest area of the department will reduce anxiety and distress. Providing space for the carer or family member to remain is also important. Ideally the patient should be situated near a toilet to minimise confusion when returning to the cubicle. Removing or covering unnecessary equipment can also reduce confusion and aid orientation. Ensuring lighting is similar to day and night, and providing adequate light in corridors are recommended.

It is also advisable to place the patient in an area that will ensure the fewest moves around the department. When this is not possible, explicitly communicating the process to the patient and carer is essential to aid understanding and minimise distress. The use of pictures and diagrams is useful when patients are in a waiting room or other areas with large groups of people.

Fast-tracking the patient to the ward is recommended if they are to be admitted. As with all patients, it is good practice to discharge a patient with dementia into the care of a responsible adult, and ideally during daylight hours.

Screening for dementia in the ED

Early identification of dementia ensures that interventions are initiated early. It is good practice to screen for cognitive impairment all patients over the age of 65 who present to the ED. A diagnosis of dementia is too complex for an ED but steps can be taken to ensure early referral. A number of screening tools exist and each department should have an agreed tool. Examples include the Mini-Mental State Examination (MMSE) and the 4-item Abbreviated Mental Test (AMT4).

43 The patient with an intellectual disability

Figure 43.1 The hospital passport

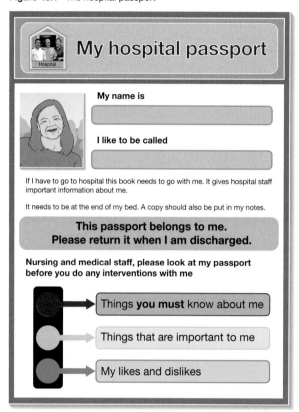

Figure 43.2 Communication board

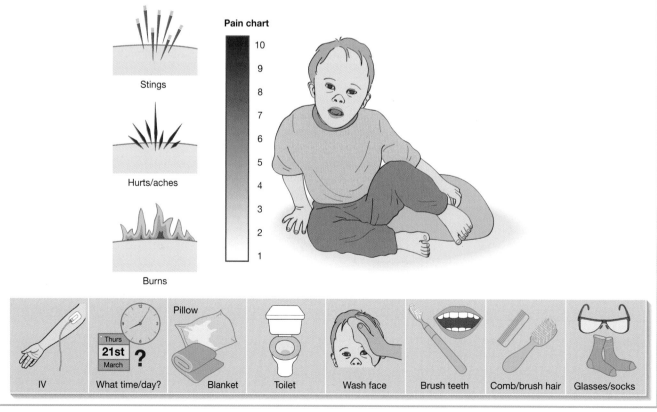

Emergency Nursing at a Glance, First Edition. Natalie Holbery and Paul Newcombe.
© 2016 John Wiley & Sons, Ltd. Published 2016 by John Wiley & Sons, Ltd. Companion website: www.ataglanceseries.com/nursing/emergencynursing

ntellectual (learning) disability has been defined by the World Health Organization (2010) as:

a condition of arrested or incomplete development of mind, which is characterised by impairment of skills manifested during the developmental period, which contribute to the overall level of intelligence and of adaptive functioning that occurs before adulthood.

Emergency departments (EDs) can be noisy, scary and unusual places for people with intellectual (learning) disabilities. Patients with an intellectual disability in an ED can become highly distressed and their behaviour may be difficult to interpret and support. Health professionals often experience anxiety and uncertainty as to how to assess and treat them, and how to ensure that they receive safe and reasonable care.

One of the greatest challenges for ED nurses caring for patients with an intellectual disability is avoiding diagnostic overshadowing (i.e. making assumptions that certain behaviours are linked to a patient's intellectual disability and not their clinical condition). Diagnostic overshadowing is most common when new behaviours evolve or existing ones increase. In an ED it can be difficult to determine which behaviours are new or increased, and involving family and carers is therefore essential. The hospital passport (Figure 43.1) is a vital tool to aid understanding and assessment of the person with an intellectual disability, and may help to reduce diagnostic overshadowing.

Hospital passport

A hospital passport is a document completed by an individual or their family or carers. It contains core information such as allergies, how the person experiences and responds to pain, and their usual behaviours. Such information can assist in eradicating diagnostic overshadowing and it provides a benchmark for ongoing assessments. If a patient does not present to an ED with a hospital passport, the family, carers or GP should be contacted and asked for a copy.

Communication

Effective communication with a patient with an intellectual disability is key to ensuring that they understand hospital procedures and feel safe. Introduce yourself by name and profession in a relaxed and calm manner. Such patients often require more time to process information; therefore, allowing more time to communicate with them is essential. Give them time to process information on one subject before moving on to the next .Time is also required for talking with family or carers.

Speak clearly, using simple language. Avoid jargon, sarcasm or metaphors. Use positive language rather than words such as 'no' and 'don't'. Maintaining open, positive body language will reduce fear and anxiety in patients with an intellectual disability. Talk to them face to face and on the same level. Look for and interpret their non-verbal communication as cues for understanding or distress. Some patients will not use words, especially if they are scared or anxious. Using picture boards or other communication aids may help (Figure 43.2).

Mental capacity

Assessing capacity to consent to treatment takes time and ED nurses should carry their assessments in a quiet area whenever possible. Each decision requires a separate capacity assessment because it is possible for someone to have capacity in relation to one aspect of care but not another. Mental capacity is outlined further in Chapter 39.

If capacity is in question, carry out the following four-point test. Is the person able to:

1 **Understand** the information relevant to the decision?
2 **Retain** the information long enough to make the decision?
3 **Use** or **weigh up** the information?
4 **Communicate** their decision?

Four key points to remember when assessing mental capacity in a patient with an intellectual disability are:

1 Everyone has capacity until assessed otherwise.
2 A person's capacity is not necessarily linked to their appearance.
3 Do not make assumptions based on a person's appearance, condition, disability or behaviour.
4 Involve the patient (and family or carers when relevant) in discussions about their care.

Practical tips

If a patient with an intellectual disability presents to an ED, the following practical tips will assist communication, assessment and treatment:

Use the hospital passport

This provides vital information about a person's needs and behaviour.

Find the best way to communicate

Remember that not all people with an intellectual disability will speak. Using photos, signs, symbols and pictures alongside speech may help.

Beware of missing serious illness

Do not ignore medical symptoms by seeing them as part of the person's disability.

Make reasonable adjustments to care

Whenever possible, minimise waiting times or move the patient away from areas that may cause distress (e.g. the waiting room) and into a private cubicle. Try to adapt the environment (e.g. by using dimmer switches to reduce the impact of bright lights). Assess and treat the patient in a quieter space with room for family or carers.

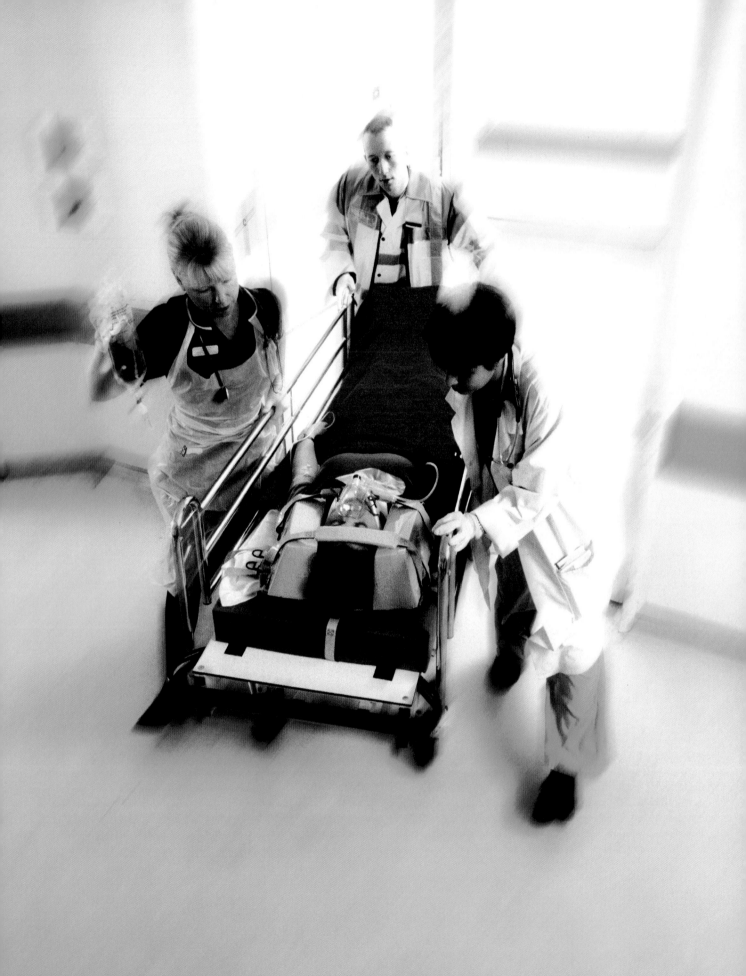

Children in the emergency department

Chapters

44 Children in the emergency department (ED)

Figure 44.1 Unique considerations of children

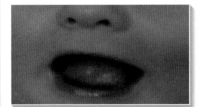

Airway – easily obstructed

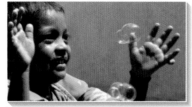

Emotionally driven

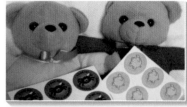

Communication

Breathing – distress occurs quickly

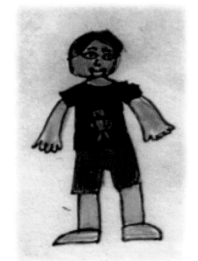

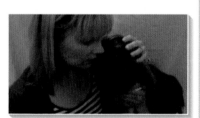

Importance of play

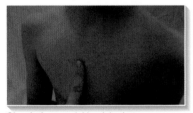

Circulation – quickly dehydrate

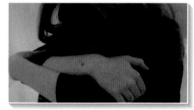

Parental/carer anxiety

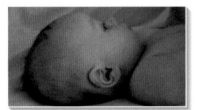

Body temperature – rapid heat loss

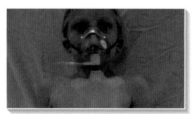

Compensatory mechanisms

Safeguarding

Figure 44.2 The United Nations Convention on the Rights of the Child (some of the articles relevant to hospital care)

Article 1 – Definition of the child

Everyone under the age of 18 has all the rights in the convention.

Article 3 – Best interests of the child

The best interests of the child must be a top priority in all actions concerning children.

Article 19 – Protection from all forms of violence

Governments must do all they can to ensure that children are protected from all forms of violence, abuse, neglect and mistreatment by their parents or anyone else who looks after them.

Article 24 – Health and health services

Every child has the right to the best possible health. Governments must provide good quality health care, clean water, nutritious food and a clean environment so that children can stay healthy.

Article 31 – Leisure, play and culture

Every child has a right to relax, play and join in a wide range of cultural and artistic activities.

Figure 44.3 Summary of safeguarding recommendations: The Children's Act 2004 and *Working together to safeguard children* (Department for Education, 2015)

• Safeguarding children is a priority for everyone

• Children are central to all decision-making and their needs and wishes are prioritised

• All professionals working with children are trained to understand and spot the risks of harm to them

• Concerns regarding a child's safety are shared at an early stage to encourage preventative actions before needs become more acute

• All professionals share information or concerns about a child in a timely way with colleagues and other agencies including social care

• Experienced professionals are available to ensure that solutions are individualised for each child

• All professionals understand the role of the Local Safeguarding Children Board and contribute regularly to actions and regular reviews of care

• Serious case reviews are published if errors occur – allowing lessons to be learned

Emergency Nursing at a Glance, First Edition. Natalie Holbery and Paul Newcombe.
© 2016 John Wiley & Sons, Ltd. Published 2016 by John Wiley & Sons, Ltd. Companion website: www.ataglanceseries.com/nursing/emergencynursing

The current trend

The attendance of children at urgent and emergency care facilities in England is now increasing by approximately a quarter of a million patients each year. With technological and clinical advances improving care, children and young people (CYP) are continuing to live longer and healthier lives. Yet we are still considered to be failing children: there is still evidence of an obvious health divide whereby children born into disadvantaged circumstances live shorter and unhealthier lives. More help and support are also needed for the increasing mental health problems in CYP.

Special considerations

In the past, children and young people have been treated as 'little adults'. However, in recent years research has highlighted how children need treatment that encompasses their unique anatomical, physiological and psychological differences (Figure 44.1).

Airway

The young child has a large head with a pronounced occiput, a small mouth and a large tongue. When laid supine, the head flexes at the neck, compressing the soft tissues of the mouth and causing an obstruction of the airway. In addition, the narrow airway of young children is easily obstructed from oedema and swelling associated with respiratory infections. The obligatory nose breathing of infants (up to 6 months) predisposes them to respiratory distress if any obstruction of the nasal passages occurs (e.g. by secretions).

Breathing

Respiratory distress occurs quickly in children due to a rapid fall in their blood oxygen levels as a result of their low oxygen reserve. They also have a high metabolism, oxygen demand and carbon dioxide production that causes their faster age-related respiratory rates. In addition, young children have a pliable chest wall because their ribs are predominantly made of cartilage. This soft structure easily recesses in respiratory compromise, which then further decreases the efficiency of breathing. Diaphragm breathing is normal in the under-fives because their intercostal muscles are weak. Anything impeding diaphragmatic movement causes respiratory distress.

Circulation

The small circulating volume of young children predisposes them to rapid dehydration during illnesses such as diarrhoea. Faster age-related heart rates maintain a high cardiac output even in mild dehydration. Blood pressure (BP) readings are also age related but are a late sign in determining the degree of illness. Owing to the compensatory abilities of a child's body, the BP only drops once the child is peri-arrest. Capillary refill time (CRT), skin colour and warmth change with increasing hypoxia. A CRT >2 seconds (over the sternum) and pale, mottled, cool skin are reliable indicators of an unwell child.

Difficulty regulating body temperature

Young children have a larger head and body surface area and less subcutaneous tissue for insulation. This results in children (in particular, infants), losing vast amounts of heat when exposed to the environment.

Compensatory mechanisms

Children have physiological responses to illness that enables them to survive (Chapter 46). Although initiated to protect the heart and brain from hypoxia, if these mechanisms are not recognised and treated while in the compensatory stage, children decompensate into cardiorespiratory arrest.

Communication

Children of all ages and their parents need honest, clear explanations about their plans of care in order to allay fear. Older children often feel ignored and undervalued in decisions regarding their treatment, resulting in a lack of trust in the healthcare professional. The inability of the young to effectively communicate heightens anxiety in both the parent and child. Using verbal praise and rewards such as stickers and specially designed teddies positively reassures children that they are coping well with their situation.

Emotionally driven

Attending ED is a traumatic and stressful experience for a child and their parents. The unknown situation causes fear and anxiety and children often regress to behaviour similar to that of a younger child. Distraction with animated conversations, use of bubbles, and pointing to pictures on the wall of animals or cartoons is known to alleviate the distress experienced by children during treatment.

Importance of play

Play is seen as a right for all children (Figure 44.2) and access to age-appropriate toys and visual equipment ensures that any anxiety and distress caused by their hospital attendance is minimised.

Parental or carer anxiety

Parental anxiety often exceeds the concern of the health professional, primarily because parents have less experience of dealing with seriously ill children. Anxiety can also be caused if a parent is confused about where their child should be treated (the changing roles of individual facilities) if they have difficulty accessing primary care (such as the GP) for advice or if unsympathetic staff label the parent as 'panicky'.

Importance of safeguarding

Children have the right to the best possible health care and protection from maltreatment (Figure 44.3). After the tragic deaths of Victoria Climbié in 2000 and Peter Connelly in the UK in 2007, it was highlighted that too many agencies including NHS staff had concerns about these children and yet failed to communicate with each other. Because ED staff may be the first professionals whom children who have been maltreated come into contact with, they need to be clear on what their role is in ensuring that children stay safe, remain healthy, enjoy and achieve, make a positive contribution to society and have economic well-being to achieve their full potential (Figure 44.3). See also Chapter 45.

45 Safeguarding children

Figure 45.1 Signs of maltreatment in children (NICE, 2009)

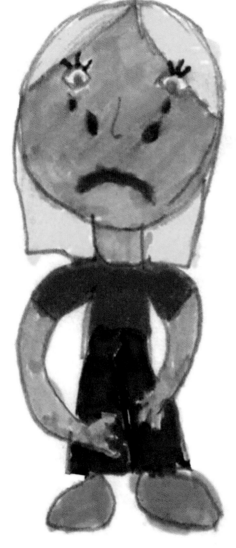

Neglect

- Infestations of scabies or head lice
- Inappropriate clothing or footwear for weather or child's size
- Persistently smelly or dirty child
- Failure to thrive (malnutrition)
- Bites or burns in a young child (lack of supervision)
- Persistent dental caries or unimmunised child (parental failure to participate in health promotion activities for child)
- Non-attendance at healthcare appointments
- Scavenging or stealing food
- Near-drowning incidents
- Abandonment

Physical abuse

- Injury with unknown or implausible explanation
- Injury to an immobile child
- Injury to an area usually covered by clothes
- Frequent attendance for treatment
- Bruising (clusters)
- Bites (particularly adult sized)
- Lacerations or abrasions (multiple)
- Burns or scalds (in certain shapes and places)
- Cold injuries (hypothermia, reddened and swollen hands or feet)
- Fractures (multiple, of different ages or of ribs and long bones)
- Poisoning (deliberate or repeated presentations in a child or siblings)
- Apparent life-threatening events

Sexual abuse

- Genital, anal or peri-anal injury
- Foreign body in anus or vagina
- Vaginal discharge
- Dysuria
- Recurrent abdominal pain
- Sexually transmitted infections such as warts, gonorrhoea or chlamydia
- Pregnancy in a child <15 years
- Sleeping problems
- Behaviour changes (aggression or withdrawal)
- Sexualised behaviour (sexual talk and actions in a young child)
- Poor school attendance
- Self-harm

Emotional and behavioural abuse

- Recurrent nightmares
- Fearful, withdrawn behaviour
- Episodes of aggression (temper tantrums)
- Overaffectionate, friendly towards strangers
- Excessively good behaviour in front of parent or carer
- Inappropriate response to medical examinations (passive or resisting)
- Wetting and soiling
- Self-harm
- Hostile parent–child interactions (lack of comfort)
- Fabricated illness

Figure 45.2 Gillick competency and Fraser guidelines (NSPCC, 2015)

Gillick competency

- Approved in 1983 and re-enforced in 1985, in the High Court
- Involved a mother (Mrs Victoria Gillick) attempting to stop her local health authority and doctors from giving contraceptive advice or treatment to children under 16 without parental consent
- Relevant to children aged under 16
- Aims to determine:
  - if a child has sufficient maturity and intelligence to understand treatment choices, implications and risks
  - if a child can use the information given, to decide and communicate that they wish to consent to the treatment

Should be the principal guidance used to judge a child's legal capacity to consent to medical tests and treatment

Fraser guidelines

- Created in 1985 by Lord Fraser, in the House of Lords
- Relates only to contraceptive advice and treatment
- Combines the Gillick test of competence with the following specific criteria:
  - a girl understands the contraceptive advice given to her
  - she cannot be persuaded to inform her parents
  - she is likely to continue having sexual intercourse with or without contraception
  - her physical and/or mental health will suffer is she does not receive contraceptive advice

It is in the girl's best interests to receive contraceptive advice and/or treatment with or without her parents' consent

Emergency Nursing at a Glance, First Edition. Natalie Holbery and Paul Newcombe
© 2016 John Wiley & Sons, Ltd. Published 2016 by John Wiley & Sons, Ltd. Companion website: www.ataglanceseries.com/nursing/emergencynursing

Key principles

Safeguarding children incorporates two main areas of action: first, the protection of children and the prevention of child maltreatment (abuse); second, it involves the promotion of children's health and development through safe and effective individualised care.

Identifying maltreatment

Nurse's role

With at least one child a week dying from maltreatment, emergency department (ED) nurses play a vital role in safeguarding children. As well as detecting potential cases of concern presenting to an ED, nurses also have a duty to ensure they that know the processes and guidance in place for sharing concerns about a child early. Early sharing of information prevents risks from escalating and thereby prevents harm from occurring (Chapter 44). Although neglect is the most prevalent form of maltreatment in children, followed by physical violence, emotional and sexual abuse (Figure 45.1), in the ED, maltreatment most commonly presents as physical non-accidental injuries (NAIs).

Indicators of NAI

It is estimated that at least 1% of all child attendances at an ED are for physical injuries caused by hitting, slapping, shaking, throwing, poisoning, burning, drowning, suffocating and even the fabrication of symptoms. Infants are the most at risk of abuse, and most commonly the perpetrator is a parent or person known to the child.

NAI should be suspected when the mechanism of any injury is unknown or unclear, in multiple injuries and those found on a child <1 year who is not independently mobile. Bruising over the knees and shins is normal in active children; however, injuries (such as wounds, bruises and scarring) found in unusual areas (e.g. around the eyes and ears, the dorsum of hands, soles of feet or areas usually covered by clothes, such as back, chest, buttocks and genital area) are highly suspicious. Furthermore, injuries shaped like fingers or hands, ligatures, cigarette ends or bites (particularly large human bites or animal bites) strongly indicate NAI.

In addition, burns and scalds, if observed on buttocks, hands and feet in a linear, glove or stocking distribution, indicate forced immersion into hot water. Intracranial head injuries (particularly in children <3 years) and/or retinal haemorrhages without known accidental trauma indicate purposeful injury from shaking or hitting. Fractures of one or more bones (in the absence of known medical problems), multiple fractures of different ages, occipital skull fractures and rib or long bone fractures in young children are also highly suggestive of NAI.

Assessment

During triage, consider:

- **History of the injury** – does the mechanism of injury fit the presenting problem? Is the story consistently repeated by both carer and child? Are there any unexplained injuries?

- **Repeated ED attendances** – suggestive of ongoing abuse
- **Delay in injury presentation to the ED** – indicating a lack of parental concern or interest in the child
- **Physical appearance of child** – is clothing smelly with ingrained dirt or inappropriate for the weather? Any infestations of scabies or severe nappy rash?
- **Child's behaviour** – are they fearful and watchful or relaxed and playful?
- **Child–carer interactions** – appropriately affectionate or hostile?
- **Any known parental factors** – poverty, domestic violence, drug or alcohol misuse, mental health issues?
- **In a high-risk group** – are they an infant, child with a disability, asylum seeker, in foster care?
- **Medical history of child** – document known conditions affecting bone formation or blood clotting
- **Social history of child** – is the child on a child protection plan (CPP) or do they have a social worker?

Management

When suspecting child maltreatment, staff must always share their concerns with a more experienced colleague – never assume that someone else will report a concern. The child should always be assessed by a senior paediatric doctor and any injuries or markings recorded on a body map chart. X-rays of the skull, chest, abdomen, spine and limbs are usually taken to scrutinise for any other 'hidden' injuries. The child is usually admitted to a ward awaiting any further treatment and social services assessment. All observations, verbal interactions and treatment given to the family and child must be documented in the child's notes in a concise and factual manner. Verbal discussions with social services immediately after treating the child should be followed by the completion of paperwork to share information about the child and their injuries with their GP, health visitor or school nurse. The child and parent should also be involved in and consent to (if appropriate) all plans of care and referrals made.

Consent

Safeguarding children requires nurses to provide care that encompasses every child's individual needs, views and wishes. In an ED, this includes enabling children, when appropriate, to consent to their own assessment and treatment. In younger children, consent is usually given by the accompanying adult with parental responsibility (e.g. a parent or foster carer). However, older children under 16 years can consent to their own medical treatment as long as health professionals feel it is in their best interests and that they have the maturity and capacity to understand the available treatment options and outcomes of the proposed care. This is called being 'Gillick competent'. In addition, children attending on their own for sexual health advice and treatment should be assessed using the Fraser guidelines. 'Gillick competence' and 'Fraser guidelines' (Figure 45.2) are separate terms not to be used interchangeably. However, both guidelines should be applied in practice when dealing with under-16s attending an ED for treatment.

46 Recognising the sick child

Figure 46.1 Consequences of progressive respiratory or circulatory failure

Compensated respiratory failure
- Tachypnoea
- Recession
- Accessory muscle use
- Position/visibly distressed child
- See-saw breathing
- Inspiratory/expiratory noises
- Peripheral SpO_2 <90% in room air

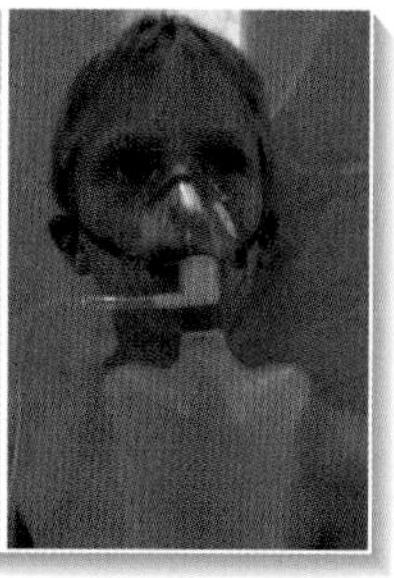

Compensated circulatory failure
- Tachycardia
- Pale, mottled skin
- Prolonged CRT
- Drowsiness
- Decreased urine output

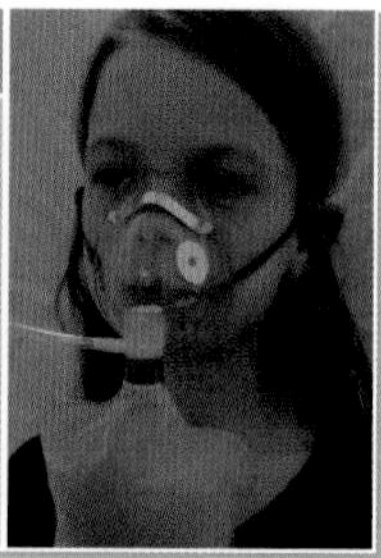

Decompensated respiratory failure
- Silent chest
- Exhaustion
- Cyanosis (central)

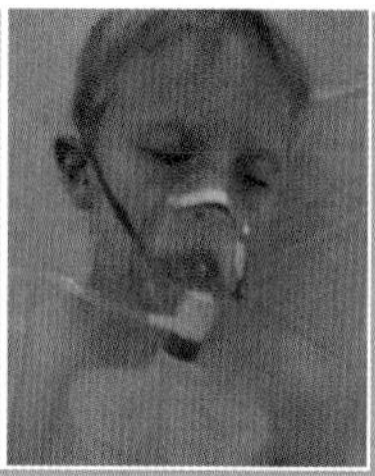

Decompensated circulatory failure
- Diminished central pulses
- Bradycardia
- Hypotension
- Cyanosis (peripheral)

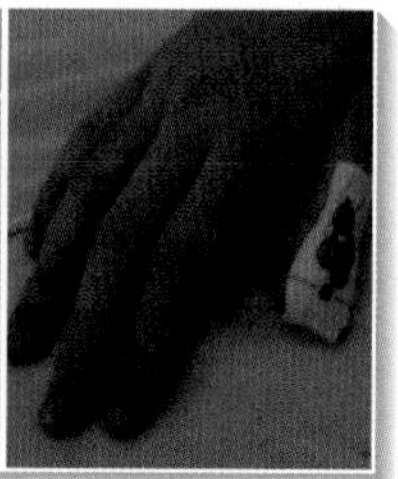

CARDIORESPIRATORY FAILURE

CARDIORESPIRATORY ARREST

Figure 46.2 Pulse and respiratory rates: Age-related parameters

Age in years	<1	1–2	2–5	5–12	>12
Respiratory rate/min	30–40	25–35	25–30	20–25	15–20
Heart rate/min	110–160	100–150	95–140	80–120	60–100

Figure 46.3 Paediatric Early Warning Score (PEWS) tool

Score	0	1	2	3
Behaviour	• Playing • Appropriate for age	• Sleeping • Irritable but consolable	• Irritable/agitated • Inconsolable	• Lethargic/floppy • Confused • Reduced pain response
Cardiovascular	• Pink and well-perfused skin • CRT <2 seconds	• Pale skin • CRT 3 seconds	• Grey skin • CRT 4 seconds • Tachycardia of 20 breaths per minute (bpm) above normal parameters	• Grey or mottled skin • CRT ≥5 seconds • Tachycardia of 30 bpm above normal limits • Bradycardia
Respiratory	• Rate within age-related limits • No recession or accessory muscle use	• Rate ≥10 respirations above normal parameters • Accessory muscle use • Oxygen (O_2) therapy ≤4 litre per min (L/min) • Initiation of O_2 therapy	• Rate ≥20 respirations above normal parameters • Accessory muscle use, tracheal tug and/or recession • O_2 therapy 5–7 L/min	• Rate 5 respirations below normal parameters • Accessory muscle use, recession, tracheal tug, and/or grunting • O_2 therapy ≥8 L/min

Emergency Nursing at a Glance, First Edition. Natalie Holbery and Paul Newcombe.
© 2016 John Wiley & Sons, Ltd. Published 2016 by John Wiley & Sons, Ltd. Companion website: www.ataglanceseries.com/nursing/emergencynursing

Assessment

When children become unwell, internal physiological responses enable them to initially compensate for their illness or injury (Figure 46.1). Hypoxia is the main cause of collapse in children and if not treated promptly in the compensatory stage, will cause vital organs to fail and the child to decompensate into a secondary cardiorespiratory arrest. In hospital, just over a quarter of children survive cardiorespiratory arrest without any neurological impairment. Preventing cardiorespiratory arrest in children relies on nurses completing a thorough assessment to enable:

• Early recognition of a seriously ill child
• Effective management of the child's condition and prompt treatment to prevent deterioration.

Rapid initial check of child

An initial inspection of each child as they arrive must be completed to allow immediate identification of critical illness. Is the child clean, is their skin pink and warm, and are they interacting appropriately with their carer? A pale, floppy child with poor interaction indicates one requiring immediate emergency treatment.

Airway – is it patent?

A child who is conscious and talking has a patent airway. However, partial obstruction should be considered in a conscious child displaying visible distress, an increased respiratory rate and work (effort) of breathing. Any respiratory noises should also be recorded. A high-pitched stridor (inspiratory and/or expiratory) is characteristic of upper airway obstruction. Wheezing tends to be expiratory and indicates a narrowing of the lower airways.

Breathing – is it adequate?

Breathing effort

Increased work of breathing is initially indicated by tachypnoea – above the child's age-related parameters (Figure 46.2). Additional signs in younger children include recession (sternal, subcostal or intercostal), nasal flaring and head-bobbing (from use of the sternocleidomastoid muscles in the neck). Grunting indicates severe respiratory distress as the infant or young child attempts to exhale while maintaining their resting lung volume (preventing alveolar collapse). See-saw breathing (where the abdomen expands as the pliable chest wall retracts) is also a sign of severe respiratory failure. Older children may adopt a forward position resting on their arms in order to maximise the use of respiratory muscles. As their chest wall is more rigid than that of a younger child, any recession is a sign of severe respiratory failure.

Breathing efficacy

The efficacy of breathing can be assessed by observing chest movement, the volume (tidal), rate and symmetry of chest expansion. Palpation can reveal areas of deformity or crepitus. Percussion enables identification of areas of collapse (dullness) or over-inflation (hyper-resonance) such as a pneumothorax. Auscultation enables the confirmation of equal air entry in all lung areas on both sides of the chest. Inefficient respiration can be identified by diminished or absent chest sounds. Pulse oximetry should always be used with children in respiratory distress. Readings of peripheral oxygen saturations below 90% on room air or below 95% on supplemental oxygen is indicative of a child in respiratory failure.

Circulation – is it adequate?

A well child has skin that is pink and warm. Hypoxia causes vasoconstriction and pallor, which, as a child's condition deteriorates, can change to mottling and peripheral cyanosis. In addition, assessment of a child's capillary refill time (CRT) should be used to identify early signs of circulatory failure. By applying finger pressure to the sternum for 5 seconds, blanching of the skin occurs that should disappear within 2 seconds (when the pressure is released). Prolonged CRT indicates decreased tissue perfusion and circulatory inadequacy. In addition, a decreasing urine output (less than 4–6 nappies) over 24 hours is also indicative of reduced renal perfusion and increasing circulatory failure.

Appropriate cardiac and blood pressure monitoring should always be used on a child in circulatory failure. Tachycardia – above age-related parameters (Figure 46.2) is the initial compensatory response to circulatory failure. A faster heart rate increases a child's cardiac output to maintain their blood pressure and tissue perfusion. However, if prolonged, inadequate tissue perfusion and increasing hypoxia result in bradycardia and hypotension. In addition, peripheral and central pulses must be palpated and compared for rate and volume. Diminishing central pulses, bradycardia and hypotension are worrying signs indicating severe circulatory failure and imminent cardiorespiratory arrest.

Disability – is the child conscious?

Hypoxia initially leads to agitation and drowsiness, but if ongoing ultimately results in loss of consciousness. A parent may report that their child is less responsive and hypotonic (floppy). Using AVPU, a quick assessment of whether a child is ALERT, responsive only to VOICE, responsive to PAINFUL stimuli or UNRESPONSIVE (unconscious) can be achieved. In addition, their pupil size, equality and reactivity to light should be recorded to ascertain brain perfusion and function. A baseline blood glucose (BG) should also be taken from a finger or toe for prompt exclusion of hypoglycaemia.

Exposure

While maintaining the dignity of a child and conserving their body heat, all skin areas must be observed for any signs of blood loss, bruises, rashes or wounds. Recording of a child's body temperature should also be completed (the axilla route is recommended for babies and children of all ages but the tympanic route is only suitable in children >4 weeks).

Paediatric Early Warning Score (PEWS)

Once a child has been assessed according to the 'ABCDE' approach (Chapter 4) all observations are compared with a tool (see Figure 46.3) and a score given to the child's condition. PEWS encourages all staff to fully assess a child, enabling them to recognise serious illness (= high score) early on and initiate prompt treatment before a child deteriorates.

47 Common illnesses in children

Figure 47.1 Common respiratory illness in children

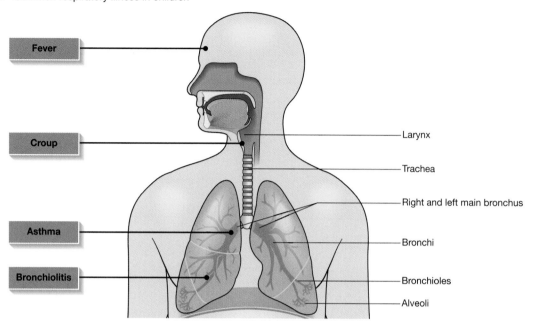

Fever

Croup

Asthma

Bronchiolitis

Larynx

Trachea

Right and left main bronchus

Bronchi

Bronchioles

Alveoli

Figure 47.2 Child using an inhaler via a spacer device

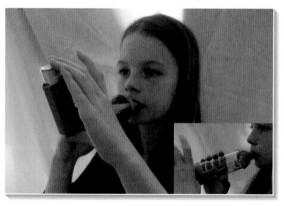

Figure 47.4 Non-blanching rashes signifying septicaemia

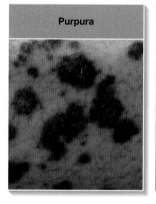

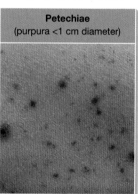

Purpura	Petechiae (purpura <1 cm diameter)

Figure 47.3 Croup scoring system

Symptom	0	1	2	3	4
Distress	None	Child comfortable	Child agitated	Child exhausted	NA
Oxygen saturations	95–100%	92–94%	89–91%	86–88%	<86%
Stridor	None	Only when agitated	Mild at rest	Moderate at rest	Severe at rest
Air entry	Normal	Reduced	Greatly reduced	NA	NA
Recession	None	Mild	Moderate	Severe	NA

Possible score 0–16:

0–3 = Mild croup (observe)

4–7 = Moderate croup (consider oral steroid administration and observe)

>8 = Severe croup (administer oral steroid or budesonide nebuliser, refer to paediatrician)

Emergency Nursing at a Glance, First Edition. Natalie Holbery and Paul Newcombe
© 2016 John Wiley & Sons, Ltd. Published 2016 by John Wiley & Sons, Ltd. Companion website: www.ataglanceseries.com/nursing/emergencynursing

Childhood illness accounts for over a third of attendances for urgent and emergency care. Respiratory problems (Figure 47.1) are the most common presentations, followed by fever, rashes and vomiting. Children presenting with illness should be assessed as discussed in Chapter 46, in order to receive appropriate early treatment and make a prompt recovery.

Asthma

Asthma is the most common, chronic illness in children. It is generally caused by an infection or allergen, which irritates the smooth muscle of the lower airways causing bronchospasm, mucosal swelling and increased mucus production. Owing to their narrow airways (Chapter 44), at least a third of children up to 2 years of age will have a 'wheezy episode' requiring hospital treatment. Only after identifying a family history of asthma, in addition to monitoring medication usage and asthma symptoms, will a child be diagnosed as 'asthmatic'.

Management

- Child and parental reassurance.
- Assessment of 'ABCDE' (Chapter 4; administer oxygen if required).
- Weigh child (for medication doses) and administer bronchodilators via spacer and inhaler – recommended whenever possible instead of nebuliser use (Figure 47.2).
- Give oral steroids (usually dispersible prednisolone).
- The child is then observed until discharge home, unless further treatment is required.

Croup (acute laryngotracheobronchitis)

Generally caused by a viral infection, typically the parainfluenza virus, croup affects the upper airways and is common in younger children during autumn and winter. The virus causes mucosal oedema and inflammation of the larynx and vocal chords, resulting in a hoarse voice, stridor and a classic 'barking' cough.

Management

- Reassurance and calmness (because the barking cough often frightens the child and parent).
- Assessment of ABCDE (administer oxygen if required) and croup severity using a scoring system (Figure 47.3)
- Record weight (for medication dose). Give analgesia (for the sore throat and fever) and steroids (dexamethasone) to reduce the oedema. Bronchodilators are not usually indicated because mucosal swelling affects the upper airways. Nebulised adrenaline may be needed if a child develops respiratory failure.
- Allow the child to find a comfortable position (often sitting up on a trolley bed or on a parent's lap).
- Monitor the child until discharged home (most common).

Bronchiolitis

In children under 1 year, bronchiolitis is a common winter respiratory infection usually caused by the respiratory syncytial virus (RSV). This virus inflames and constricts the lower airways (bronchioles) and increases mucus production, resulting in a moist cough, runny nose and mild fever.

Management

- Reassurance and assessment of ABCDE.
- Babies who appear happy, are feeding well and without signs of respiratory distress are usually allowed home.

- However, a baby who is not feeding is fatigued and at risk of dehydration. They need admission for supportive care, nursed in a head-up position, airway kept clear of secretions, oxygen administration and assistance with hydration (usually via nasogastric tube feeds).
- Antipyretics can be administered if a child is feverish and distressed. Bronchodilators (ipratropium bromide) rarely improve a baby's condition.
- A nasopharyngeal aspirate should be collected from every baby admitted to identify the cause of their illness (RSV is highly contagious and needs isolation on a ward).

Fever

Although fevers are generally caused by a self-limiting viral infection, serious causes of fever can include pneumonia, urinary tract infections (UTIs) and meningococcal disease (meningitis, septicaemia). Using an electronic thermometer in the axilla is the recommended route for taking a temperature in all children. Any child who appears unwell with a temperature ≥38°C (especially babies ≤6 months) should always be reviewed by a doctor.

Management

- Parental reassurance (many parents fear that their child has meningitis or will experience a febrile convulsion).
- Assessment of ABCDE and removal of clothing to cool the child – observe skin for non-blanching rash (Figure 47.4).
- Record weight and administer antipyretics only if the child is distressed as a result of the fever. Paracetamol and ibuprofen should only be alternated if one medication alone fails to improve the child's condition.
- In children under 1 year with a fever and no apparent source, the following should be collected – bloods (including blood gas and blood cultures), urine sample (clean catch if possible to rule out UTI), stool sample if experiencing diarrhoea and chest X-ray if in respiratory compensation. A lumbar puncture (LP) may also be performed if meningitis is suspected.

Non-blanching rash

The classic rash signifying septicaemia has a non-blanching, pin-prick or blood blister appearance (Figure 47.4). The child will be unwell with a fever, symptoms of circulatory failure (Chapter 46) and limb pain. Early recognition of the symptoms and rash is vital because death can occur within 24 hours of symptom onset. Any child with a non-blanching rash and fever needs continuous ABCDE monitoring, immediate senior medical assessment and intravenous antibiotics.

Febrile convulsions (FCs)

Approximately a fifth of all children (up to 5 years of age) will experience a clonic–tonic seizure associated with their pyrexia. FCs cannot be prevented (not even by antipyretic use) and generally occur when a fever suddenly spikes above 37.8°C. Parents often report that they think their child is dying during an FC, so reassurance that the seizure does not cause brain damage and is not a sign of epilepsy is paramount. Any child experiencing an FC should be nursed on their side, given high-flow oxygen with ABCDE, continually monitored and have an immediate medical assessment.

48 Paediatric advanced life support

Figure 48.1 Head positioning for airway patency

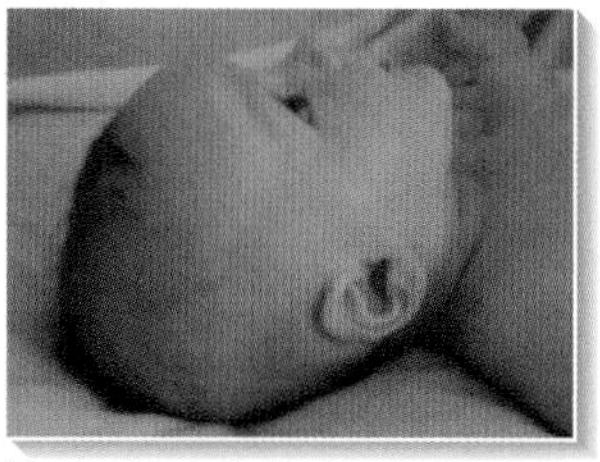

Neutral in infants (under 1 year)

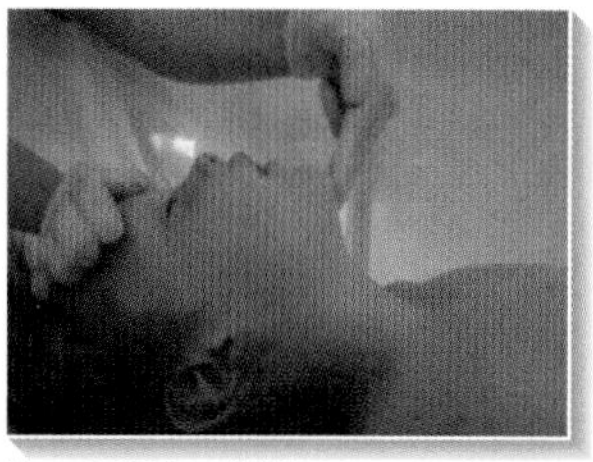

Head-tilt in child

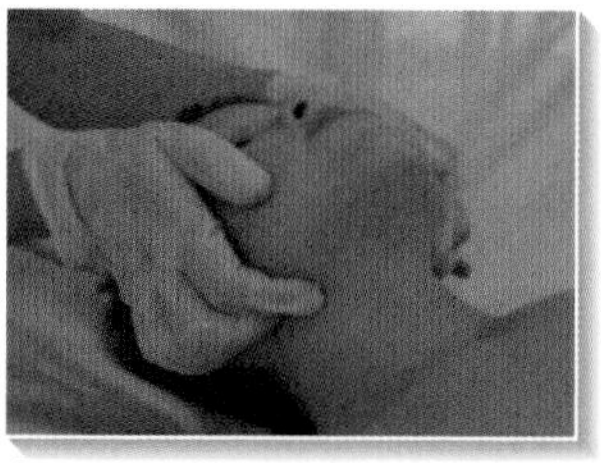

Jaw-thrust in child

Figure 48.2 Airway and breathing adjuncts

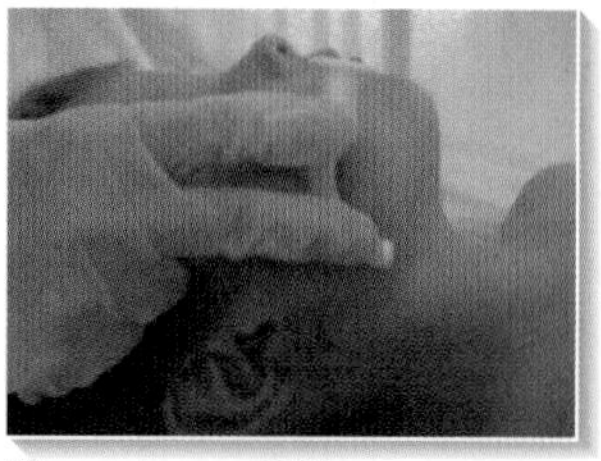

Measuring an OPA

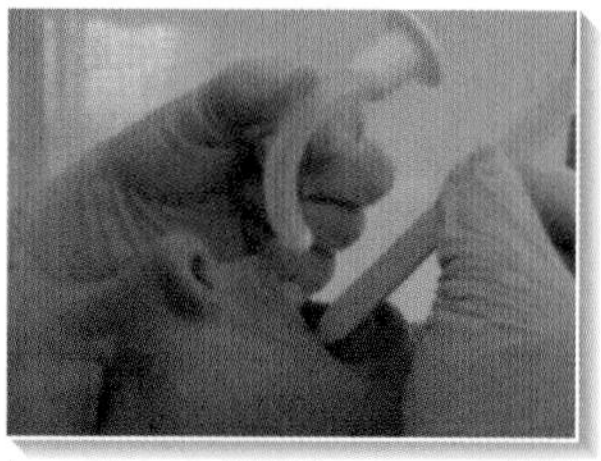

Inserting an OPA in a young child

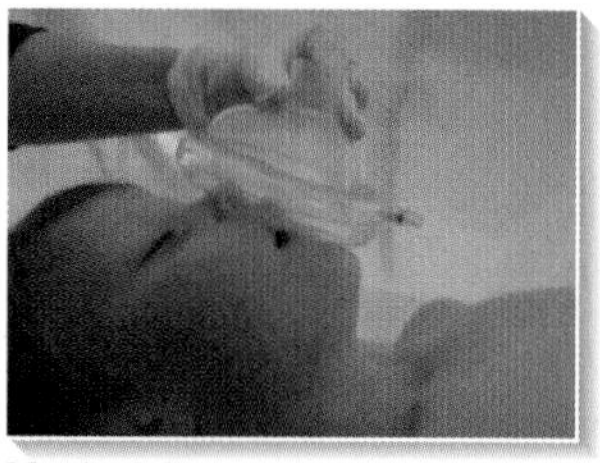

Mask sizing

Figure 48.3 Positioning for chest compressions

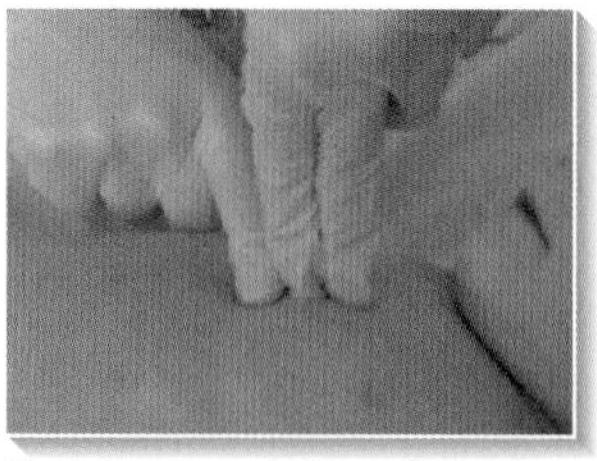

Two-finger technique (infant)

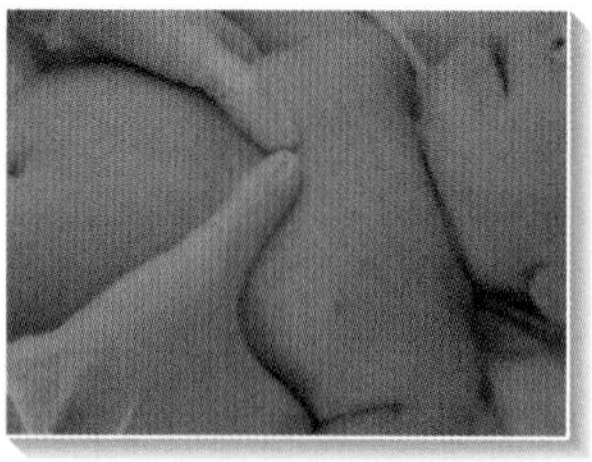

Two-thumb technique (infant)

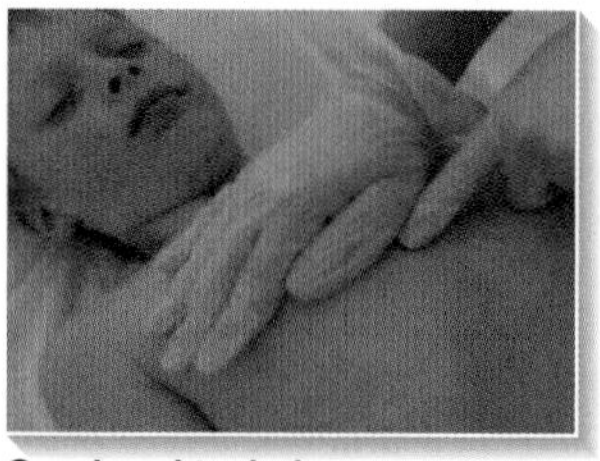

One-hand technique

Figure 48.4 Paediatric advanced life support algorithm

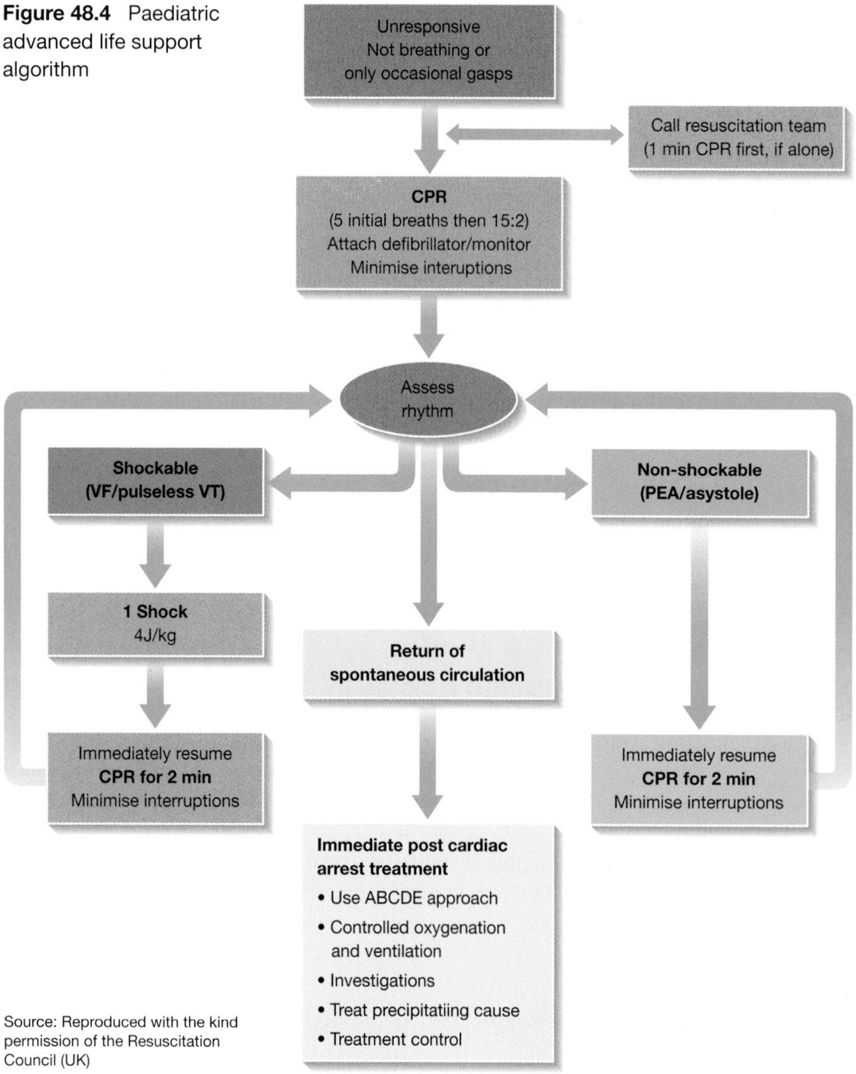

Unresponsive
Not breathing or
only occasional gasps

Call resuscitation team
(1 min CPR first, if alone)

CPR
(5 initial breaths then 15:2)
Attach defibrillator/monitor
Minimise interuptions

Assess rhythm

Shockable
(VF/pulseless VT)

Non-shockable
(PEA/asystole)

1 Shock
4J/kg

Return of
spontaneous circulation

Immediately resume
CPR for 2 min
Minimise interruptions

Immediately resume
CPR for 2 min
Minimise interruptions

Immediate post cardiac
arrest treatment
• Use ABCDE approach
• Controlled oxygenation
  and ventilation
• Investigations
• Treat precipitatiing cause
• Treatment control

Source: Reproduced with the kind permission of the Resuscitation Council (UK)

During CPR
• Ensure high-quality CPR rate, depth, recoil
• Plan actions before interrupting CPR
• Give oxygen
• Vascular access (IV, IO)
• Give adrenaline every 3–5 min
• Consider advanced airway and capnography
• Continuous chest compressions when advanced
  airway in place
• Correct reversible causes
• Consider amiodarone after 3 and 5 shocks

Reversible causes
• Hypoxia
• Hypovolaemia
• Hypo-/hyper-
  kalaemia/metabolic
• Hypothermia

• Thrombosis – coronary
  or pulmonary
• Tension pneumothorax
• Tamponade – cardiac
• Toxic/therapeutic
  disturbances

Figure 48.5 IO drill, needle and giving set

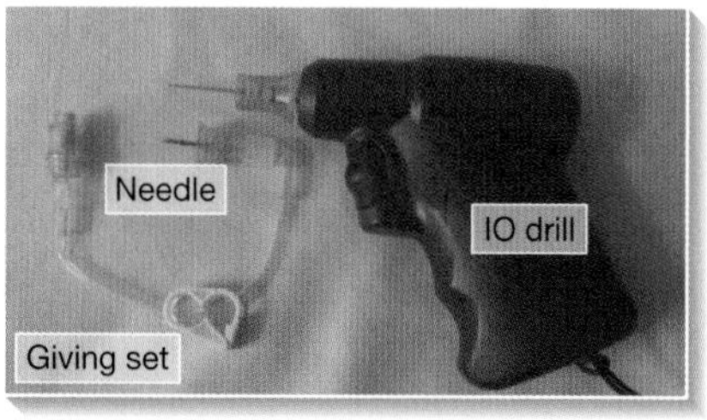

Needle

IO drill

Giving set

Emergency Nursing at a Glance, First Edition. Natalie Holbery and Paul Newcombe.
© 2016 John Wiley & Sons, Ltd. Published 2016 by John Wiley & Sons, Ltd. Companion website: www.ataglanceseries.com/nursing/emergencynursing

Cardiorespiratory arrest

• Children who experience cardiorespiratory arrest are usually hypoxic; therefore immediate life support with 5 rescue breaths is vital to provide adequate oxygenation and prevent organ damage.

• The most common arrhythmia in paediatric cardiorespiratory arrest is bradycardia progressing into asystole. Effective cardiopulmonary resuscitation (CPR) is therefore more important when treating a collapsed child than using a defibrillator.

Safety, stimulation and summoning help

Before approaching any child, assess the area for obvious hazards. Ensure that help is summoned by shouting or asking a colleague to dial 2222 (in-hospital resuscitation team). The child should be transferred to the resuscitation room ensuring that the cervical spine (c-spine) is immobilised if neck trauma is suspected. Establish whether the child responds to vocal stimulation or gentle shaking of their arms. If responsive, place them in a position maintaining c-spine immobilisation and airway patency. If unresponsive, commence paediatric advanced life support (PALS) until further help arrives.

Airway management

Airway patency can be achieved using a head-tilt position (with one hand on the forehead and 1–2 fingers on the bony area of the chin) in the child and a neutral head-tilt in infants (Figure 48.1). However, a jaw-thrust is the most effective action to open a child's airway (particularly if c-spine injury is suspected). The mouth should be checked for any foreign object and, if visible, this should be removed with a single finger sweep. An oropharyngeal airway (OPA) measuring from the angle of the child's jaw to the incisors can then be inserted (Figure 48.2). However, owing to the delicate structures of the palate in young children, OPAs should be introduced over the tongue the correct way up and not with the 180° rotation used in older children and adults. Nasopharyngeal airways (NPAs) can also be used and should reach from the child's ear tragus to their nostril tip. Once lubricated, NPAs should fit into the nostril without causing pallor. Age-appropriate advanced airways such as a laryngeal mask airway (LMA) or tracheal tube can be prepared, but must only be inserted by competent professionals.

Breathing – effective ventilation

Assessment of breathing over 10 seconds must include looking for chest movement, listening and feeling over the mouth for breath sounds. If the child is breathing effectively and within age-related parameters (Chapter 46), high-flow oxygen (15 litres) should be administered via a non-rebreathing oxygen mask. Ineffective breathing or irregular gasping requires 5 rescue breaths to be given using a self-inflating bag mask device (BMD) with an appropriately sized facial mask (Figure 48.2). The BMD should then be attached to 15 litres of oxygen (to deliver >90% oxygen to the child). Each rescue breath should last approximately 1 second and must be accompanied by the chest rising and falling at a ventilation rate of 12–20 min^{-1}. If no chest movement is seen, despite suctioning and head repositioning, the presence of a foreign body must be suspected and chest compressions started.

Circulation – determining signs of life

Assessment of an adequate spontaneous circulation via a central pulse (brachial for infant, carotid for child) and signs of life (such as crying) should take no more than 10 seconds. If no signs of life are observed and a pulse is not felt, then chest compressions should be started. These should be administered over the lower half of the sternum, one finger width above the xiphisternum. In infants, compressions can be applied using two fingers or a two-thumb technique (Figure 48.3). For the younger child (under 8 years), a single hand may be used to administer compressions progressing to two hands in the older child. The chest should always be compressed by one-third of its diameter at a rate of between 100 and 120 beats per minute. When combined with ventilations, a ratio of 2 ventilations to 15 chest compressions should be maintained.

Paediatric advanced life support (PALS)

A defibrillator should be attached as per algorithm guidelines (Figure 48.4) and the child's cardiac rhythm checked. Most commonly, a non-shockable rhythm (pulseless electrical activity [PEA] or asystole) is detected. Adrenaline (epinephrine) must be administered via the intravenous (IV) or intraosseous (IO) route followed by CPR. Brief checking for rhythm change every 2 minutes with repeated doses of adrenaline every 3–5 minutes should continue.

If a child is in a shockable rhythm – ventricular fibrillation (VF) or pulseless ventricular tachycardia (VT) – then one shock should be delivered (either 4 joules/kg shock from a manual defibrillator or one shock from an adult automated external defibrillator (AED), attenuated to a lower energy level if the child is less than 8 years old). CPR should be resumed for 2 minutes before the rhythm is re-checked. If three shocks are required, adrenaline and amiodarone should be administered (to improve the success of defibrillation) and CPR continued.

The reversible causes of cardiorespiratory arrest (Figure 48.4) must always be considered and corrected. CPR should continue until the return of spontaneous circulation is observed or a decision to stop treatment occurs.

Circulatory access

IO needles are the preferred access route in emergency situations and are inserted using a specialised drill (see Figure 12.5) usually 2–3cm below the tibial tuberosity on the medial aspect of the leg. As IO needles are introduced through the bone cortex and into the marrow cavity, they enable the rapid administration of multiple drugs and fluids. Fluid resuscitation begins with a bolus of 20mls/kg of 0.9% saline, which can be repeated twice more before a surgical opinion is required.

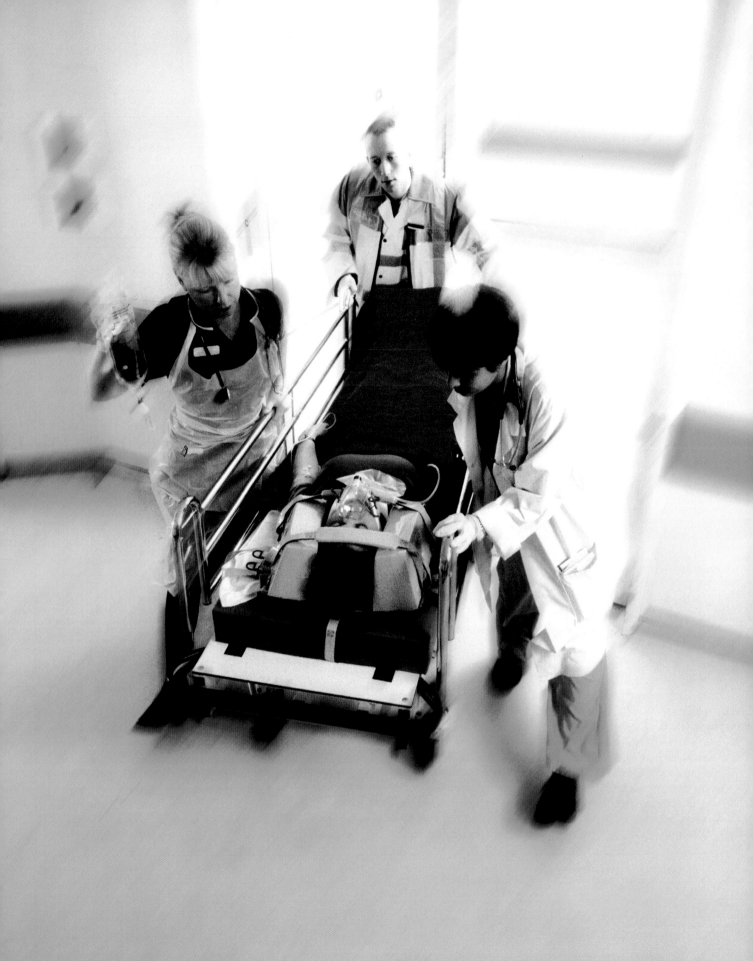

Minor injuries and conditions

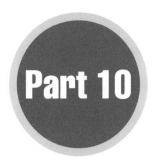

Part 10

Chapters

49 # Minor injuries in children

Figure 49.1 Paediatric Glasgow Coma Scale

			<5 years	>5 years
Eye opening	E4		Spontaneous	
	E3		To voice/speech	
	E2		To pain	
	E1		No response	
Verbal	V5	Smiles, coos, babbles, follows objects, interacts		Orientated and appropriate
	V4	Cries but consolable		Confused
	V3	Cries to pain, moaning		Inappropriate words
	V2	Inconsolable, agitated		Incomprehensible sounds
	V1		No response	
Motor	M6	Moves spontaneously and purposefully		Obeys commands
	M5	Withdraws from touch		Localises pain
	M4	Withdraws from pain		Withdraws from pain
	M3	Abnormal flexion to pain		Abnormal flexion to pain
	M2	Abnormal extension to pain		Extension to pain
	M1		No response	

Figure 49.2 Head injury (NICE, 2014)

Worrying symptoms

- GCS ≤14 at triage
- Witnessed loss of consciousness >5 min
- Irritability/behavioural changes
- Abnormal drowsiness
- Any focal neurological deficit (visual, speaking, walking difficulties)
- Visible head injury (bruising, wounds >5 cm, open/depressed skull fracture/tense fontanelle in infants)
- Amnesia >5 min (of events pre- and/or post-head injury)
- Headache
- More than 3 vomiting episodes since injury
- History of seizure (no known epilepsy)
- Dangerous mechanism of injury (high-impact road traffic collision, fall from height greater than 1 metre)
- Bleeding or clotting disorders
- ?Non-accidental injury

Figure 49.3 'Pulled' elbow

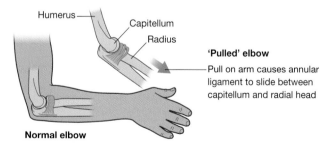

'Pulled' elbow
Pull on arm causes annular ligament to slide between capitellum and radial head

Figure 49.4 Salter Harris Type 2 growth plate fracture

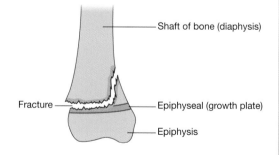

Figure 49.5 Torus 'buckle' fracture

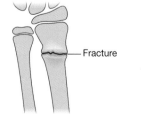

Figure 49.6 Greenstick fracture

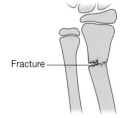

Figure 49.7 Displaced supracondylar fracture

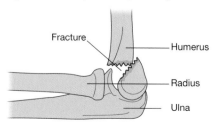

Emergency Nursing at a Glance, First Edition. Natalie Holbery and Paul Newcombe.
© 2016 John Wiley & Sons, Ltd. Published 2016 by John Wiley & Sons, Ltd. Companion website: www.ataglanceseries.com/nursing/emergencynursing

Injury prevalence

Injuries account for over half of all child attendances at an emergency department (ED). Head injury and limb injuries are the most common presentations, followed by lacerations, burns or scalds, foreign body-related issues, eye problems, bites and stings, and accidental ingestions. Infants and young children sustain more harm through non-accidental injuries (NAIs) (Chapter 45) and falls while older children incur injuries from road traffic collisions (RTCs) and sports-related accidents.

Head injury

Younger children are the most at risk of head injuries because of their large and heavy head (in relation to their body size), causing them to lose balance more readily. Most children sustain mild swelling and bruising to the forehead and recover without any problem. However, those who present with a Glasgow Coma Scale (GCS)score of 12 or below are at risk of serious complications.

Management

Ideally, head injuries should be triaged within 15 minutes of arrival at an ED in order to determine injury severity and the requirement for a computed tomography (CT) head scan. ABCDE (Chapter 48) should be assessed, followed by the use of a head injury proforma in addition to an age-appropriate GCS chart to guide treatment (Figure 49.1). If worrying symptoms are highlighted (Figure 49.2), the child should be reviewed immediately by a clinician and considered for a CT scan within the hour. Analgesia should be administered orally or intravenously to reduce the risk of raising intracranial pressure. In children with a GCS of 15, observations should be recorded every 30 minutes for 2 hours, then every hour for 4 hours. If discharged home, the advice given should include a clear diagnosis, indications of when the child should return for re-assessment and a recovery prognosis.

Pulled elbow

A pulled elbow or radial head subluxation is a common soft tissue injury affecting children under 6 years (in particular 1–2 year olds). It is caused by a sudden pull on a child's extended arm during activities such as lifting. The resultant tear or stretching of the annular ligament causes the radial head to slip out and the ligament to move between the radius and capitellum (Figure 49.3). Post-incident, the child will generally hold their arm in a semi-flexed position by their side.

Management

If a classic pulling history is described in a young child and there is no suspicion of a fracture (no direct trauma, swelling or deformity), treatment is by manual reduction. During triage, an experienced professional will either supinate (turn palm upwards) or hyperpronate (turn palm downwards) the forearm with elbow flexion. A 'clunk' is then felt, which signifies that the ligament and radial head have returned to their correct positions. Although the child may cry initially, within 30 minutes of the reduction full arm movement is usually observed. To prevent reoccurrence of a pulled elbow, discharge advice to the carers should emphasise not to pull on the child's arms in activities until the child is over 6 years.

Fractures

Children's bones differ from adult bones in three main ways:

1 Faster healing (younger children heal the quickest).
2 Bones are softer and tend to buckle rather than break.
3 Epiphyseal plates (growth plates) are located at the ends of long bones to enable bone growth until adulthood. Any disruption to the growth plate can result in limb length discrepancies.

With all fractures, the first-line treatment at triage is the assessment of pain (using an age-appropriate pain scale) and administration of analgesia (e.g. paracetamol, oral morphine or intranasal diamorphine – dependent on individual hospital trust policies).

Epiphyseal fractures

Growth plate fractures (Salter Harris fractures) commonly occur in the wrist, elbow or ankle. They are classified into five different types with type 2 being the most common injury (see Figure 49.4). Management of these fractures range from application of a backslab (a cast made of half plaster of Paris that allows for swelling) to requiring an orthopaedic opinion.

Distal radius and ulna fractures

The wrist is the most prevalent area for children to injure and accounts for almost half of all childhood fractures. Compression forces cause a torus (buckle) fracture (Figure 49.5) however a greenstick fracture (Figure 49.6) – where the bone cortex breaks on one side while the other side creases – is caused by a force to the side of the bone. Non-displaced fractures are generally treated with a below-elbow backslab and elevation in a sling. Displaced fractures may require manipulation under general anaesthetic.

Supracondylar fractures (SCFs)

These are the most common elbow fractures in children, predominantly occurring in the 5–7 year age group and in boys. Caused by a FOOSH (fall onto an outstretched hand), SCFs occur at the distal end of the humerus and are often displaced (Figure 49.7) requiring orthopaedic referral. Treatment can vary from immobilisation in a collar and cuff or above-elbow backslab cast (non-displaced) to reduction and internal fixation in theatre (if displaced). In all SCFs, neurovascular observations are paramount because of the high risk of circulatory impairment from damage to the brachial artery (which crosses the distal humerus).

Lacerations and gluing

In children, traumatic lacerations to the forehead, chin and scalp are common presentations to an ED. Most of these wounds are linear, superficial and <5cm in length. Tissue glue is the primary closure method; it is dripped onto opposed wound edges after cleaning with sterile saline or tap water.

Discharge advice should include keeping the laceration clean and dry for 5 days, and allowing the glue to flake off naturally once the laceration has healed.

50 Lower limb injuries

Figure 50.1 Buddy strapping

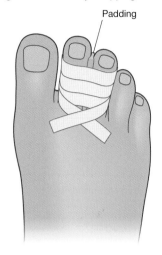

Padding

Figure 50.2 Ankle fracture dislocation

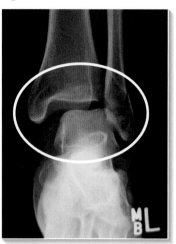

Source: By James Heilman, MD (own work) [GFDL by CC BY-SA 3.0] via Wikimedia Commons

Figure 50.3 Base of fifth metatarsal fracture

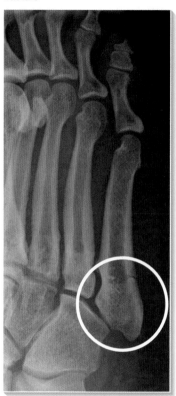

Source: Boundless. 'Fractures of the Metatarsals'. *Boundless Anatomy and Physiology*. Boundless, 02 Jul. 2014. Retrieved 22 Apr. 2015 from https://www.boundless.com/physiology/textbooks/boundless-anatomy-and-physiology-textbook/the-skeletal-system-7/appendicular-skeleton-diseases-disorders-injury-and-clinical-cases-90/fractures-of-the-metatarsals-506-994/

Figure 50.4 Ottawa ankle rules

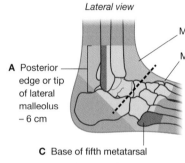

Lateral view *Medial view*

Malleolar zone

Mid-foot zone

A Posterior edge or tip of lateral malleolus – 6 cm

B Posterior edge or tip of medial malleolus – 6 cm

C Base of fifth metatarsal

D Navicular

A series of ankle X-ray films is required only if there is pain in the malleolar zone and any of these findings:
• Bone tenderness at **A**
• Bone tenderness at **B**
• Inability to bear weight both immediately and in ED

A series of ankle X-ray films is required only if there is pain in the mid-foot zone and any of these findings:
• Bone tenderness at **C**
• Bone tenderness at **D**
• Inability to bear weight both immediately and in ED

Source: Bachmann LM et al. BMJ 2003;326:417 (22 February). Reproduced with permission of *BMJ* Publishing Group Ltd

Figure 50.6 Undisplaced patella fracture

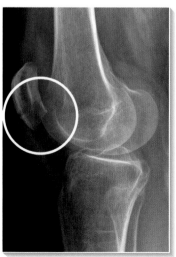

Source: By Hellerhoff (own work) [GFDL by CC BY-SA 3.0] via Wikimedia Commons

Figure 50.5 Knee anatomy

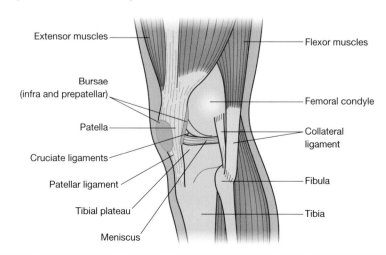

Extensor muscles

Flexor muscles

Bursae (infra and prepatellar)

Femoral condyle

Patella

Collateral ligament

Cruciate ligaments

Patellar ligament

Fibula

Tibial plateau

Tibia

Meniscus

Emergency Nursing at a Glance, First Edition. Natalie Holbery and Paul Newcombe
© 2016 John Wiley & Sons, Ltd. Published 2016 by John Wiley & Sons, Ltd. Companion website: www.ataglanceseries.com/nursing/emergencynursing

Lower limb injuries are a common presentation to an emergency department (ED). They can cause considerable pain and be disabling to otherwise independent patients.

It is important to obtain an accurate history from a patient. Understanding the mechanism of injury (MOI) is of vital importance and provides clues to the extent of the injury. Further assessment will determine the need for an X-ray.

Toes

If the toe has no clinical deformity, then an X-ray is not indicated because it does not affect the management of the injury. Treatment consists of analgesia (paracetomol or non-steroidal anti-inflammatories), ice packs, sensible supportive shoes and buddy strapping (Figure 50.1). With any limb injury, the time it takes to recover should not be underestimated. The recovery time for a toe injury may be several weeks.

A dislocated fracture of the toe should be reduced. This involves a local ring block, reduction of the fracture, X-ray to confirm the joint has been relocated and follow-up in the fracture clinic.

Ankle injuries

Dislocated ankles are a true orthopaedic emergency (Figure 50.2). Patients should go straight to the resuscitation area for a senior review.

History taking should include MOI, time of injury, ability to weight bear, first-aid measures, analgesia and its effectiveness, previous ankle injuries, past medical history and any allergies.

When assessing the ankle it is important to expose both ankles, so that the degree of swelling can be compared against the non-injured ankle. The joint below and above the injured ankle should be examined. A commonly associated injury is a base of the fifth metatarsal fracture (Figure 50.3). On examination, the limb should be palpated for tenderness and the range of movement should be assessed. Ottawa ankle rules (Figure 50.4) are used to decide if an X-ray is necessary.

If there is a bony injury, it is classified as either an undisplaced or a displaced fracture. If displaced, specialist advice should be sought from the orthopaedic team. An undisplaced fracture needs to be immobilised with a backslab. The patient will need crutches, advice about analgesia and referral to the fracture clinic.

If there is no bony injury, it is likely that there has been a sprain to the ligaments surrounding and supporting the movement of the ankle. In the acute stage, it is often difficult to make an accurate diagnosis as to the severity of the sprain. The history and assessment of the clinical signs can provide an idea of the severity of the sprain. Grade 1 is the lowest grade sprain, involving micro tears of the ligament. Signs and symptoms include mild pain and local swelling. Treatment consists of RICE (rest, ice, compression and elevation), early mobilisation and advice about ankle exercises.

A grade 2 sprain involves partial tearing of the ligaments with no joint instability. Pain is moderate and swelling is diffuse. The range of motion is reduced due to swelling. Treatment is similar to a grade 1 sprain and includes early mobilisation, RICE, analgesia and possibly crutches for short-term use only.

Grade 3 sprains involve a complete rupture of one or more ligaments. The patient is unable to weight bear, has marked bruising, severe pain and the joint may be unstable. Treatment consists of non-weight bearing movement with follow-up review in the fracture clinic or another relevant outpatient setting. Physiotherapy should also be considered.

Knee injuries

The knee is a load-bearing hinge joint. Structures within the knee that can sustain damage are outlined in Figure 50.5.

The MOI gives a strong indication of the likely structural damage. When assessing patients with knee injuries, the look, feel, move approach should be used. A knee examination should be undertaken on a trolley, exposing both knees. X-rays are indicated if the patient is >55 years old, tender at the head of the fibula, tender over the patella, cannot flex to 90 degrees or cannot walk four steps after injury.

Common knee injuries consist of a collateral ligament sprain. The medial ligament is more easily sprained than the lateral and can be caused by a blow to the lateral aspect of the knee that stretches and tears the medial ligament. Knee sprains are classified as grade 1, 2 and 3. Grades 1 and 2 are treated with RICE, regular anti-inflammatories and crutches for 48 hours before gradual mobilisation. A grade 3 sprain is classified as an unstable joint. Often there is also an intra-articular fracture. Treatment consists of analgesia and referral to the orthopaedic team.

Anterior cruciate ligament rupture is most commonly seen as a result of sporting injuries. The posterior cruciate can be ruptured by direct impact when the knee is flexed or by hyperextension. If there is no haemarthrosis (bleeding in the joint), the patient should be provided with crutches and booked in for follow-up.

Patients may also present with a 'locked knee', a condition that prohibits full extension of the knee. It is usually due to a torn meniscus being caught between the articular surfaces. Providing analgesia such as entonox and gradually straightening the leg is first-line treatment. If this is not successful, then the orthopaedic team needs to be involved.

A fractured patella is caused by a direct blow or a fall onto the knee. There is usually swelling and an effusion over the knee cap. If the X-ray reveals an undisplaced fracture (Figure 50.6), treatment includes analgesia, an above-knee plaster and crutches with fracture clinic follow-up.

51 Upper limb injuries

Figure 51.1 Shoulder joint

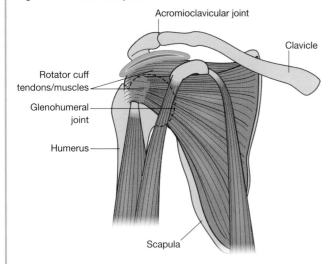

Acromioclavicular joint

Clavicle

Rotator cuff tendons/muscles

Glenohumeral joint

Humerus

Scapula

Figure 51.2 X-ray of dislocated shoulder

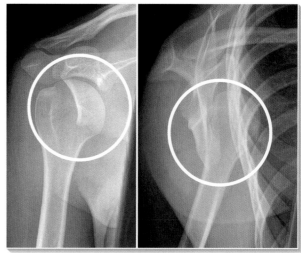

Source: By Hellerhoff (own work) [GFDL by CC BY-SA 3.0] via Wikimedia Commons

Figure 51.3 Fractured clavicle

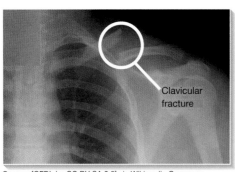

Clavicular fracture

Source: [GFDL by CC BY-SA 3.0] via Wikimedia Commons

Figure 51.4 Broad arm sling in situ

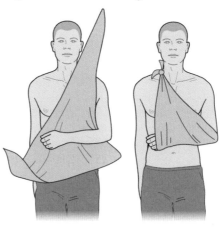

Figure 51.5 Elbow anatomy

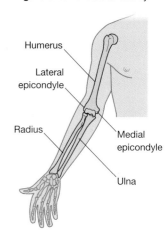

Humerus

Lateral epicondyle

Radius

Medial epicondyle

Ulna

Figure 51.6 Elbow (olecranon) fracture

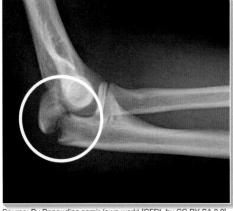

Source: By Benoudina samir (own work) [GFDL by CC BY-SA 3.0] via Wikimedia Commons

Figure 51.7 Wrist and hand anatomy

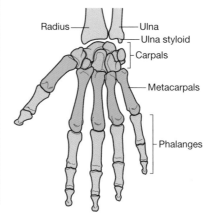

Radius

Ulna

Ulna styloid

Carpals

Metacarpals

Phalanges

Figure 51.8 Distal radius (colles) fracture (with incidental ulna styloid fracture)

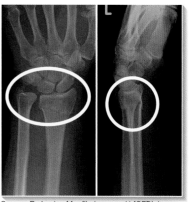

Source: By Lucien Monfils (own work) [GFDL by CC-BY-SA-3.0,2.5,2.0,1.0] via Wikimedia Commons

Emergency Nursing at a Glance, First Edition. Natalie Holbery and Paul Newcombe.
© 2016 John Wiley & Sons, Ltd. Published 2016 by John Wiley & Sons, Ltd. Companion website: www.ataglanceseries.com/nursing/emergencynursing

The neck

The neck supports the head and allows it to move. It is also the communication channel between the head and the rest of the body, with the spinal cord passing through it. Most people will experience neck pain at some point in their lives. Severe and acute neck pain may be due to many factors including acute disc prolapse, muscle spasm, injury to an osteoarthritic facet joint, inflamed lymph nodes or an undiagnosed cervical dislocation. Common causes of neck pain in people presenting to an emergency department (ED) are torticollis (wry neck), whiplash and osteoarthritis. During the assessment, it is important to exclude trauma. If there is a history of trauma and definitive central cervical spine (C-spine) tenderness, a hard collar should be applied and the patient should be reviewed by a senior doctor urgently (Chapter 57). Check for local sepsis including tonsillitis, quinsy or a submandibular abscess. All these illnesses can cause neck pain. Chapter 54 covers ear, nose and throat conditions in more detail.

Neck pain origin can be difficult to diagnose and many patients may suffer from reoccurrence or prolonged pain and disability. For most, the treatment is rest, simple analgesia and avoidance of strenuous exercise including lifting.

The shoulder

The shoulder joint consists of the glenohumeral joint and the acromioclavicular joint, but movement also occurs between the scapula and the posterior chest wall. It is very mobile and allows the arm to move in all directions. The humerus is stabilised and pulled into the glenoid by a group of strong muscles and their associated tendons called the 'rotator cuff', which facilitates the movement of the most mobile joint in the body (Figure 51.1).

Patients can present with traumatic or non-traumatic pain. During the assessment, it is important to check for swelling, muscle wasting, deformity, and the size and position of the scapula. It is always important to assess the injured limb for blood supply and sensation. This can be done by checking for a distal pulse, assessing capillary refill, the temperature of the injured limb and if there is any sensation deficit in comparison to the opposite limb. If there is suspicion of a dislocation or neurovascular compromise, the patient must be seen by a clinician urgently.

Common conditions affecting the shoulder are rotator cuff syndromes, adhesive capsulitis (frozen shoulder), tendonitis and rheumatoid arthritis.

Common conditions as a result of trauma are rotator cuff tear, glenohumeral dislocation (Figure 51.2), acromioclavicular dislocation, fracture of the clavicle (Figure 51.3) and fracture of the head or neck of the humerus. Clavicle fractures are one of the most common long bone fractures seen in an ED. Unless there is obvious protruding of the bone, clavicle injuries are managed in a broad arm sling. Patients should then have a follow-up appointment arranged for the fracture clinic. All other shoulder injuries are usually rested in a sling (Figure 51.4).

The elbow

The elbow is a synovial hinge joint between the humerus in the upper arm and the radius and ulna in the forearm. The elbow allows hand movement away from and towards the body. There are three bones at the elbow: the distal humerus, the head of the radius and the proximal end of the ulna (olecranon). The medial and lateral epicondyles are the flexor and extensor origins for the forearm muscles (Figure 51.5).

The mechanism of injury provides clues as to the type of injury and can assist in diagnosing a fracture. During examination, assess the overall alignment of the elbow. Inspect for swelling, infection or deformities. The lack of function in an acute elbow joint injury is normally caused by swelling in the joint, which may indicate a fracture.

Most elbow injuries including fractures are managed in a sling. Olecranon fractures require surgical fixation (Figure 51.6). Pulled elbows are typical in children under 5 years of age following traction on the arm (Chapter 49).

The wrist

The wrist joint and hand are complex with a wide range of possible movements. There are also many underlying structures that initially can be difficult to assess. There are many bones and joints to consider (Figure 51.7). Patients presenting to an ED will often complain of localised pain, stiffness, loss of function and trauma.

During the assessment look for colour change. Erythema (redness) suggests acute inflammation caused by soft tissue infection, septic arthritis, tendon sheath infection or crystal-induced disease (gout). Swelling and deformity suggest fracture if there is a history of trauma. Deformity can be an indication of dislocation at a joint or tendon injury.

A patient's age, hand dominance and profession are all considered in the management of hand and wrist injuries. The most common cause for a wrist fracture is due to patients falling onto an outstretched hand to break the fall, which is common in the winter months with the increased risk of slipping, especially in the elderly population. Distal radius (Colles) fracture is common in older patients (Figure 51.8); scaphoid fracture is common in younger patients. All patients with hand and wrist injuries should be offered analgesia at triage and the injured limb should be elevated. Most wrist fractures will be put into a temporary cast and sling. It is important to assess elderly patients' mobility with a cast to establish if it is safe for them to be discharged.

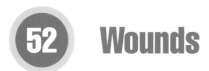

52 Wounds

Figure 52.1 Chronic and acute wounds

Chronic wounds	Acute wounds
• Pressure ulcers	• Abrasions
• Diabetic ulcers	• Lacerations
• Venous ulcers	• Puncture
• Radiation poisoning	• Incisions
• Surgical wounds	• Gunshot
	• Burns and scalds

Figure 52.2 Types of wounds

(a) **Cut**	(b) **Abrasion**	(c) **Laceration**	(d) **Skin flap**	(e) **Bites**
Incision to skin, usually straight edges	Scraping to skin	Tear to skin, usually uneven edges	Separation of skin layers, often due to friction	Caused by human, animal or insect

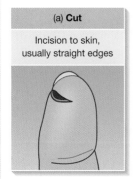
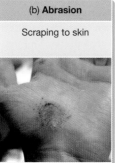
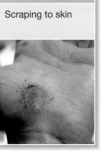
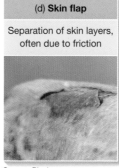
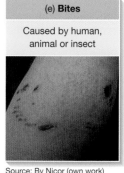

Source: via Wikimedia Commons

Source: By tandemracer [GFDL by CC-BY-2.0] via Wikimedia Commons

Source: Pixaby.com

Source: By Nicor (own work) [GFDL by CC BY-SA 3.0] via Wikimedia Commons

Figure 52.3 Sutured wound

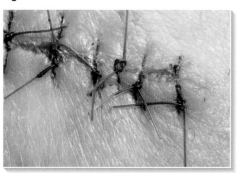

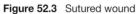

Figure 52.4 Wound closed with glue and steristrips

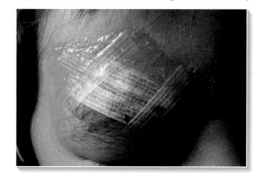

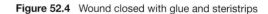

Emergency Nursing at a Glance, First Edition. Natalie Holbery and Paul Newcombe

A wound is any break in the skin. Wounds can be acute or chronic (Figure 52.1) and heal by either primary or secondary intervention. Most patients with wounds that present to an emergency department (ED) are of a traumatic nature and, as a result, patients are often anxious or distressed by the sudden unexpected interruption to their normal activity, especially if this has happened at work. The mechanism of the injury gives important clues as to the type of wound being dealt with. A penetrating wound with a knife or a laceration with a saw will likely require exploring to rule out damage to any underlying structures that might not be obvious on initial examination. Acute wounds from trauma normally have a short and uneventful healing time. Chronic wounds such as leg ulcers, pressure sores and malignant wounds tend to have longer healing times and be prone to infection. Most patients with chronic wounds will be referred to the tissue viability team, some requiring secondary intervention.

Common wounds in an ED

Common wound presentations to an ED are cuts, abrasions, lacerations, skin flaps and bites (Figure 52.2). Elderly patients are at risk of pre-tibial (shin) lacerations and skin tears due to their skin breaking easily. All shin lacerations should be cleaned and soaked as soon as possible to ensure optimum tissue viability. Wounds that often require specialist input are penetrating wounds of the hand or finger involving nerve, tendons, joint space and vascular damage.

Wound assessment

Wound management commences with an assessment and a plan of care with patient-specific aims that include diagnosing wound aetiology and promoting an environment to encourage wound healing and prevent further deterioration of the wound. It is important to document the time and date of injury, mode and mechanism of injury, first aid applied and any relevant illnesses, medications and allergies. Inadequate assessment of the wound can often lead to incorrect and inadequate treatment with potentially serious consequences. The patient's temperature and pulse should be checked and analgesia offered. X-rays should always be requested for injuries that are suggestive of glass, metal or tooth fragments. This is usually done by the clinician who will see, treat and discharge the patient.

The registered nurse assessing the wound is responsible for including the following in the assessment:

Wound appearance
- Overall location, shape, size and position of the wound
- Types of tissue visible in the wound bed (i.e. necrotic; sloughy; granulating; over-granulating; epithelialising; fungating)
- The presence of foreign bodies (e.g. glass)

Exudate
Amount, consistency, colour and odour.

Surrounding skin
Evidence of inflammation, maceration, oedema or excoriation.

Pain
Assess pain before and after dressing wounds.

Infection prevention and control

Every effort must be made to prevent contamination of wounds by micro-organisms that may cause infection and delay healing. All dressing techniques should employ a no-touch technique. Although the terms 'no-touch' and 'aseptic' are often used interchangeably, the aseptic technique requires a higher level of precaution. Both techniques aim to ensure that fingers or hands do not contaminate the patient or the equipment used. The purpose of cleansing is to remove debris and reduce the potential for infection.

Warmed saline 0.9% is recommended as the solution of choice to clean wounds. Debris and non-viable tissue should be removed (debridement) as soon as possible. Patients may have to be seen by a specialist for this, depending on the size and depth of the wound.

For heavily contaminated wounds or wounds from a dirty source, tetanus immunisation status should be noted. Patients who present to an ED with wounds more than 8 hours old should have them cleaned and irrigated immediately and an iodine dressing applied until they are seen by a clinician, because they are more prone to developing an infection.

Dressings
Every wound is different and there is no product that can be ideal for every wound type. Dressing selection should be based on the wound assessment and referral to local wound management policies.

Burns
Burns and scalds are damage to the skin caused by heat. Burns can be very painful, especially on the hands, and can cause blistering. It is important that all patients are offered adequate analgesia and their burn cooled immediately in cool water. It should then be dressed with a non-adherent dressing or wrapped in cling film until the patient is seen by a clinician. Burns are covered in more detail in Chapter 62.

Bites
All human or animal bites should be seen as a priority because they are at increased risk of infection. The wounds should be cleaned with one litre of normal saline with 5 mls of added iodine to minimise the risk of infection.

Lacerations
Most lacerated wounds are closed by either suturing (Figure 52.3), applying adhesive skin closure strips (sterstrips) (Figure 52.4) or using a tissue adhesive (glue). Aftercare is normally application of a non-adherent dressing, educating the patient regarding wound management at home and informing them when to see their GP or return for removal of sutures (as required).

Patient advice

All patients should be given written advice on caring for their wound at home before being discharged and follow-up should be organised if appropriate.

53 Eye conditions

Figure 53.1 Eye anatomy

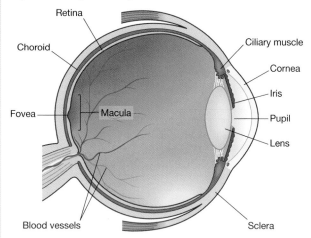

Retina
Choroid
Ciliary muscle
Cornea
Iris
Fovea
Macula
Pupil
Lens
Blood vessels
Sclera

Figure 53.2 Snellen Chart for testing visual acuity

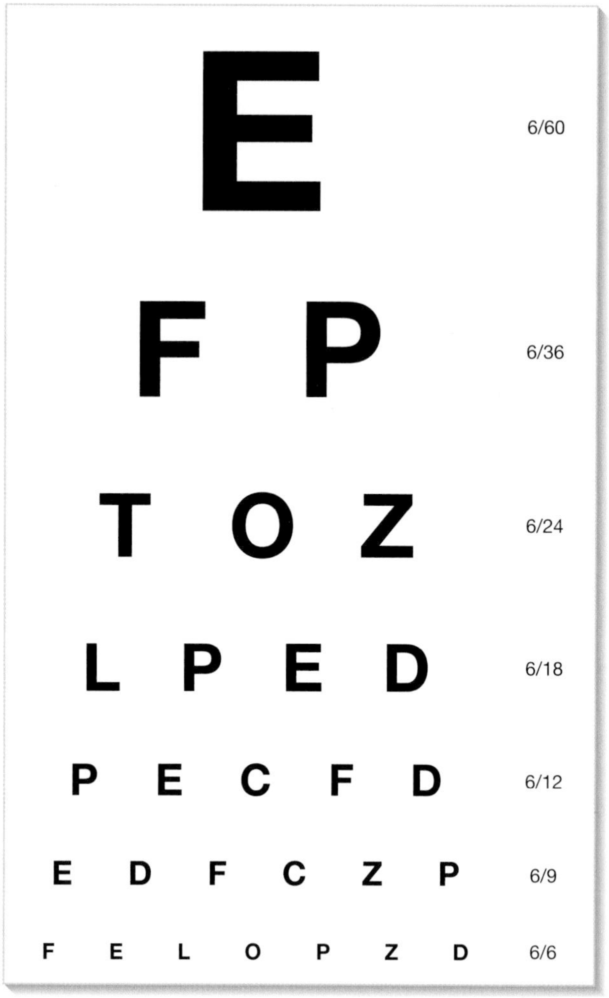

E 6/60
F P 6/36
T O Z 6/24
L P E D 6/18
P E C F D 6/12
E D F C Z P 6/9
F E L O P Z D 6/6

Source: By James Heilman, MD (own work) [GFDL by CC BY-SA 3.0] via Wikimedia Commons

Figure 53.3 Fluorescein staining

Colour	Injury/condition
No stain	No injury
Yellow/orange	Conjunctival abrasions or ulcers
Green ring	Foreign body
Bright green	Corneal abrasions

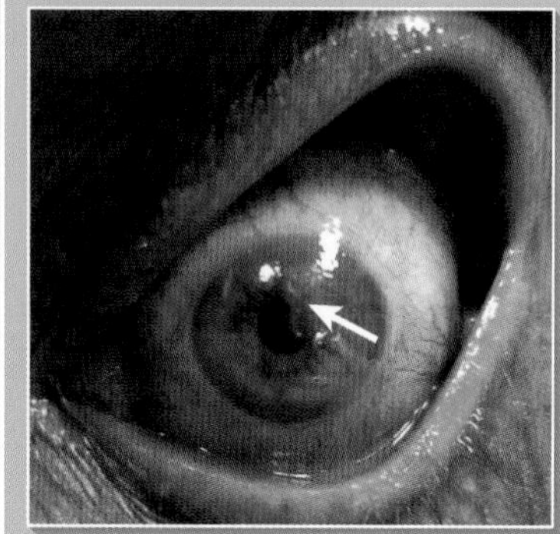

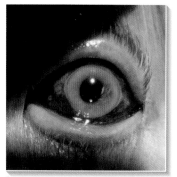

Figure 53.4 Discharge typical with bacterial conjunctivitis

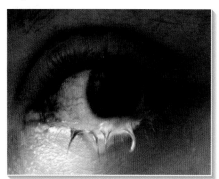

Source: By Tanalai at en.wikipedia [GFDL by CC BY-SA 3.0] via Wikimedia Commons

Figure 53.5 Subconjunctival haemorrhage

Source: By James Heilman, MD (own work) [GFDL by CC BY-SA 3.0] via Wikimedia Commons

Figure 53.6 Chemical (alkali) eye injury

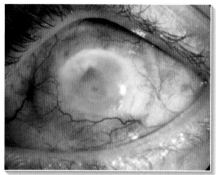

Source: © 2009 Genevieve A. Secker and Julie T. Daniels [CC BY-SA 3.0] via Wikimedia Commons

Emergency Nursing at a Glance, First Edition. Natalie Holbery and Paul Newcombe.
© 2016 John Wiley & Sons, Ltd. Published 2016 by John Wiley & Sons, Ltd. Companion website: www.ataglanceseries.com/nursing/emergencynursing

There is a spectrum of eye problems that range from mild, non-sight threatening to serious, sight threatening injuries and conditions. Most eye problems are minor, affecting the pre-orbital structures or the ocular surface. Only 2% of eye injuries require admission. Anatomy of the eye is displayed in Figure 53.1.

With all eye problems an accurate history should be obtained. This should include the mechanism of injury (MOI), time of onset or occurrence, presence of lacrimation, photophobia, discharge, itchiness, pain or grittiness. Past medical history, current medications and any allergies should also be determined.

When examining a patient with an eye injury, gloves should be worn and a systematic approach adopted. If the patient is wearing contact lenses, these should be removed before examination. Visual acuity (Figure 53.2) should be checked before any examination, apart from a chemical injury; this can be done once the eye is made comfortable. Fluorescein is applied to the cornea before the eye is illuminated with a blue light. Figure 53.3 outlines the possible findings.

Any of the symptoms listed here should be discussed with an ophthalmologist – any sudden loss of vision, flashes of light, halos, double vision, transient loss of vision, marked difference of vision between two eyes, severe pain, redness, discharge or watering, veil or curtain blocking vision and any swelling or mass in or around the eye.

The acute painful red eye

Foreign bodies or corneal abrasion

Anaesthetic drops should be instilled into the eye before the removal of the foreign body. Any visible foreign body can be removed with a moist cotton bud. If this is not successful and the foreign body appears superficial, a sterile green needle can be used.

The eyelid should be everted and cleaned with a moist cotton bud. If necessary, the eye can be washed out with a litre bag of 0.9% normal saline, particularly if there are multiple foreign bodies. Once these have been, removed the eye should be stained with fluorescein to reveal any corneal abrasions. The patient should be discharged with chloramphenicol ointment four times a day for 4 days for the affected eye. They should be given advice about eye care over the next few days. If necessary, an eye pad can be applied.

Arc eyes

This very painful condition classically affects welders who do not wear eye protection. It is caused by exposure of insufficiently protected eyes to ultraviolet rays. It can be compared to sunburn of the cornea and conjunctiva. Anaesthetic eye drops can be used if the patient has severe pain. Chloramphenicol should be applied to both eyes. A double eye pad can be applied for comfort. The patient should be given analgesia, shown how to apply eye ointment and advised to wear sunglasses. Follow-up should occur in 48 hours.

Acute uveitis

Patients typically present with photophobia, blurred vision, headache and pain when moving the eyes. On examination, the patient may have reduced visual acuity, redness around the corneal edge and the pupils may be constricted or irregular. In severe cases, white clumps can be viewed on the corneal surface. Treatment is usually with medication. Eye drops are the first-line treatment if the uveitis is not caused by infection. Steroids are also commonly prescribed.

The acute non-painful red eye

Conjunctivitis (bacterial/viral/allergic)

Bacterial conjunctivitis is one of the most common causes of a red eye. Patients present with a history of discomfort in one eye that often spreads to the other. After sleep, the eye may be difficult to open due to discharge and clumped lashes. Visual acuity is normal although engorgement of the conjunctival blood vessels and mucopurulent discharge are discerning features (Figure 53.4). Chloramphenicol ointment is the treatment of choice. The patient should be given advice about eye hygiene (not sharing face towels) and be shown how to apply the ointment.

Viral conjunctivitis is commonly associated with upper respiratory tract infections. The patient complains of gritty, uncomfortable eyes and there may be photophobia and a watery discharge. On examination, both eyes are red with diffused conjunctival injection and clear discharge. There may also be small white lumps (follicles) on the conjunctiva. This condition is generally self-limiting although it is extremely contagious. Strict hygiene measures are important for the patient and clinicians. Treatment consists of symptomatic relief and chloramphenicol ointment.

The main feature with allergic conjunctivitis is itching. Both eyes are usually affected and symptoms may have occurred at the same time in previous years. Examination reveals a diffusely injected conjunctivae, possible oedema, clear, stringy discharge and round swellings on the upper eyelid conjunctivae. Treatment involves an eyewash, oral chlorphenamine and advice to the patient to purchase Otrivine Antistin eye drops from a pharmacist.

Subconjunctival haemorrhage

This may be spontaneous or traumatic and patients are usually asymptotic. There is blood under the conjunctiva covering all or part of the eye (Figure 53.5) and visual acuity is normal. In elderly people, blood pressure should be checked because this can be associated with hypertension. The condition is self-limiting and usually takes about a fortnight to resolve.

Other eye complaints

Chemical injuries

Chemical eye injuries require a prompt and effective response. Chemical injuries require immediate repeated irrigation because damage can intensify as long as the chemical is present (Figure 53.6). If there is doubt about the chemical the local poisons unit should be contacted to clarify. Anaesthetic drops can be applied if the patient complains of pain. Such drops also assist with irrigation. The eye should be irrigated with water or normal saline 0.9%. If an alkaline burn, irrigation should continue for 30 minutes. Five minutes post-irrigation, the pH of the eye should be checked. If the pH has not returned to normal (7.4–7.8), irrigation should be repeated until the pH returns to normal. Visual acuity should be checked post-irrigation, a fluorescein stain performed and any abrasion noted.

54 Ear, nose and throat conditions

Figure 54.1 Ear anatomy

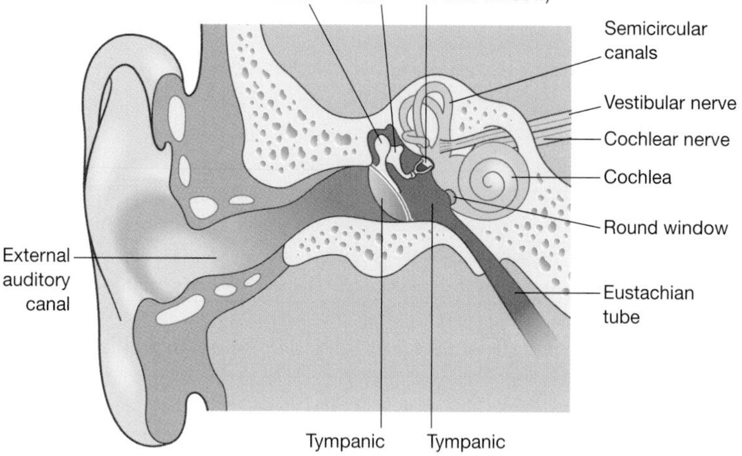

Malleus Incus Stapes (attached to oval window)

Semicircular canals

Vestibular nerve

Cochlear nerve

Cochlea

Round window

External auditory canal

Eustachian tube

Tympanic membrane Tympanic cavity

Figure 54.2 Tympanic membrane

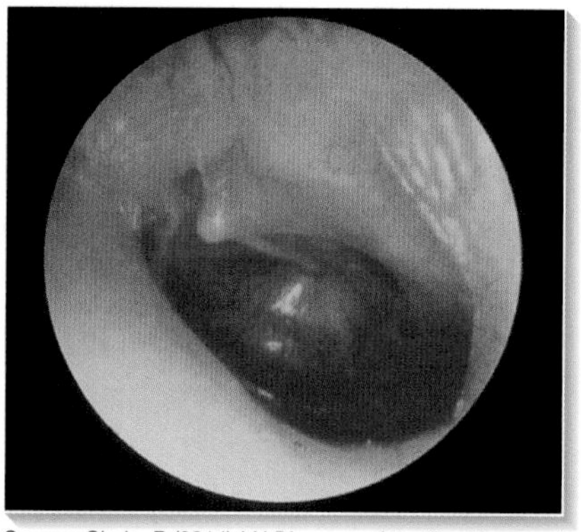

Source: Clarke R (2014) *LN Diseases of the Ear, Nose and Throat*, 11th edn. Reproduced with permission of Wiley

Figure 54.3 Nasal cavity

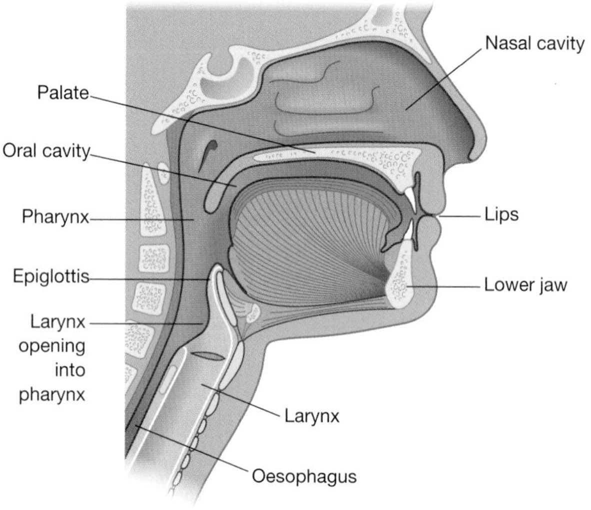

Nasal cavity

Palate

Oral cavity

Pharynx

Epiglottis

Larynx opening into pharynx

Lips

Lower jaw

Larynx

Oesophagus

Figure 54.4 Angle of nasal tampon insertion and 'common mistakes'

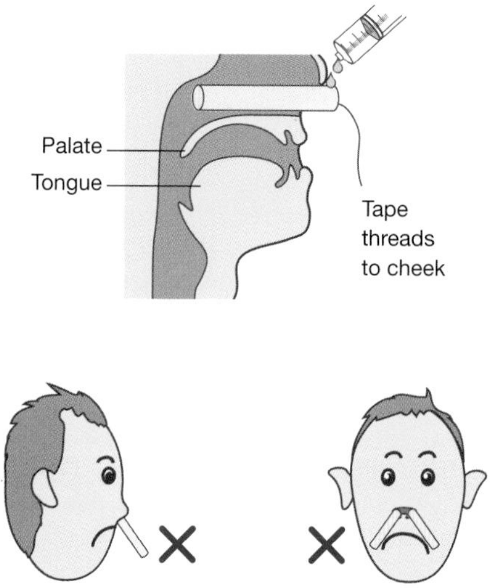

Palate

Tongue

Tape threads to cheek

Pushing tampon vertically

'Walrus sign' tampon should not protrude from nose

Source: Hughes T & Cruickshank J (2011) *Emergency Medicine at a Glance*. Reproduced with permission of Thomas Hughes and Jaycen Cruickshank

Figure 54.5 Quinsy

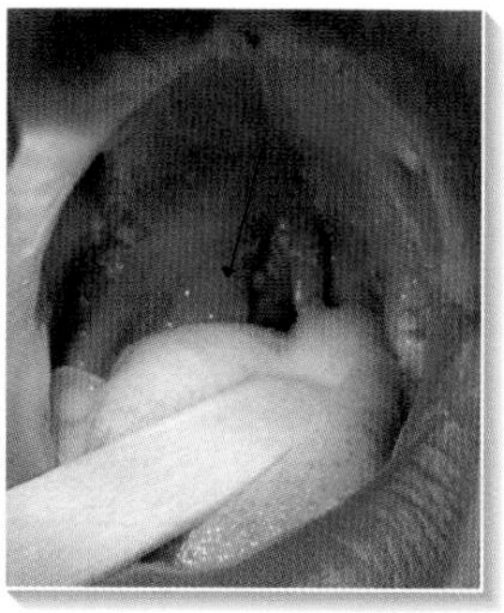

Source: By James Heilman, MD (own work) [GFDL by CC BY-SA 3.0] via Wikimedia Commons

Ear conditions

Ear problems, while not life threatening, can cause much pain and distress for patients. Figure 54.1 demonstrates the anatomy of the ear.

History and examination

Ensuring an adequate history will provide clues as to the type of condition. Assessment involves examining the ear for redness,

Emergency Nursing at a Glance, First Edition. Natalie Holbery and Paul Newcombe
© 2016 John Wiley & Sons, Ltd. Published 2016 by John Wiley & Sons, Ltd. Companion website: www.ataglanceseries.com/nursing/emergencynursing

exudate and swelling. The same assessments should be made of the inner ear using an otoscope, although this is usually performed by a doctor or nurse practitioner. As many ear conditions are painful, nurses should assess the severity of pain and provide analgesia as prescribed. The most common ear conditions that present to an emergency department (ED) are as follows.

Otitis externa

This condition is a generalised infection of the auditory canal. Symptoms include pain, itchiness in the ear canal and some degree of hearing loss. On examination, a whitish, offensive-smelling discharge may be present. It is more common in adults than children. Treatment usually consists of antibiotic- or steroid-based eardrops. Nurses should provide education and advice to patients about the method and frequency of eardrop administration.

Acute otitis media

Acute otitis media is an infection of the middle ear (Figure 54.2). It often occurs in children and is commonly associated with respiratory infection. Signs and symptoms in young children include fever, pulling, tugging or rubbing the ear, irritability, poor feeding or diminished hearing. An older child or adult will complain of ear pain, possible discharge (pus or blood) and diminished hearing. Treatment consists of oral analgesia and oral antibiotics.

Ruptured tympanic membrane (eardrum)

The tympanic membrane can be perforated following direct trauma (inserting an object into the ear canal), indirect trauma (slap or explosion) or infection. Infection such as otitis media can also cause perforation. The patient will usually present with a sudden pain in the ear. They may also report bleeding from the ear and hearing loss. Treatment consists of analgesia, antibiotics (if an infective cause) and follow-up with the ear, nose and throat (ENT) team. Nurses should advise the patient to keep the ear clean and dry.

Foreign body in ear

Children are the main group of patients who present with foreign bodies in the ear. In adults, the most common presentation is a cotton bud stuck in the ear canal. Removal is dictated by the type of object but usually involves a pair of fine forceps. Referral to ENT should occur if the object cannot be removed or has sharp edges.

Nose problems

The nose filters the air breathed and removes dust, germs and irritants. The nose also contains the nerve cells that are responsible for smell. Figure 54.3 highlights the nasal cavity. The most common nasal condition in an ED is epistaxis.

Epistaxis

Epistaxis, also known as nose bleed, can be very distressing for patients and their relatives. It can rapidly become life threatening if major bleeding is not halted. It commonly occurs in adults with hypertension, patients on anticoagulants, alcohol-dependent patients and patients who have sustained recent nasal trauma. Nurses should establish the location and severity of bleeding and assess for signs of shock. Further assessments include vital signs and estimated blood loss.

Priorities of care are stopping the bleeding and replacing lost fluid, usually with blood products. If the patient is shocked they should be moved to the resuscitation area. Stopping the bleeding involves applying pressure to the bleeding point. The patient should be sat upright and asked to apply pressure to the anterior aspect of their nose. If they cannot perform this independently, the nurse will need to assist. They should be encouraged to spit blood out of their mouth to reduce the likelihood of vomiting. Ice packs can be applied to the nose to encourage vasoconstriction. Nurses should provide reassurance for what can be a frightening condition.

Ongoing management involves packing the nose and cauterising the bleeding point. Cauterising is performed by a doctor or nurse practitioner but all ED nurses should be familiar with applying a nasal bolster and inserting a nasal tampon (Figure 54.4).

If the bleeding is resolved in the ED and the patient is fit for discharge, then nurses should advise the patient to avoid the following: blowing their nose, strenuous activity for 4–6 weeks and medication containing aspirin. Patients who require nasal packing should be referred to the ENT team.

Nasal injury

Nasal injury is often caused by blunt trauma. Assessment should include the mechanism of injury, presence of epistaxis, previous injury to the nose, deformity and previous nasal surgery. The nasal passages should be inspected for septal haematoma or deviation of the septum. Referral to ENT should occur if there is a septal haematoma, septal deviation or marked deformity.

Foreign body in nose

This is most commonly seen in children. The child may not tell their parents and the first sign may be when the child has a purulent nasal discharge. Assessment involves trying to establish the type and size of the object, how long it has been in the nostril and if there has been any bleeding or discharge. Removing the foreign body in a child requires distraction. A play specialist may be involved; however, children are often most content sitting on a parent's lap. A doctor or nurse practitioner will attempt to remove the foreign body. Referral to ENT should be made if the foreign body cannot be removed.

Throat problems

Most patients presenting with a throat problem will complain of a sore throat. Most sore throats are not considered urgent or emergent and can be seen in minors or referred to a primary care provider in line with local systems. Outlined here are the most concerning throat problems encountered in an ED.

Quinsy (peritonsillar abscess)

Quinsy is a potentially serious complication of tonsillitis. It is characterised by a collection of pus in the peritonsillar region and usually only forms on one side of the throat (Figure 54.5). It can occur in any age but commonly affects young adults. Signs and symptoms include unilateral sore throat, fever, difficulty in swallowing and drooling. Patients may also find it difficult to open their mouth (trismus). Quinsy can be life threatening if not treated because the airway may become compromised. Patients will require admission to hospital, drainage of the abscess, antibiotics, analgesia, fluids and antipyretics as needed.

Epiglottitis

Epiglottitis is an inflammation of the epiglottis (Figure 54.2) usually caused by a bacterial infection. It is relatively rare and affects children more than adults. As the airway can rapidly become obstructed, it is considered a medical emergency. Signs and symptoms include stridor, fever, drooling and a stiff neck. Patients who present with epiglottis should be cared for in the resuscitation area and nurses should call for immediate help. An anaesthetist should also be alerted. Antibiotics will be required to treat the infection and patients will often require intravenous fluids.

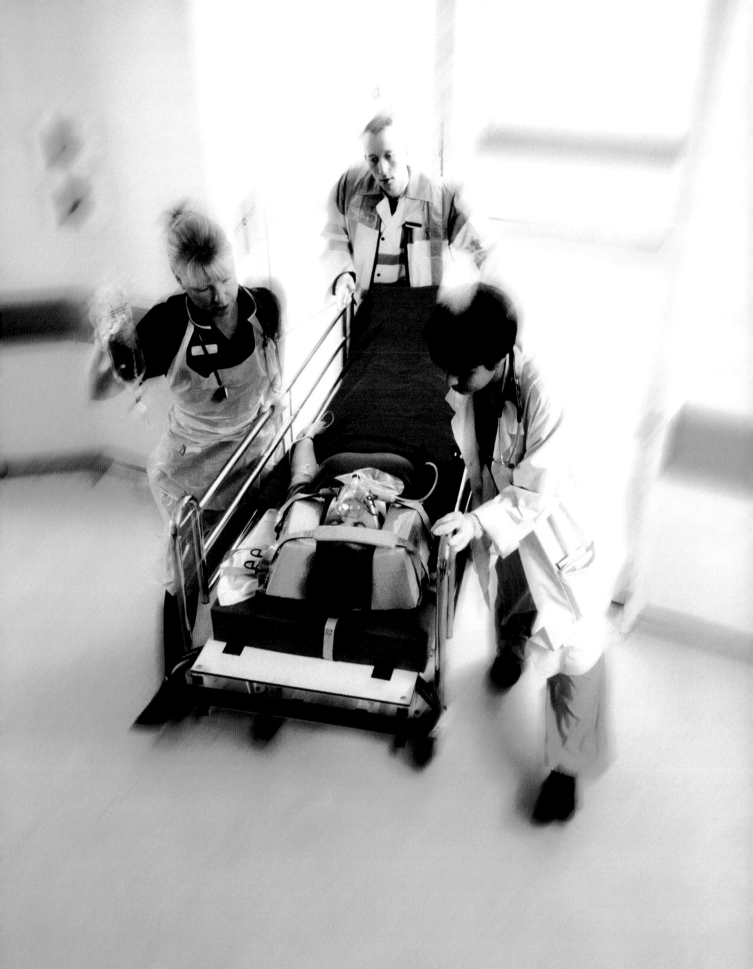

Major Trauma

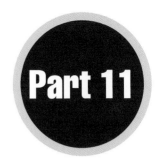

Part 11

Chapters

55 Trauma in context

Figure 55.1 Types of trauma assessment

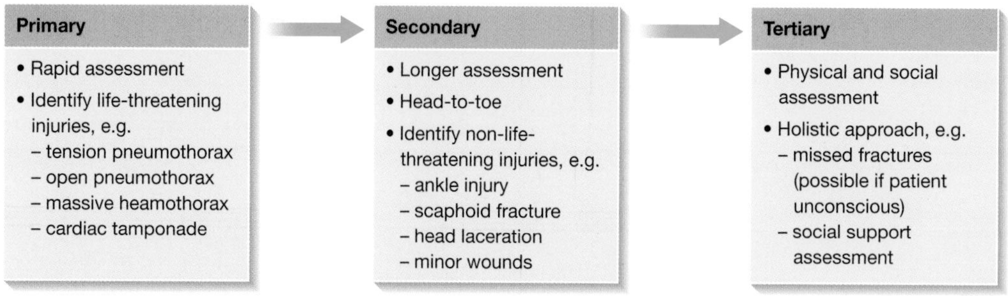

Primary	Secondary	Tertiary

• Rapid assessment
• Identify life-threatening injuries, e.g.
  – tension pneumothorax
  – open pneumothorax
  – massive heamothorax
  – cardiac tamponade
	• Longer assessment
	• Head-to-toe
	• Identify non-life-threatening injuries, e.g.
	  – ankle injury
	  – scaphoid fracture
	  – head laceration
	  – minor wounds
		• Physical and social assessment
		• Holistic approach, e.g.
		  – missed fractures (possible if patient unconscious)
		  – social support assessment

Figure 55.2 The trauma team

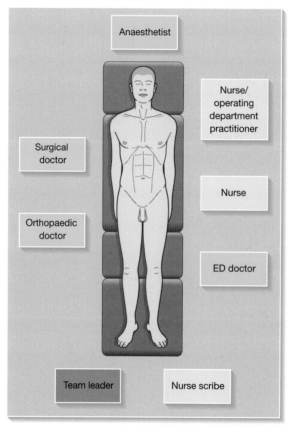

Figure 55.3 Example of trauma call criteria

Mechanism of injury	Injuries	Physiological parameters
• Ejection or entrapment >20 mins • Death of vehicle occupant • Bullseye windscreen • Damage to 'A' post of vehicle • Motorcyclist separated from bike • Vehicle rollover • Fall >3 m (or x2 height)	• Chest injury • Pelvic injury • Penetrating injury to chest, abdomen, groin, neck, back • Suspected skull fracture • Traumatic amputation of limb • Spinal trauma • Facial and circumferential burns	• Glasgow Coma Scale <14 • Respiratory rate <10 or >29 • Systolic Blood pressure (BP) <90 • Pulse >systolic BP

Emergency Nursing at a Glance, First Edition. Natalie Holbery and Paul Newcombe
© 2016 John Wiley & Sons, Ltd. Published 2016 by John Wiley & Sons, Ltd. Companion website: www.ataglanceseries.com/nursing/emergencynursing

Trauma is the leading cause of death in people aged under 40 years. In adults it is the fourth leading cause of death behind cancer, heart disease and stroke. Worldwide there are estimated to be 5.8 million deaths per year as a result of trauma. It is generally considered to be a disease affecting young men, with three-quarters of trauma patients being male. Road traffic collisions (RTCs) are the most common mechanism of injury in the UK.

'Polytrauma' is the term used to describe trauma that affects more than one system. Polytrauma equates to an injury severity score (ISS) of greater than 15. The ISS is a measure of anatomical injury and is calculated retrospectively on a scale of 0–75. The greater the number, the more severe the injury. The assessment and management of various trauma injuries are covered in Chapters 56–64.

Types of trauma

Three terms are used to describe the types of trauma: blunt, penetrating and burns. Burns are covered in Chapter 62. Blunt trauma relates to any non-penetrating or blunt force trauma resulting in injury. It is the most common type of trauma in the UK. Injuries can be numerous and occult bleeding is the main concern. RTCs, falls and assault are common examples.

Penetrating trauma results from any object penetrating the skin. Penetrating injuries are more commonly seen in wartime and countries where knife and gun crime predominate. Although commonly linked to stabbing and gunshot wounds, penetrating trauma can result from impalement on any object (e.g. a fence post, spear or pole).

Trauma systems

A trauma system is a network of hospitals where one is the main provider and equipped to deal with the most severely injured while the other hospitals provide care for the less severely injured. Trauma systems have been shown to improve outcomes and reduce mortality. The terminology used in the UK is 'major trauma centres' and 'trauma units'.

Pre-hospital trauma

Trauma care provided at the scene of injury is delivered by pre-hospital staff. Paramedics, technicians, doctors and occasionally nurses provide pre-hospital care. Trauma patients may present to hospital in a number of ways (Chapter 2). Pre-hospital staff follow a standard approach for assessment and initial management (Chapter 56). The goal is to transfer the patient to hospital as soon as possible. This requires rapid assessment and minimal intervention at the scene. Once the patient arrives at hospital, the crew hand over the patient using a systematic approach. It is important for all members of the trauma team to listen to the handover to avoid missing key information.

Assessment

There are three types of trauma assessments: primary, secondary and tertiary (Figure 55.1). The primary survey is the first and is a rapid assessment, usually no longer than 5 minutes. The goal is to identify and treat life-threatening injuries. This is performed initially by pre-hospital staff and again on arrival at the emergency department (ED). Pre-hospitally, the primary survey is performed using a vertical approach whereas in an ED a horizontal approach is adopted. A vertical approach involves assessing and managing each aspect of the primary survey before moving on. This approach is ideal for an individual clinician or a two-person team. A horizontal approach, however, is used when a larger team is available, and is characterised by numerous assessments and interventions being carried out simultaneously. The layout of an ED trauma bay is designed to support a horizontal approach.

The secondary survey is a head-to-toe assessment of non-life threatening injuries. This is performed in the ED or sometimes in a definitive care setting. The tertiary survey is performed after resuscitative and/or operative interventions, usually 24 hours after arrival at the ED. It is often carried out in intensive care or on a ward. The goal is to detect any injuries not identified during the primary and secondary surveys.

Mechanism of injury

Mechanism of injury is defined as circumstances in which an injury occurs. It can provide clues as to the location and extent of injury. Factors such as force, energy, velocity and the biological response to injury should be considered. Examples include fall from height, pedestrian hit by car and stabbing to chest. Mechanism of injury is one criterion used to determine the need for a trauma call.

The trauma team

The trauma team consists of a number of specialties including ED nurses (Figure 55.2). Each member of the team has a dedicated role and the team is led by a trauma team leader. In order to prepare for the arrival of the trauma patient, the pre-hospital crew alerts the ED via a priority phone. This allows the team to gather before the patient's arrival so that equipment can be prepared and the team members can introduce themselves. It is not uncommon for members of a trauma team to be unfamiliar to each other. Occasionally the patient self-presents or is transported by friends and there is no opportunity for a pre-alert. In this situation, local trauma call criteria will determine the need for a trauma call (Figure 55.3).

56 Primary survey

Figure 56.1 Trauma assessment

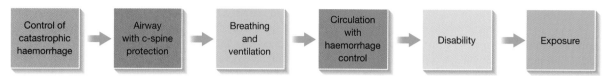

Control of catastrophic haemorrhage → Airway with c-spine protection → Breathing and ventilation → Circulation with haemorrhage control → Disability → Exposure

Figure 56.2 Breathing and ventilation assessment

Look, listen and feel		
R	Respiratory rate	What is the respiratory rate?
I	Inspection	What can you see on the chest? (e.g. wounds, bruising, symmetry)
P	Palpation	What can you feel? (e.g. crepitus, does this elicit pain?)
P	Percussion	What can you hear? (e.g. normal resonance, dull, hyper-resonant)
A	Auscultation	Can you hear breath sounds? They may be present, reduced or absent
S	Saturations	What is the peripheral oxygen saturation?

Figure 56.3 Common bleeding sites in the trauma patient

'On the floor and four more'	
Floor	Is there blood on the floor or at the scene?
Chest	Is there blood in the chest (massive haemothorax)? Clues include shock, dull note on percussion, absent air entry (to affected side)
Abdomen	Is there blood in the abdomen? Clues include shock, bruised, tender or distended abdomen
Pelvis	Is there blood in the pelvis? Clues include bruised, deformed, painful pelvis
Long bones	Is there blood in the long bones (femur, humerus)? Clues include bruised, deformed, swollen, painful limb

Figure 56.4 Warming device in trauma

Emergency Nursing at a Glance, First Edition. Natalie Holbery and Paul Newcombe

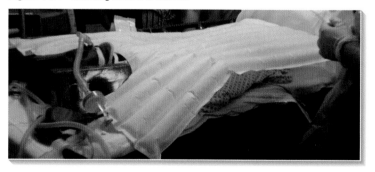

For trauma care to be safe and efficient, it is important to follow a systematic approach. Assessment of the trauma patient requires a common language familiar to healthcare professionals across the globe. Known as the primary survey, the purpose of this assessment is to identify and treat life-threatening injuries. The approach is outlined in Figure 56.1.

Catastrophic haemorrhage

Catastrophic haemorrhage is defined as uncontrolled external bleeding, often from limb amputation. The need to address catastrophic haemorrhage before airway is common in military situations but rare in civilian populations.

Airway with cervical spine control

Airway with cervical spine control is the next step in the assessment of the trauma patient. Assessing airway patency involves seeking a verbal response from the patient. This is best achieved by using their name and asking an open-ended question. If the patient responds verbally the airway is considered patent. It is important to note that airway assessment should be a dynamic process because the airway may become compromised if the patient deteriorates.

If the patient does not respond verbally, it must be assumed that the airway is not patent and therefore at risk. Further assessment involves listening for upper airway sounds such as gurgling and snoring. Gurgling in trauma patients is often due to blood or vomit and requires suctioning. Snoring indicates a partial airway obstruction.

Cervical spine control is usually commenced pre-hospitally based on mechanism of injury. On arrival, the cervical spine precautions remain until imaging confirms no injury.

Breathing and ventilation

Assessment of breathing and ventilation in the trauma patient ensures not only that the patient is breathing but that gaseous exchange is effective. Assessment of breathing and ventilation using the RIPPAS acronym is outlined in Figure 56.2.

Respiratory rate is measured as the number of breaths per minute. Performing this manually is generally more accurate than relying on cardiac monitors. Inspecting the chest involves assessing depth of breathing, symmetry and use of accessory muscles. Assessing for wounds, bruises and other signs of injury should be comprehensive enough to also include the patient's back.

Palpation involves feeling the chest for obvious fractures, crepitus and surgical emphysema. Percussion is used to assess the presence of fluid or excess air in the chest. Percussion is a key indicator in a number of chest injuries (Chapter 58).

Auscultation, or listening for breath sounds, is used in trauma to denote the presence or absence of breath sounds and thus to determine if there are any chest injuries. Ongoing recording of peripheral oxygen saturations is vital in trauma patients to assess for adequacy of breathing. However, peripheral oxygen saturations may be unreliable in the shocked trauma patient.

Circulation with haemorrhage control

The purpose of assessing circulation and haemorrhage is to determine the presence of bleeding and shock. Assessing pulse (rate, volume and regularity), blood pressure, capillary refill and skin (pallor and temperature) is key in this step. The most common bleeding sites are 'on the floor and four more' (Figure 56.3). 'On the floor' relates to external blood loss at the scene or in the resuscitation area. 'Four more' relates to internal bleeding sites: abdomen, chest, pelvis and long bones. Each of these internal bleeding sites can account for massive blood loss and shock. Assessing each of these areas for pain, swelling, bruising, wounds and deformity will provide clues as to the likelihood of such injuries. A focused assessment with sonography in trauma (FAST) scan is often used to detect the presence of free fluid in the abdomen. The FAST scan can also be used to assess for free fluid in the pelvic and cardiac regions. Free fluid in trauma generally equates to blood.

Disability

Disability relates to assessment of neurological function and factors that may cause neurological impairment. The key assessment here is AVPU (Alert, Voice, Pain, Unresponsive) followed by the Glasgow Coma Score (GCS) (Chapter 19). AVPU is designed to be quick and easy while a GCS provides a more comprehensive assessment. A blood glucose reading should also be recorded because alterations in blood glucose may also cause neurological impairment. It is important to note that a slightly elevated blood glucose level is expected as part of a stress response.

Drugs, both prescribed and non-prescribed, can alter a patient's physiologic response to traumatic injury and therefore should be considered during this stage of the primary survey. Although the patient's medication and drug history may not be known initially, it is important to assess the likelihood of such factors playing a part in the patient's response to injury.

Exposure

Exposing the patient allows for assessment of further injuries. This may involve a log-roll to examine the back; however, this should be deferred until after computed tomography (CT). Minimising patient movement will reduce the risk of further bleeding and pain.

When exposing the patient, privacy and dignity should be maintained by only exposing areas requiring assessment and ensuring that curtains are closed. Hypothermia must be avoided to prevent coagulopathy, a deranged clotting state. Regularly assessing temperature and reducing heat loss by keeping the patient covered is recommended. A warming device is required for patients who are hypothermic (Figure 56.4).

57 Head and spinal injury

Figure 57.1 Subarachnoid and skull fracture

Subarachnoid haematoma

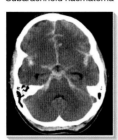

Skull fracture

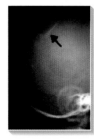

Source: By James Heilman, MD (own work) [GFDL by CC BY-SA 3.0] via Wikimedia Commons

Figure 57.2 High risk for head injury

- GCS less than 15
- Focal neurological deficit
- More than 1 episode of vomiting
- Suspected open or depressed skull fracture
- Sign of basal skull fracture ('panda' eyes)
- Cerebrospinal fluid leakage from the ear or nose, blood from ear (Battle's sign) concerning mechanism

Figure 57.3 Indications for CT in head injury

Adults	Children
• GCS less than 13 in ED	• Suspected non-accidental injury
• GCS less than 15 at 2 hours after the injury (in ED)	• Post-traumatic seizure (with no history of epilepsy)
• Suspected open or depressed skull fracture	• GCS less than 14 in ED, or for children under 1 year paediatric GCS less than 15
• Suspected basal skull fracture (signs include blood from ears, 'panda' eyes, cerebrospinal fluid leaking from ears or nose, Battle's sign)	• GCS less than 15 at 2 hours after the injury
• Post-traumatic seizure	• Suspected open or depressed skull fracture or tense fontanelle
• Focal neurological deficit	• Suspected basal skull fracture (signs include blood from ears, 'panda' eyes, cerebrospinal fluid leaking from ears or nose, Battle's sign)
• More than 1 episode of vomiting	• Focal neurological deficit
	• Infants (children under 1 year): any bruising, swelling or laceration greater than 5 cm to the head

Figure 57.4 Measures to reduce intracranial pressure

- Nurse patient at 30 degree head-tilt
- Maintain neutral neck position
- Provide adequate analgesic
- Insertion of bolt (where indicated)
- High-flow oxygen
- Reduce restrictive equipment around neck
- Appropriate fluid therapy to reduce oedema
- Control environmental stimulation

Figure 57.5 Discharge information and advice

- Type and severity of injury and treatment provided
- Risk factors and situations when to return to the ED
- The need for a responsible adult for 24 hours post-injury
- What to expect from recovery (e.g. headaches, tiredness)
- ED contact details
- Information regarding activities (work, school, sport)
- Local support organisations

Figure 57.6 Common causes of neck injury

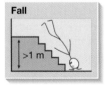
Fall
>1 m

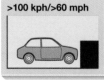
>100 kph/>60 mph

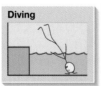
Diving

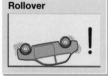
Rollover
!

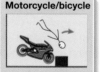
Motorcycle/bicycle

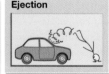
Ejection

Figure 57.7 Risk factors for neck injury

Low risk	High risk
• None listed in high-risk category	• Loss of consciousness
• Pain that radiates to shoulder and arm	• Focal neurological deficit
• Headache	• Concerning mechanism of injury
• Muscular spasm	• C-spine tenderness
	• Sudden pain after incident/event
	• Age >65

Figure 57.8 Hard collar

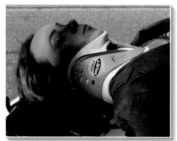

Source: By Alexisrael (own work) [GFDL by CC BY-SA 3.0] via Wikimedia Commons

Figure 57.9 Miami J collar

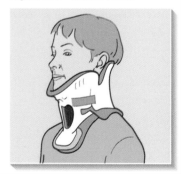

Emergency Nursing at a Glance, First Edition. Natalie Holbery and Paul Newcombe

Head and neck injury commonly occurs from blunt trauma such as road traffic collisions (RTCs), sports incidents and falls. As a general rule, neck injuries should be suspected in patients with a head injury and vice versa until proven otherwise. Regardless of the type of injury, assessment should follow the '<C>ABCDE' approach as outlined in Chapter 56.

Head injury

Head injury after trauma is the leading cause of death in both adults and children. Head injury is defined as any trauma to the head, excluding superficial lacerations and injuries to the face. It is a relatively common presentation to an emergency department (ED) with approximately 1.4 million people presenting each year. Up to half of these are children. Non-accidental injury and abusive head injury should be considered in all children and vulnerable adults. Types of head injuries seen in trauma include extradural haematomas, subdural haematomas, subarachnoid haemorrhage, skull fractures and contusions (Figure 57.1).

While most patients present with a mild head injury (95%), patients with moderate or severe head injuries can deteriorate rapidly and ED nurses must be familiar with assessment and management principles.

Assessment

Neurological observations are performed to detect changes in brain function. Assessment of the patient with a head injury is outlined in Chapter 19. All patients with a head injury should have a neurological assessment on arrival. The triage nurse should identify patients at high risk of head injury (Figure 57.2) and prioritise and allocate treatment area accordingly. High-risk patients should be cared for in the resuscitation area to allow for close monitoring of neurological function and airway compromise. Low-risk patients can generally be cared for in minors or urgent care.

Neurological observations should be performed in the ED every 15–30 minutes until the GCS returns to 15 (or is normal for the patient). After this, neurological observations should be performed hourly for 4 hours and 2-hourly thereafter. These later observations are likely to occur in a clinical decision unit or observation area if the patient is to be observed overnight or beyond 4 hours.

Management

Regardless of the severity or type of head injury, management should be in line with the <C>ABCDE approach. The overarching goal is early detection of primary brain injury and prevention of secondary brain injury. Primary injury is the initial insult; secondary brain injury is further injury caused by hypoxia. Computed tomography (CT) is recommended as key to detecting brain injury, for which there are clear guidelines (Figure 57.3). Patients who do not meet the criteria for CT may require continued observation in the ED. Nurses should perform and record neurological observations as discussed earlier and report any abnormalities to the doctor.

For patients with moderate or severe brain injury, interventions to minimise secondary brain injury focus on reducing intracranial pressure. Such interventions are outlined in Figure 57.4.

While some patients will require admission to a ward or intensive care, most have a mild head injury and are discharged home. On discharge, all patients and carers should receive verbal and printed discharge advice and education. Advice and education should be appropriate to their age and cognitive ability. Figure 57.5 outlines the requirements of such advice.

Neck injury

As with head injuries, patients may present with minor or severe life-threatening neck injuries. RTCs and sport injuries are common causes of neck injuries seen in an ED (Figure 57.6).

Assessment

The triage nurse should assess for high- and low-risk factors and allocate priority and treatment area accordingly (Figure 57.7). Neck injuries may involve soft tissue injury, bony (vertebrae or transverse process) fractures, spinal cord injury or a combination.

Management

Patients with suspected neck injuries and a concerning mechanism of injury should initially be immobilised using manual inline immobilisation before a hard collar is fitted (Figure 57.8). Soft tissue injury alone (whiplash) is not life threatening and patients with this type of injury can be cared for in minors or urgent care. Whiplash is a minor yet painful condition caused by excessive hyperextension or hyperflexion of the neck resulting in soft tissue injury. It can also be associated with headache. Analgesia should be offered and patients can return home with advice to continue paracetamol and ibuprofen as required. They should be reassured that the injury is self-limiting and advised to return to normal activities. They can also be advised to consult their GP for a referral to a physiotherapist if pain persists.

Patients with high-risk factors or severe neck injuries should be cared for in the resuscitation area to monitor for neurological deterioration and shock, which may result in breathing or ventilation difficulties (Chapter 13). Inline immobilisation using a hard collar should be applied to reduce neck movement. Nurses should provide analgesia as required and perform and record neurological observations, reporting any abnormalities to a doctor. Patients may be extremely anxious, especially if they are aware of neurological changes. ED nurses should provide reassurance that they are being cared for in the right place, and involve the family whenever possible. CT is indicated in these patients and nurses should prepare equipment to ensure a safe transfer (Chapter 66).

Depending on the type of injury, a patient may have surgery or conservative treatment with a cervical collar such as a Miami J (Figure 57.9). Patients with a cervical fracture without cord injury (and no other injuries) are permitted to mobilise in a Miami J collar and are often discharged home from the ED. ED nurses should provide discharge advice about activities of daily living, signs of deterioration, collar maintenance and follow-up appointments.

58 Chest trauma

Figure 58.1 Types of chest injuries

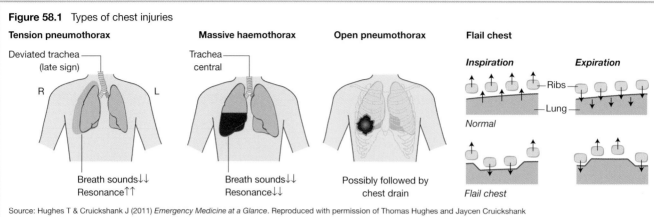

Tension pneumothorax

Deviated trachea (late sign)

R   L

Breath sounds↓↓
Resonance↑↑

Massive haemothorax

Trachea central

Breath sounds↓↓
Resonance↓↓

Open pneumothorax

Possibly followed by chest drain

Flail chest

Inspiration   *Expiration*

Ribs
Lung

Normal

Flail chest

Source: Hughes T & Cruickshank J (2011) *Emergency Medicine at a Glance*. Reproduced with permission of Thomas Hughes and Jaycen Cruickshank

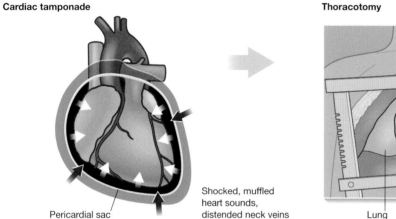

Cardiac tamponade

Pericardial sac

Shocked, muffled heart sounds, distended neck veins

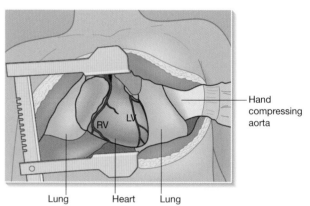

Thoracotomy

Hand compressing aorta

RV   LV

Lung   Heart   Lung

Figure 58.2 Assessment of breathing

Look, listen and feel		
R	Respiratory rate	What is the respiratory rate?
I	Inspection	What can you see on the chest? (e.g. wounds, bruising, symmetry)
P	Palpation	What can you feel? (e.g. crepitus, does this elicit pain?)
P	Percussion	What can you hear? (e.g. normal resonance, dull, hyper-resonant)
A	Auscultation	Can you hear breath sounds? They may be present, reduced or absent
S	Saturations	What is the peripheral oxygen saturation?

Figure 58.3 Chest drains

Before   After   Before   After

Chest drain   Chest drain

Pneumothorax   Re-inflated lung   Massive haemothorax   Re-inflated lung

Emergency Nursing at a Glance, First Edition. Natalie Holbery and Paul Newcombe.
© 2016 John Wiley & Sons, Ltd. Published 2016 by John Wiley & Sons, Ltd. Companion website: www.ataglanceseries.com/nursing/emergencynursing

A chest injury is a relatively uncommon presentation to an emergency department (ED); however, they are responsible for up to 25% of all trauma deaths. It is common for patients with a chest injury to have associated trauma, necessitating an advanced trauma life support (ATLS) approach to assessment and management (Chapter 56). The most common life-threatening chest injuries are tension pneumothorax, massive pneumothorax, open haemothorax, flail chest and cardiac tamponade (Figure 58.1). Each requires a team approach to achieve a positive outcome. General nursing responsibilities involve psychosocial support for the patient, assessment, performing or assisting with interventions, administration of oxygen, analgesia and fluids/blood, communication with the family and documentation.

Assessment of chest injuries

Assessment of breathing and ventilation in trauma is more rapid and less extensive than a comprehensive respiratory assessment. The goal is to detect life-threatening chest injuries only. A useful acronym to remember the steps of a breathing assessment in trauma is outlined in Figure 58.2.

Tension pneumothorax

A tension pneumothorax is defined as air in the pleural cavity creating extensive pressure, leading to mediastinal shift. It is a type of obstructive shock (Chapter 13) and usually seen in blunt trauma. It is characterised by tachypnoea, unequal chest movement, hyper-resonance, absent breath sounds on the affected side and low saturations. Tracheal deviation may be seen although this is a late sign and should not be relied on. Initial management involves needle decompression by inserting a large bore cannula into the second intercostal space, mid-clavicular line. This is usually performed by a doctor or an experienced nurse. Definitive management requires the insertion of a chest drain to the affected side.

Open pneumothorax

An open pneumothorax is usually caused by penetrating trauma to the chest. It is often seen in stabbings and gunshot wounds to the chest. It is defined as air in the pleural cavity with a perforation to the lung that makes contact with the atmosphere. It is characterised by tachypnoea, an open wound to the chest that may be 'sucking', hyper-resonance and reduced air entry on the affected side, as well as low saturations. Management usually involves a chest drain to the affected side and closure of the wound.

Massive haemothorax

A massive haemothorax can result from blunt or penetrating trauma. It is defined as blood in the pleural cavity exceeding 1,500 ml or greater than 200 ml/hour for 2–4 hours. It is a type of hypovolaemic shock (Chapter 13) and characterised by tachypnoea, possible bruising, hypo-resonance and absent air entry to the affected side, as well as low saturations. Management involves administration of blood products to replace lost volume and a chest drain to remove the blood from the pleural cavity. Cardiothoracic surgeons may choose to take the patient to theatre to repair bleeding vessels.

Flail chest

A flail chest alone is not a life-threatening condition; however, the pulmonary contusions usually associated with it may be. A flail chest occurs as a result of blunt trauma and is defined as two or more rib fractures in two or more places. This results in a segment of the chest wall being separated from the rest of the chest, creating a flail segment. The force involved in fracturing the ribs often extends into the lung tissue, causing the contusions. Management involves analgesia and close monitoring of ventilation. If the patient is unable to ventilate adequately due to the pulmonary contusions, a decision to intubate the patient may be made.

Cardiac tamponade

Cardiac tamponade is uncommon but can progress rapidly and if not detected will result in death. It is a type of obstructive shock (Chapter 13) and can occur as a result of blunt or penetrating trauma. It is defined as a collection of blood around the pericardium that constricts the heart, preventing effective pumping. The blood collects after disruption of a nearby vessel. The volume of blood need not be large to cause this condition. The patient will show signs of shock. A focused assessment with sonography in trauma (FAST) scan confirms the diagnosis. Management involves ultrasound-guided pericardiocentesis or thoracotomy if the patient has arrested. Cardiothoracic surgeons should also be involved.

The patient with a chest drain

Chest drains are commonly used to treat chest injuries. They allow the release of air or blood from the pleural cavity, permitting the lung(s) to re-inflate (Figure 58.3). Once the trauma team has left, the nurses become responsible for the ongoing monitoring of the patient and the chest drain. Vital signs should be recorded at least every 30 minutes to detect any deterioration in breathing or ventilation. Analgesia should be continued to ensure that the patient can breathe adequately, optimising ventilation and preventing a chest infection.

The chest drain should be monitored to ensure that it continues to swing (with each breath) and bubble (as air is released). In the case of a massive haemothorax, blood loss should be monitored and recorded on a fluid balance chart. The drain site should be covered with an opaque dressing to allow for inspection of the site. The site should be clean and dry. Any redness, ooze or swelling needs to be documented and reported to a doctor.

Chest drains should not be clamped in the ED unless the bottle is being changed. Clamping a chest drain prevents release of air or blood from the pleural cavity and may lead to a tension pneumothorax.

59 Limb injuries

Figure 59.1 Compound fracture

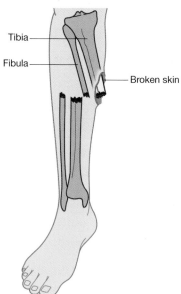

Tibia

Fibula

Broken skin

Figure 59.2 5Ps

Pain – is pain worsening?

Pallor – is skin pale or cold?

Pulse – is pulse weak or absent?

Paraesthesia – does the patient have sensation to the limb?

Paralysis – can the patient move the limb?

Figure 59.3 Patients at high risk of complications

- Unconscious
- Unable to communicate
- Increasing pain
- Crush injuries
- Anti-coagulated patients

Figure 59.4 (a, b) Traction splints

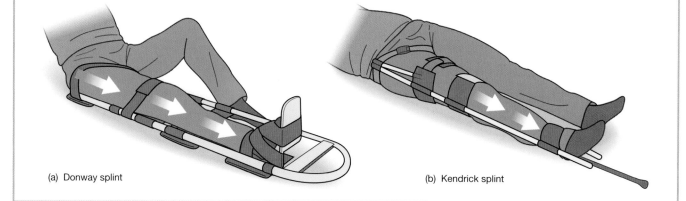

(a) Donway splint

(b) Kendrick splint

Emergency Nursing at a Glance, First Edition. Natalie Holbery and Paul Newcombe

© 2016 John Wiley & Sons, Ltd. Published 2016 by John Wiley & Sons, Ltd. Companion website: www.ataglanceseries.com/nursing/emergencynursing

Limb trauma occurs in up to 80% of all trauma patients. It is rare for these injuries to be life threatening, although at times they are limb threatening. Unless massive external haemorrhage is present, the assessment and management of limb trauma is performed under 'circulation and haemorrhage control'. Clinicians must not be distracted by limb injuries at the expense of dealing with airway and breathing problems.

Limb trauma may be life changing and lead to an altered body image. The ED nurse must be aware of these issues and provide advice and psychological support to the patient and family when required. The management of specific minor injuries to upper and lower limbs is discussed in more detail in Chapters 50 and 51.

Open and closed fractures

A closed fracture is any break to a bone where the skin remains intact. An open or compound fracture is a break to a bone with an associated wound (Figure 59.1).

Assessment of limb trauma

Nurses should assess a patient's neurovascular status using the '5Ps' (Figure 59.2). Warmth and capillary refill should also be assessed. A full neurovascular assessment should occur immediately after the primary survey and be performed at least hourly in the emergency department (ED). The frequency may need to be increased for certain patients at high risk of complications such as compartment syndrome (Figure 59.3).

Management of limb trauma

In an ED, the management of limb trauma is guided by the following principles: haemorrhage control, re-alignment, pain control and infection prevention (in open fractures).

The approach to haemorrhage control is determined by the type of limb injury. For external haemorrhage, direct pressure (or the application of a haemostatic agent) should be applied until the patient receives definitive treatment in theatre. Internal haemorrhage is managed by realigning the limb and replacing blood loss, followed by definitive treatment in theatre.

Realignment using a splinting device serves to reduce bleeding, prevent further injury, reduce pain and minimise the risk of fat embolism. Traction splints are the most common form of limb splintage in an ED (Figure 59.4). Regardless of the type of splint used, regular checks should be carried out. These include splint position, neurovascular observations, pain assessment and pressure areas. If the patient's neurovascular status or pain worsens, the splint should be removed and either reapplied or an alternative sought.

Open and closed fractures are often very painful and require appropriate assessment and analgesia. Pain assessment should be carried out with each set of observations and documented in the patient's notes. Pain assessment is covered in more detail in Chapter 6.

As most limb injury in trauma causes moderate to severe pain, opioids are commonly used. Nurses should closely monitor the patient's respiratory rate because opioids are central nervous system depressants. If the respiratory rate falls significantly (usually below 8 breaths per minute) a doctor should be informed and naloxone administered as per local policy. Increasingly, intravenous (IV) paracetamol is used with similar efficacy to morphine and fewer immediate side effects. Oral medication is avoided to ensure that the patient remains nil by mouth.

In addition, open fracture management requires IV antibiotics to be administered as soon as possible and certainly within 3 hours of injury. Open fractures carry a high risk of infection and early antibiotic use reduces morbidity. The wound should be cleaned with normal saline. A simple saline-soaked gauze dressing will suffice until the patient receives definitive treatment in theatre. Handling of the wound should be kept to a minimum to prevent infection. Photos may be taken in line with local policy to limit removal of the dressing.

Traumatic amputation

Traumatic amputation is the loss of a body part, usually a limb, following trauma. Sometimes partial amputation occurs where the goal is limb salvage; however, this is unlikely if the body part is no longer viable.

Pre-hospital clinicians initiate the management of traumatic limb amputation. This involves the application of a tourniquet if massive external haemorrhage is present or a simple saline-soaked gauze dressing and splint in the absence of massive haemorrhage. If the amputated limb is brought to the ED, it should be cleaned to remove any large debris, wrapped in saline-soaked gauze, placed in a sealable plastic bag and inserted in cold water. It should not be placed directly on ice because this can cause a cold burn and reduce the likelihood of salvage.

Compartment syndrome

Compartment syndrome is a condition where pressure, due to swelling or bleeding, exceeds normal levels in the limb fascia and results in nerve, vessel or muscle damage. Limb trauma is a common cause of compartment syndrome. Although regular neurovascular observations are advised, many of the 5P's (Pain, Pulselessness, Pallor, Paresthesia, Paralysis) are late signs. Pain is the best indicator. Pain that is greater than expected for the type of injury, or is increasing at an unusual rate, is a sign of compartment syndrome.

Management involves a fasciotomy, an incision to the fascia to release pressure. Neurovascular observations, analgesia and wound care are ongoing nursing responsibilities.

60 Abdominal and pelvic trauma

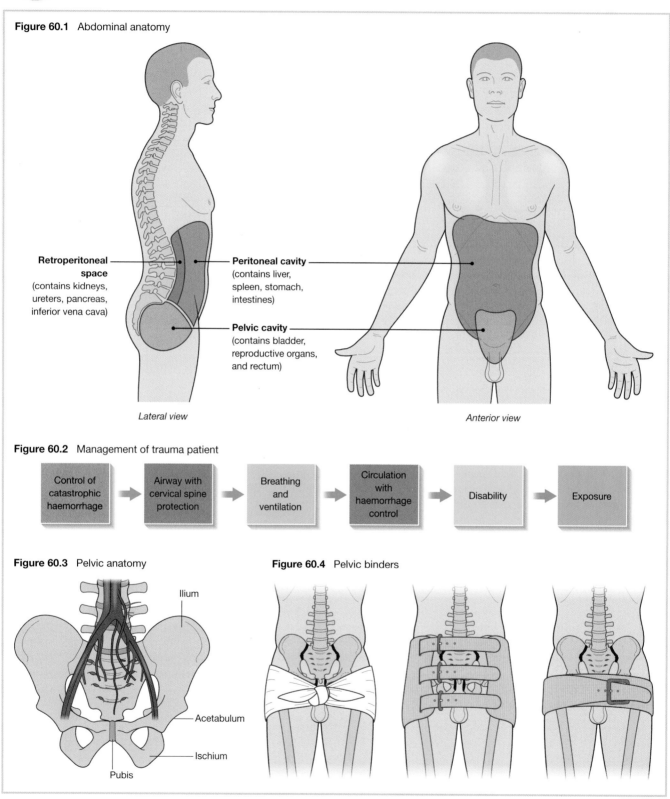

Figure 60.1 Abdominal anatomy

Retroperitoneal space
(contains kidneys, ureters, pancreas, inferior vena cava)

Peritoneal cavity
(contains liver, spleen, stomach, intestines)

Pelvic cavity
(contains bladder, reproductive organs, and rectum)

Lateral view

Anterior view

Figure 60.2 Management of trauma patient

Control of catastrophic haemorrhage → Airway with cervical spine protection → Breathing and ventilation → Circulation with haemorrhage control → Disability → Exposure

Figure 60.3 Pelvic anatomy

Ilium

Acetabulum

Ischium

Pubis

Figure 60.4 Pelvic binders

Emergency Nursing at a Glance, First Edition. Natalie Holbery and Paul Newcombe
© 2016 John Wiley & Sons, Ltd. Published 2016 by John Wiley & Sons, Ltd. Companion website: www.ataglanceseries.com/nursing/emergencynursing

Abdominal and pelvic trauma account for significant mortality among trauma patients. The mortality rate for pelvic injuries is up to 50% with abdominal trauma being 10–30%. Haemodynamic instability in abdominal trauma is associated with a greater mortality rate. Unless massive external haemorrhage is present, see 'Circulation with haemorrhage control' (Chapter 56) for the assessment and management of abdominal and pelvic injuries.

Abdominal trauma

Abdominal trauma can be either blunt or penetrating. Penetrating injuries are generally associated with knife or gunshot wounds whereas blunt trauma is mostly caused by road traffic collisions (RTCs). Abdominal injuries due to blunt trauma can be associated with missed injuries due to occult bleeding. Understanding the abdominal anatomy, principles of assessment and diagnostic tools available will increase the likelihood of detecting injury.

The abdomen comprises three main sections: peritoneal cavity, retroperitoneal space and pelvic cavity (Figure 60.1). Organs in the retroperitoneal space may be difficult to detect clinically. Typical signs such as a distended abdomen may not be present. Highly vascular, solid organs such as the liver and spleen bleed profusely if injured.

Diagnostic tools

Focused assessment of sonography in trauma (FAST) is commonly used to detect free fluid in the abdomen. FAST scans are non-invasive and allow for rapid assessment; however, a negative FAST scan (no free fluid) is not an absolute indicator of the absence of abdominal injury or bleeding.

Computed tomography (CT) is the diagnostic tool of choice today because it allows for rapid screening with high diagnostic safety. Haemodynamically unstable patients are increasingly being transferred to CT. Nurses should treat this as any other transfer and ensure that equipment is prepared and transported securely with the patient, accompanied by clinicians as appropriate (Chapter 66).

Diagnostic peritoneal lavage (DPL) is an invasive technique to detect abdominal bleeding. It is considered sensitive to bleeding but non-specific to the site of injury. As a result it has been superseded by FAST and CT in the UK.

Management of abdominal trauma

The goal of abdominal assessment in trauma is to detect injuries that are life threatening and expedite the patient to theatre or interventional radiology. Occasionally the decision may be made to conservatively management the patient's injury. In this situation, nurses should monitor the patient closely for signs of deterioration. Analgesia should be administered as required.

Patients with abdominal trauma who stay more than 90 minutes in an emergency department (ED) have an increased mortality rate. ED nurses need to work efficiently as part of the trauma team to assess abdominal trauma and initiate interventions such as blood transfusions and analgesia. Management of abdominal trauma follows the same principles for all trauma patients (Figure 60.2).

In the case of extensive bleeding and haemodynamic instability, the massive haemorrhage protocol should be initiated (Chapter 61) and tranexamic acid administered. Movement of the patient should be kept to a minimum to avoid dislodging clots. Caring for a patient on a trauma mattress avoids the need to slide or roll them when moving them on and off CT and theatre tables.

Pelvic trauma

Pelvic injury commonly results from blunt trauma. Common mechanisms include RTCs and falls. RTCs involving pedestrians or motorcyclists may also be associated with open or compound fractures (Chapter 59).

The pelvis is made up a number of bones that are in close proximity to an extensive vascular supply (Figure 60.3). Severe pelvic fractures are associated with high energy force. The posterior aspect of the pelvis is highly vascular and as a result pelvic fractures are often associated with massive haemorrhage. Pubic rami fractures are associated with low energy force, usually as isolated injuries in older adults. Significant bleeding is rare with this type of injury.

Diagnostic tools

Severe pelvic fractures can often be detected clinically. Signs include deformity, bruising, pain and shortening or rotation of the legs. Manipulation of the pelvis should not occur because this causes more pain for the patient, increases the risk of further bleeding and offers no further clinical information. As severe pelvic fractures are associated with haemorrhage, it is advisable to obtain a pelvic X-ray before transferring a patient. An X-ray will confirm the presence of a fracture and the likelihood of bleeding based on the type of fracture. Patients who present with a significant mechanism or signs of injury will have a CT to confirm the presence of bony injury and detect damage to vessels and nearby organs.

Management of pelvic trauma

As with abdominal trauma, the management of a patient with a pelvic fracture is the same for any trauma patient (Chapter 56). Specific priorities of in managing severe pelvic injury, however, are haemorrhage control, pain relief and definitive treatment. Patients with suspected pelvic injury usually have a pelvic binder applied pre-hospitally. Binders minimise bleeding, assist with re-alignment and reduce pain (Figure 60.4). They are a temporary device until the patient receives definitive treatment such as surgical fixation.

In the presence of haemorrhage, blood products and tranexamic acid should be administered. If bleeding is severe, the massive haemorrhage protocol should be activated (Chapter 61). Pelvic fractures are associated with severe pain. Analgesia should be prompt and adequate for the pain score. Opioids such as morphine are recommended. Intravenous paracetamol is also used as an effective analgesia in trauma patients.

Management of pubic rami fractures consists of analgesia and early mobilisation. Nurses should consider the patient's social situation, including home access, ability to carry out activities of daily living and social support.

61 Massive haemorrhage

Figure 61.1 Lethal triad

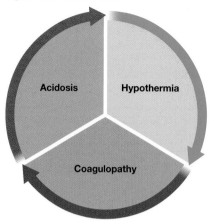

Acidosis

Hypothermia

Coagulopathy

Figure 61.2 Control of catastrophic haemorrhage

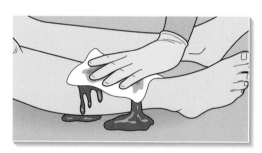

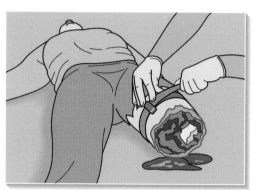

Figure 61.3 Massive haemorrhage protocol example

- **Trauma/team leader/clinician must initiate massive haemorrhage protocol if:**
  – systolic blood pressure <90
  – poor response to initial fluid resuscitation
  – suspected active haemorrhage

- **Nominated team member must contact blood bank immediately and declare 'massive haemorrhage'. Baseline samples to be taken prior to transfusion:**
  – FBC
  – group and save
  – clotting screen
  – fibrinogen
  – send immediately to laboratory

- **Request one pack A (contains 6 units of red cells, 6 units of fresh frozen plasma (FFP). Send porter/nurse to collect immediately.** If there is an immediate need for transfusion, collect 'flying squad' units from ED resus (satellite) fridge. If bleeding continues request one **pack B (contains 6 units of red cells, 6 units of FFP, 1 unit of platelets and 2 pools of cryoprecipitate).**
  Continue to request pack B until bleeding stops

- **Anticipate coagulopathy**

- **When bleeding is controlled, repeat FBC and clotting screen**

- **If bleeding persists, contact on-call haematology registrar**

Emergency Nursing at a Glance, First Edition. Natalie Holbery and Paul Newcombe
© 2016 John Wiley & Sons, Ltd. Published 2016 by John Wiley & Sons, Ltd. Companion website: www.ataglanceseries.com/nursing/emergencynursing

Massive haemorrhage in trauma is the leading cause of preventable death. It leads to haemorrhagic shock and can be the result of internal or external bleeding. Blunt trauma can cause massive haemorrhage from widespread damage to multiple vessels and organs. Massive haemorrhage from penetrating trauma, such as gunshot or stab wounds, usually results in more localised damage.

Early recognition of massive haemorrhage, rapid interventions to stem bleeding and replace blood loss are key to improving outcome. In the UK, all major trauma centres have protocols for the management of massive haemorrhage in adults and children. These protocols recognise the need to rapidly replace volume that is as near to whole blood as possible. However, replacing blood volume in a patient with massive haemorrhage is only the first step. In most cases, severe bleeding can only be stopped with surgical intervention. The goal is therefore to administer blood products and expedite the patient to theatre.

Coagulopathy

Coagulopathy is a deranged clotting state where the body's ability to form clots is impaired. Coagulopathy forms part of the lethal triad in trauma (Figure 61.1), along with hypothermia and acidosis. Removing at least one of these factors will reduce mortality.

Tissue trauma, inflammation, shock, dilution, hypothermia and acidosis all contribute to coagulopathy. Up to 25% of trauma patients are thought to arrive in an emergency department (ED) already in a state of coagulopathy. Ensuring that all bleeding trauma patients receive high-flow oxygen, are prevented from getting cold and receive warmed blood products will reduce mortality.

Management of massive haemorrhage

Control of catastrophic haemorrhage is the first step in the approach to a trauma patient. This step relates only to external haemorrhage and requires application of direct pressure to the wound. In some cases a tourniquet may be indicated (Figure 61.2). Some EDs will stock haemostatic agents that form a gel-like substance to halt bleeding. For all types of blunt trauma, when there is no external haemorrhage, other interventions are required.

All trauma patients with massive haemorrhage should have two large-bore cannulas inserted into the antecubital fossa. If intravenous access is difficult, a central trauma line will be required. Intraosseous access is another option, although it is more commonly used in children and pre-hospital settings. Bloods should also be drawn for urea and electrolytes, full blood count (FBC), clotting and crossmatch. Depending on the mechanism of injury and history, the team leader may also request a toxicology screen.

The fluid of choice for bleeding trauma patients is blood. Administering crystalloids leads to dilution, a factor that contributes to coagulopathy. Blood should be warmed using a medical device and ideally administered via a rapid infuser. Rapid infusers in trauma can administer up to 500 ml/min if required; however, boluses of 250 ml/min are generally recommended.

Addressing and, whenever possible, halting the bleeding in the ED will prevent further shock and coagulopathy. Common bleeding sites are chest, abdomen, pelvis and long bones. Chest injuries such as massive haemothorax are managed with the insertion of a chest drain, administration of blood products and cardiothoracic intervention to stop the bleeding. The management of chest injuries is covered in Chapter 58.

Management of abdominal bleeding in the ED is limited. Using a focused assessment of sonography in trauma (FAST) scan can help to determine the likelihood of free fluid (blood) in the abdomen, although computed tomography (CT) is more accurate and reliable. The patient would ideally have a CT scan before theatre to determine the location and extent of the bleeding.

Pelvic trauma can lead to significant haemorrhage. Pelvic binders reduce the volume of the pelvis and attempt to realign vessels, reducing haemorrhage. Most patients suspected of a pelvic fracture usually arrive with a binder applied pre-hospitally. Abdominopelvic trauma is covered in more detail in Chapter 60.

Long bone fractures require traction splinting to reduce bleeding (Chapter 59).

Minimising movement of a trauma patient will also reduce further bleeding. Movement can dislodge clots and should be avoided whenever possible. Using a specially designed trauma mattress allows for easy transfer of the patient without rolling or shearing.

Massive haemorrhage protocol

Known in some EDs as a 'Code Red', massive haemorrhage protocols allow a coordinated response to severe bleeding (Figure 61.3). Most of these protocols derive from military experience where massive haemorrhage is all too common. The underlying principle is to replace 'like for like'. This usually includes red blood cells, fresh frozen plasma (FFP) (or equivalent) and cryoprecipitate. Tranexamic acid is also administered because it has been shown to significantly reduce mortality with its antifibrinolytic effects (i.e. it prevents clot breakdown).

Massive haemorrhage protocols allow for a significant amount of blood and blood products to be available for as long as a patient requires a transfusion. This can be in excess of 60 units for the most severely injured. A ratio as near to 1:1 of red blood cells to fresh frozen plasma has been shown to reduce mortality. Patients should receive o-negative (females of child-bearing age) or o-positive (males) blood while the massive haemorrhage pack is being prepared.

Pre-hospital crews can request a 'Code Red' to ensure that blood is ready for when the patient arrives in the ED. Helicopter emergency medical service crews in the UK carry red blood cells on board and may have already administered a couple of units. It is important to consider this when calculating ratios of red blood cells to fresh frozen plasma. Tranexamic acid is also increasingly administered pre-hospitally.

62 Burns

Figure 62.1 Types of burn

Thermal
- Hot – flame, flash, scald
- Cold – frostbite

Chemical
- Household or industrial
- Acid
- Alkali

Electrical
- Low or high voltage

Radiation
- Sunburn
- Radiotherapy

Figure 62.2 Burns classification and characteristics

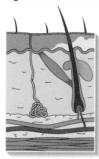
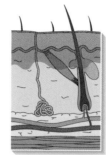
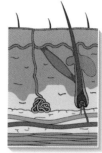
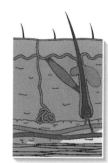

Superficial epidermal
Red and painful, but not blistered

Partial thickness (superficial dermal)
Pale pink and painful with blistering

Partial thickness (deep dermal)
Dry or moist, blotchy and red, and may be painful. There may be blisters

Full thickness
Dry, painless, no blisters, white/brown/black/leathery/waxy

Source: Hughes T & Cruickshank J (2011) *Emergency Medicine at a Glance*. Reproduced with permission of Thomas Hughes and Jaycen Cruickshank

Figure 62.3 Estimated body surface area by burns

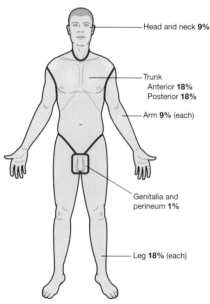

Head and neck **9%**

Trunk
Anterior **18%**
Posterior **18%**

Arm **9%** (each)

Genitalia and perineum **1%**

Leg **18%** (each)

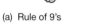

(a) Rule of 9's

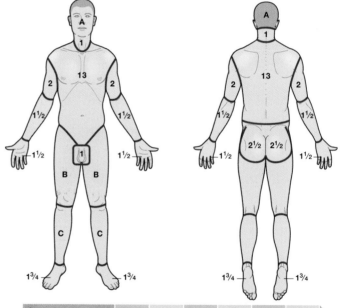

Area	Age 0	1	5	10	15	Adult
A = ½ of head	9½	8½	6½	5½	4½	3½
B = ½ of one thigh	2¾	3¼	4	4½	4¼	4¾
C = ½ of one lower leg	2½	2½	2¾	3	3¼	3½

(b) Lund-Browder diagram for estimating extent of burns

Figure 62.4 Burns referral criteria example

Adults	Children
• >3% partial thickness burn	• >1% partial thickness burn
• All deep dermal and full thickness burns	• All deep dermal and full thickness burns, circumferential burns
• All burns associated with electrical shock	• Burns involving the face, hands, feet and perineum
• All burns associated with chemical burn	• Burns associated with smoke inhalation or electrical shock
• All burns associated with non-accidental injury	• Severe metabolic disturbance
• All burns to face, hands, perineum, feet	• Burn wound infection
• All circumferential burns to limbs or trunk or neck	• Unhealed burns after 2 weeks
• All burns with inhalation injury	• All neonatal burns
• All burns not healed within 2 weeks	• All burns associated with non-accidental injury

Emergency Nursing at a Glance, First Edition. Natalie Holbery and Paul Newcombe

Each year in the UK around 175,000 people attend an emergency department (ED) with a burn injury. Approximately 13,000 of these require admission and further treatment. Causes of burns are varied and tend to be categorised according to general management principles: thermal, chemical, electrical and radiation (Figure 62.1). Thermal burns are the most common, with scalds being the most common in children. Radiation burns are the least commonly seen in EDs and are not covered within this chapter.

Classification

In the UK, burns are classified according to their depth: superficial, mid dermal, deep dermal and full thickness. The characteristics of each vary and it is possible to have a combination for each burn injury (Figure 62.2). Classifying burns is essential to guide ongoing management. Burns cause a significant fluid shift, resulting in shock in the most severe cases. Intravenous (IV) fluid replacement is determined by the depth and extent of the burn, therefore assessing this on the patient's arrival is key to optimal management.

Total body surface area burned

The extent of the burn is known as the 'total body surface area' (TBSA). There are various tools available to determine TBSA; however, the Lund and Browder chart is considered the most accurate and is used by most burns units in the UK (Figure 62.3). It is appropriate for both adults and children.

When calculating TBSA superficial burns are not included. Superficial burns tend not to be associated with significant fluid shifts and are therefore not included in the calculation. It is good practice to calculate TBSA with a colleague to avoid miscalculation.

Fluid requirements

The Parkland Formula is used to calculate IV fluid requirements: 4 ml/kg/TBSA. The fluid of choice is Hartmann's. The total volume is to be administered over 24 hours: the first half given in the first 8 hours from the time of the burn injury, and the other half to be completed by 24 hours from the time of the burn injury. Children may also require additional maintenance fluid that includes glucose to address their increased metabolic demand.

Management of burns

Regardless of burn type, patients will experience pain. Full thickness burns eliminate sensation due to nerve damage; however, these patients experience pain at the burn edges where burn depth is superficial or partial thickness. All further movement and interventions will cause pain and analgesia should be provided as a priority of care.

A patient should be assessed for an inhalation burn. Signs include hoarse voice, sore throat and singed nasal hairs. The team should have a low threshold for early intubation because the patient's airway can become compromised rapidly.

Two large cannulas should be inserted if not already sited pre-hospitally. Ideally these would be inserted into large veins and through non-burned skin. If IV access is difficult, intraosseous or central line access may be required.

The burn will need to be washed and covered if not already done so. Washing with saline or soap and water is adequate. In an ED, cling film is the dressing of choice because it prevents contamination, reduces pain by preventing air contact with the burn and allows for easy inspection.

Patients should have an indwelling catheter inserted to monitor hourly urine output. The goal in adults is a minimum of 0.5 ml/kg/hour. In children this is increased to a minimum of 1 ml/kg/hour. Urine should also be assessed for colour, with the goal being straw coloured. Too dark suggests dehydration (or haemoglobinuria/myoglobinuria in electrical burns) and requires an increase in fluid administration. Pale urine suggests excessive fluid resuscitation, increasing the risk of oedema. In this situation, fluid should be slowed or halted according to a doctor's instruction. Fluid replacement is generally a significant volume and care needs to be taken with older patients and those with congestive heart failure or other cardiac conditions.

Electrical burns

Electrical burns result in injuries requiring care as discussed earlier; however, other factors also need to be considered. A patient with an electrical injury may have associated trauma, requiring an advanced trauma life support (ATLS) approach (Chapter 56).

The voltage causing the burn injury may cause arrhythmias. The patient should have an early electrocardiogram(ECG) and be placed on a cardiac monitor.

Concealed muscle damage may occur in patients with electrical burns. This results in myoglobinuria (myoglobin in urine), a condition that can cause kidney failure. Increasing IV fluids is essential if the urine is dark in colour.

Chemical burns

Chemical burns are commonly seen as eye injuries in EDs (Chapter 53). Occasionally patients present with chemical burns to the face, chest or limbs. In this case, copious irrigation may still be required before management as discussed earlier.

Definitive care

Some patients will require admission to a burns unit and Figure 62.4 outlines general referral criteria for adults and children. It is good practice to make early contact with the unit to alert the staff to the patient's arrival and seek advice regarding ongoing management. Most burns units will require completion of a proforma that details the patient's demographics, history, mechanism of injury, burn details and current care. Providing as much information as possible will support the burns unit to prepare for the patient.

Consideration needs to be given to the transfer to ensure that it is safe for the patient and staff. If the patient is intubated, an anaesthetist will also need to escort them. Nurses should ensure that all documentation, analgesia, fluids and emergency equipment are checked and prepared for transfer. Chapter 66 covers transfer in more detail.

63 Trauma: Special circumstances

Figure 63.1 Anatomical and physiological changes during pregnancy

Airway – reflux, oedema	A
Breathing – raised diaphragm, respiratory distress from growing uterus, increased oxygen demand (15–20%)	B
Circulation – increased circulating volume (30–50%), dilutional anaemia, decreased resistance to flow = vasodilatation, heart rate increases (10–20 beats per minute), blood pressure decreases, may see fetal distress first, gravid uterus compresses aorta and vena cava	C
Disability – seizures may occur if woman has eclampsia	D
Exposure – screen for domestic abuse, fetal assessment	E

Figure 63.2 Left lateral tilt and manual displacement

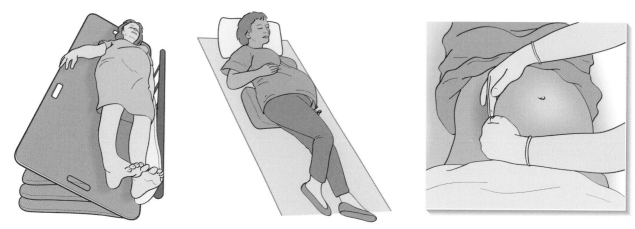

Figure 63.3 Physiological changes in the older adult

Airway – Increased risk of airway obstruction due to reduced airway tone	A
Breathing – increased sensitivity to hypoxia and hypercarbia	B
Circulation – decreased cardiac output, increased vascular resistance, decreased renal function,	C
Disability – increased likelihood of cognitive impairment (use appropriate tools to assess pain), decreased metabolism and poorer excretion of medicines	D
Exposure – screen for elder abuse	E

Emergency Nursing at a Glance, First Edition. Natalie Holbery and Paul Newcombe

All trauma patients should be assessed and managed using the advanced trauma life support (ATLS) model (Chapter 56). There are certain groups of patients, however, who may require special attention because of their age or altered physiology. Such groups include pregnant women, older adults and children. Trauma in children is covered in Chapter 64.

The pregnant trauma patient

Trauma during pregnancy is relatively uncommon; however, it remains the leading cause of non-obstetric mortality. The most common mechanism is road traffic collisions (RTCs) followed by falls and assault. The latter is usually related to domestic abuse.

Various changes during pregnancy, particularly the third trimester, result in an altered response to injury (Figure 63.1). These changes require a modified approach to the pregnant trauma patient. All approaches are guided by the following premise: resuscitating the mother will resuscitate the foetus. Nursing responsibilities involve providing psychological support to the patient and family, assisting with assessments and procedures, and administering medicines and blood when required. There should be a team approach to screening for domestic abuse and any concerns should be reported in line with local policy.

Owing to potential difficulties with a patient's airway, nurses should anticipate the need for difficult airway equipment, ideally stored on a dedicated trolley. The patient may complain of difficulty in breathing, dizziness or nausea when lying supine due to aortal compression. If spinal precautions are in place, preventing her sitting up, the woman should be positioned at a 30-degree angle on her left side. This is often achieved with a wedge or tilting a spinal board (Figure 63.2). Frequent observations, perhaps every 5–10 minutes, but at a minimum of every 30 minutes, will detect any haemodynamic changes.

The increased circulating volume will often result in a normal blood pressure (BP) until the point of deterioration. Foetal distress may be detected before signs of shock in the mother. For this reason, early midwifery and obstetric involvement is key. The midwife will assess foetal function and should stay with the mother at least until the trauma team has left.

If a blood transfusion is required, the nurses should alert the blood bank and ensure that o-negative blood is administered until group-specific blood is available. Administering o-negative blood in women of child-bearing age is mandatory to avoid a reaction to possible RhD antigen.

In some cases an emergency caesarean may need to be performed. These are rarely successful, with most foetuses being delivered stillborn. This is a very distressing situation for staff and the team should be attuned to each other's reactions. A team debrief may be helpful after such an event.

Older adults

The most common cause of injury in older adults is falls. This is often due to syncope but may also be caused by mechanical falls. Compared with the younger person, older adults are more likely to require admission and have an increased length of stay and increased mortality rate following trauma. Staff should screen for elder abuse in all cases of older adult trauma.

Injuries commonly include fractures, especially of the cervical spine and hip, and head injuries. Some older adults have comorbidities and take regular medication, whereas others may be fit and well. It is important to establish a patient's medical history early to determine whether any comorbidities or medicines are likely to affect their management. For example, if the patient is on a beta-blocker, they will be unable to mount a tachycardia, masking shock. If the patient is unable to reliably provide this information, staff will need to contact a family member, carer or the patient's GP.

If the patient wears dentures, it is best to keep these in situ. Dentures allow for easier bag or mask ventilation if the patient deteriorates, and encourage good nutrition when the patient is permitted to eat.

The primary survey is completed as per Chapter 56; however, a medical assessment is also recommended to identify a medical cause. Assessing for chest pain, shortness of breath, back pain, dizziness, palpitations and other medical signs should be included. An electrocardiogram (ECG) may be required.

Physiological changes in the older adult result in a decreased ability to compensate during shock (Figure 63.3). The patient is likely to deteriorate more rapidly than a younger adult. Frequent observations, perhaps every 5–10 minutes, but at a minimum of every 30 minutes, is required. Nurses should also assess for pain, bruising, external bleeding, oxygenation and neurological status (Chapter 19). If the Glasgow Coma Score (GCS) is low, it is important not to assume that the patient has dementia or other cognitive impairment. Any new confusion or altered GCS may be a sign of shock or head injury, and must be documented and reported to the team leader.

64 Trauma in children

Figure 64.1 A pad beneath the shoulders creates a neutral airway position

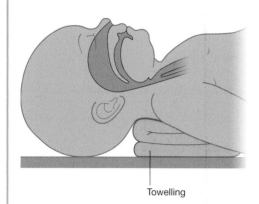

Towelling

Figure 64.2 Airways

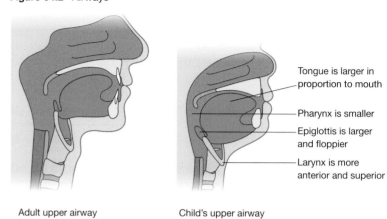

Adult upper airway

Child's upper airway

Tongue is larger in proportion to mouth

Pharynx is smaller

Epiglottis is larger and floppier

Larynx is more anterior and superior

Figure 64.3 Paediatric Glasgow Coma Scale

		<5 years	>5 years
Eye opening	E4	Spontaneous	
	E3	To voice/speech	
	E2	To pain	
	E1	No response	
Verbal	V5	Smiles, coos, babbles, follows objects, interacts	Orientated and appropriate
	V4	Cries but consolable	Confused
	V3	Cries to pain, moaning	Inappropriate words
	V2	Inconsolable, agitated	Incomprehensible sounds
	V1	No response	
Motor	M6	Moves spontaneously and purposefully	Obeys commands
	M5	Withdraws from touch	Localises pain
	M4	Withdraws from pain	Withdraws from pain
	M3	Abnormal flexion to pain	Abnormal flexion to pain
	M2	Abnormal extension to pain	Extension to pain
	M1	No response	

Trauma is the leading cause of death in children over the age of 12 months. Mechanism of injury is closely related to age and stage of development. In infants, the leading cause of death is non-accidental injury (Chapter 45). In children, road traffic collisions (RTCs) are the most common followed by falls. Head injuries are the most common cause of death.

Regardless of the type of injury, assessment of a child follows the same approach as that for adults (Chapter 56). Understanding the various anatomical and physiological differences will ensure that assessments and interventions are appropriate to the child, thus improving outcome.

Catastrophic haemorrhage

Catastrophic haemorrhage is defined as uncontrolled external bleeding, often from limb amputation. The need to address catastrophic haemorrhage before airway is common in military situations but rare in civilian populations.

Airway with cervical spine (c-spine) control

Children have relatively large tongues compared with adults, increasing the risk of airway obstruction. The larger occiput in infants naturally flexes the neck when lying supine, causing potential airway obstruction and preventing an aligned cervical spine. Placing a blanket, pad or towel under the shoulders is recommended to achieve a neutral position (Figure 64.1).

Intubation in younger children can be more difficult due to a higher, more anterior larynx and a soft, funnel-shaped airway (Figure 64.2). Current practice is to use cuffed endotracheal (ET) tubes for all ages. Historically, uncuffed ET tubes were advocated to avoid pressure-related necrosis of the trachea. Modern ET tubes, however, are designed to seal at lower pressures, reducing the risk of necrosis. Nurses should ensure that the correct-sized ET tube and difficult airway equipment is available, ideally on a dedicated trolley.

Immobilising the cervical spine is indicated in most cases of blunt trauma; however, it is often a daunting experience for young children. When children do not tolerate a hard collar, insisting on immobilisation only increases child and parent or carer distress and increases the risk of neck movement. In this situation, it is usually best to keep the child calm and request that the parent or carer sit with them, reducing movement and distress.

Breathing and ventilation

Children have more pliable bones compared with adults, which may result in underlying lung and thoracic injuries in the absence of rib fractures. If rib or sternal fractures are present, the force to generate such injuries is great and the team should have a low threshold for suspecting significant thoracic injuries.

The mediastinum in children is more mobile than in adults, resulting in the greater likelihood of a tension pneumothorax – a condition not well tolerated in children. Rapid assessment and ongoing monitoring will detect key signs such as tachypnoea, reduced chest wall movement and lowered oxygen saturations. Spinal cord injuries may impair breathing and ventilation and the team should be aware of a condition known as 'spinal cord injury without radiographic abnormality' (SCIWORA).

Circulation with haemorrhage control

Blunt trauma, such as RTCs, are more likely to result in multiple injuries in children. Children are more compact than adults and the same force can have an impact on many more organs. Children have a thinner abdominal wall with less protection for underlying organs. This increases the risk of haemorrhage to organs such as the liver and spleen.

Children have efficient compensatory abilities, with hypotension being a late sign of deterioration. Regular monitoring, perhaps every 5 minutes in the most severely injured, will detect changes to vital signs – in particular, respiratory rate and heart rate. In situations where intravenous access is difficult, an intraosseous line may be inserted. All fluids should be administered based on 10 ml/kg.

Disability

Children have larger heads relative to adults and therefore a greater risk of head injury. The Glasgow Coma Scale (GCS) was originally designed for adults and is often used for older children; however, it is difficult to apply to pre-verbal children. A modified GCS known as the Paediatric Glasgow Coma Scale is a more appropriate tool (Figure 64.3).

Children have decreased glycogen stores, which may warrant additional fluids containing glucose to avoid hypoglycaemia.

Exposure

Children generally have less body fat compared with adults and a larger surface area to mass ratio, both of which place them at greater risk of hypothermia. Ensuring a child is covered and actively warmed if cold will address hypothermia and minimise the risk of coagulopathy.

Routine 'top-to-toe' computed tomography(CT) scanning is avoided in children. Radiation exposure is particularly damaging to developing cells and organs. Most major trauma centres in the UK have a child-specific CT protocol.

Regardless of mechanism, attention to safeguarding is imperative. Most trauma charts contain screening tools for safeguarding children. If concerns do exist, one member of the team should take responsibility for reporting in line with local policy.

Parents or carers

Parents or carers should be given the option to stay with their child but allowed the freedom to leave if they need a break. A senior nurse should initially be responsible for communicating with them.

65 Major incidents

Figure 65.1 Major incident 'sieve and sort'

| Walking | → No → | Breathing | → Yes → | Respiratory rate | → 10–29 → | Capillary refill or heart rate | | Mass casualties with extensive injuries |

- Walking — Yes → **Priority 3** (delayed)
- Breathing — No (After airway opening) → **Dead**
- Respiratory rate — <10 >30 → **Priority 1** (immediate)
- >2 secs >120 → **Priority 1** (immediate)
- Capillary refill or heart rate — <2 secs <120 → **Priority 2** (urgent)
- Mass casualties with extensive injuries → **Expectant**

Figure 65.2 Major incident triage categories

Category	Major incident	CBRNe incident
P1	Immediate	Severe
P2	Urgent	Moderate
P3	Delayed	Mild
P4	Expectant	Expectant
Dead	Dead	Dead

Figure 65.3 Decontamination zones in a chemical, biological, radiological, nuclear and explosive (CBRNe) incident

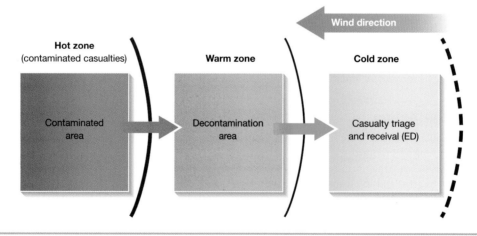

Wind direction

Hot zone (contaminated casualties) — Contaminated area → **Warm zone** — Decontamination area → **Cold zone** — Casualty triage and receival (ED)

Emergency Nursing at a Glance, First Edition. Natalie Holbery and Paul Newcombe

© 2016 John Wiley & Sons, Ltd. Published 2016 by John Wiley & Sons, Ltd. Companion website: www.ataglanceseries.com/nursing/emergencynursing

A major incident is an event that requires special arrangements to be made by pre-hospital services, emergency departments (EDs) and hospitals due to the number or types of patients (casualties) involved. It requires a predefined, coordinated response called a 'major incident plan'.

Types of major incidents

A major incident can be caused by a number of different events:

- Natural causes (e.g. floods, earthquakes, hurricane)
- Major accidents (e.g. plane crash, train derailment, building collapse)
- Health related (e.g. pandemics, swine flu)
- Hostile acts (e.g. terrorism).

A 'CBRNe' incident is a particular type of event that involves the deliberate release of chemical, biological, radiological or nuclear and explosive materials with the intention of causing harm.

Role of emergency services

Major incidents involve a multi-agency response in which all the emergency services work together to rescue those injured or affected by the event:

- Police – overall coordination, investigation of the incident, evidence gathering and liaison with families
- Fire service – detection and management of hazardous materials, search and rescue
- Ambulance – treatment and stabilisation of casualties at the scene, transport of casualties to hospital
- Hospital – assessment, stabilisation and definitive treatment of casualties.

Triage 'sieve and sort'

In incidents involving a large number of casualties, it is necessary to ensure that those most severely injured are prioritised first. At the site of the incident this is performed by ambulance personnel. It is similar to the concept of triage applied in EDs but where 'sieve' is a rapid primary assessment based on any signs of life, and 'sort' involves a more thorough secondary clinical assessment (Figure 65.1). Casualties are assigned categories or priorities based on the severity of injury, similar to in-hospital triage, using an algorithm (Figure 65.2). The 'Expectant' category is unique to major incidents and used when the number of casualties overwhelms the available resources. This means that casualties at the scene who have potentially unsurvivable injuries are triaged 'to wait' and other priority 1 casualties are treated first.

Triage is a dynamic process and casualties are re-triaged by senior clinical staff on arrival at hospital.

Hospital response

All NHS hospitals have a major incident plan detailing the hospital-wide response to any such event. This plan will include a range of departments and wards in addition to the ED. The hospital is usually notified of a major incident by the ambulance service and is either placed on 'standby' when there is preliminary advice to anticipate a major incident (in the initial stages when the number of casualties at the scene may be unclear), or 'declared' when there is implementation of the full plan.

When a major incident is declared, the hospital will activate a predetermined series of alerts to key staff and set up a command centre to coordinate the response. This involves discharging patients from the wards and stopping non-emergency surgery to ensure theatres are able to take casualties from the major incident.

The role of the ED

The primary role of the ED in a major incident is in the reception of casualties. It provides treatment to casualties according to their injuries or symptoms. In the first few hours after a major incident is declared it is the focus of the activity and a large number of clinical staff from across the hospital will arrive to assist in the management of the patients coming into the ED.

Patients who arrive at the ED who are not a casualty of the major incident are encouraged to seek treatment elsewhere. Other ambulances are diverted by pre-hospital services to hospitals not involved in the major incident.

CBRNe incidents

Incidents that are suspected of involving the deliberate release of hazardous materials require a special type of major incident response aimed at reducing the effects of exposure to the contaminant. Potential contaminants are:

- Chemical – chemical agents (e.g. cyanide, mustard gas, nerve agents)
- Biological – bacteria, viruses or toxins (e.g. anthrax, botulism, smallpox). Release can be directly into the environment or into food sources.
- Radiological – radioactive material released through an explosive 'dirty bomb', or radioactive material being left in a public place
- Nuclear – nuclear material released accidentally or through a terrorist act.

Recognising a CBRNe incident

Recognition of potential exposure to a CBRNe incident is crucial to management, treatment and preventing further spread of the contaminant. Owing to the wide variety of agents, it is possible that casualties may present to an ED with a range of non-specific symptoms, such as rashes, breathing problems and vomiting, whose onset is sometimes hours but may not occur until weeks after exposure. Emergency nurses should be aware of multiple patients arriving from the same location and presenting to the ED with similar symptoms.. Advice can be sought through the health protection or public health agencies.

Decontamination of casualties

Decontamination is a process employed to remove external traces of any hazardous substance and to avoid further spread. In a major incident this is usually carried out at the scene, but hospitals also have decontamination facilities usually in the form of a special tent with washing facilities. This is a role that requires special training and can be carried out by emergency nurses who will wear personal protective equipment (PPE). Most contaminants can be removed with soap and water as the casualties pass through a series of zones from contaminated (the 'hot' zone) to clean, ready for treatment (Figure 65.3).

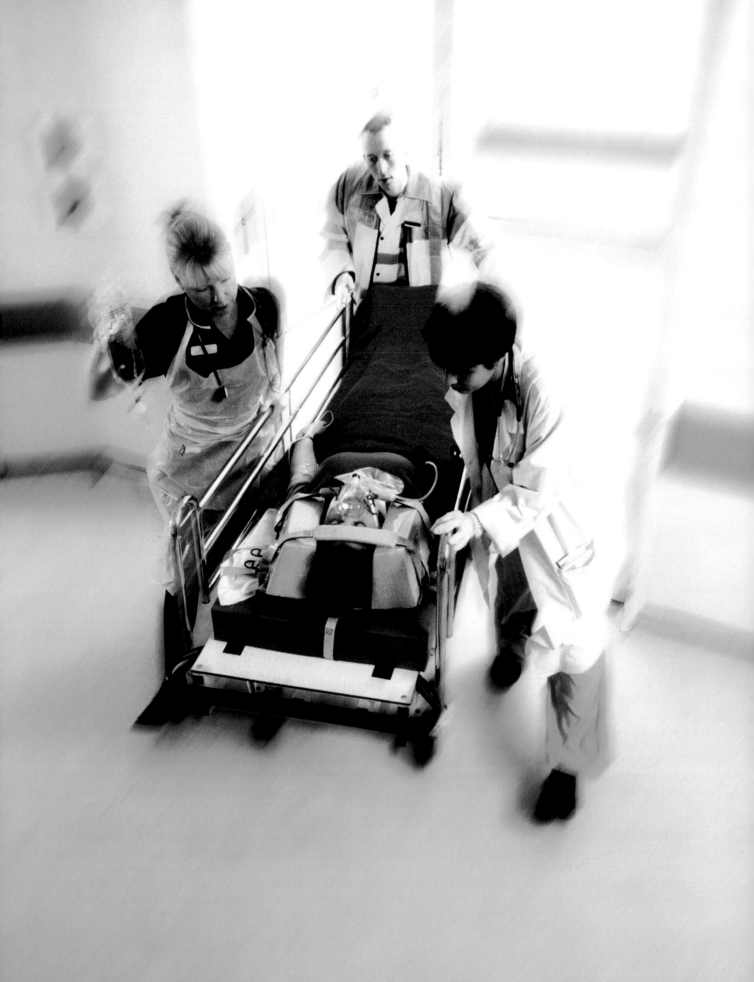

Patient transfer and end of life care

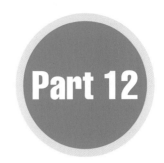

Part 12

Chapters

66 Patient transfer

Figure 66.1 Potential problems during transfer

Equipment

- Batteries lose charge
- Depleted fluid, blood products or drugs
- Depleted oxygen supply
- Disconnected ECG monitoring leads
- Tangled tubing
- Transport vehicle breaks down or is involved in a collision

Staff

- Level of training and experience not appropriate for type of transfer
- Staff suffer with travel sickness
- Staff unable to get back to place of work

Patient

- Patient deteriorates on route (desaturation, haemodynamic instability)
- Tubes/lines become dislodged on route
- Patient suffers with travel sickness

Figure 66.2 Principles of safe transfer

Preparation

- Receiving unit to be made aware of patient and estimated time of arrival
- Patient to be 'packaged' ready for transfer before transport vehicle arrives
- Equipment to be gathered and checked
- Staff to take warm clothing, money and directions back to place of work (transport vehicle not obliged to return staff to work)

Patient

- Gather notes, ensure the person/team transferring the patient is familiar with the patient's condition

Staff

- Suitably trained
- Have received handover
- Appropriate clothing
- Return plans in place
- Insurance/indemnity in place

Equipment

- Suitable equipment
- Spare batteries
- Sufficient oxygen for duration of transfer

Organisation

- Transfer checklist completed
- Notes and investigations gathered and copied as per local policy
- Patient and relatives informed
- Transport vehicle arranged

Destination

- Transfer team (and driver/pilot) aware of receiving unit name, address and phone number
- Directions available for destination

Figure 66.3 Example transfer checklist

Transfer form

Demographics	Past medical history	
Name:	❑ COAD	❑ Cancer
DOB:	❑ Asthma	❑ MI
Hospital Number:	❑ Stroke	❑ Pacer
	❑ HT	❑ Diabetes
(Or Affix Label)	❑ Other	
Next of Kin: Name:		
Phone:		

When and why?	Background
Intra or Inter Hospital:	Allergies:
Time of referral:	Medications/Infusions: ❑Inotropes ❑ Sedation ❑Other:
Referred from e.g. ICU, HDU, GCCU:	
Staff accepting referral (Name/Grade):	Infection Status:
Receiving destination e.g. CT, MRI, GCCU:	**Respiratory Support**
	❑ Face Mask ❑ Nasal Mask
Staff accepting patient on arrival:	❑ ETT ❑ Tracheostomy
	Tube size and length:
Departure from unit hh:mm:	Ventilator Model:
Arrival back on unit hh:mm:	Mode: FiO$_2$
Time LAS contacted hh:mm:	**Incident**
Time of LAS arrival hh:mm:	❑ Yes, please give details below: ❑No
Escort Personnel:	❑ Minor/Brief ❑Life Threatening ❑Fatal
Doctor (name and grade):	❑ Respiratory
	❑ Circulatory
Nurse (name and grade):	❑ Neurological
	❑ Drug related
Other Information:	❑ Equipment problem
	❑ Organisational
	❑ Trauma/injury
	❑ Battery failure
	❑ Transfer specific problem

Summary of transfer:

Signature and date:

Observations

Parameter	Key	Time:	°C
Date:			
		200	42
Parameter	Key	190	
HR	●	180	
BP	↕	170	
PAP/CVP	▲	160	40
Temp	*	140	
MAP	■	130	
Checklist		120	38
ECG	❑	110	
Oxygen	❑	100	
Venflon	❑	90	
ETCO$_2$	❑	80	36
Drugs	❑	70	
Suction	❑	60	
Pupils	❑	50	
RASS		40	34
		30	
Hb		20	
INR		10	
APTT		0	32
Pits		RR	
Urea		SaO$_2$	
Creat		ETCO$_2$	
P$_a$O$_2$		FiO2	
P$_a$CO$_2$		Paw	
		Vt	
Drugs/Fluids		Units	
Propofol		mg/hr	
Urine Output			

Telephone Numbers

Transfers of critically ill or injured patients in the emergency department (ED) occur frequently. Transfer is defined as the movement of patients between clinical care settings.

Types of transfer

Patients are transferred from the ED for a number of reasons, either to other clinical areas within the hospital (internal or intra-hospital transfers) or to other hospitals (external or inter-hospital transfers).

Intra-hospital transfers

Intra-hospital transfers are the most common type of transfer in the ED and include movement between different areas of the ED, such as transfer from the resuscitation area to the computed tomography (CT) scanner. All transfers of patients from the ED to inpatient wards or critical care areas are in this category.

Inter-hospital transfers

Inter-hospital transfers occur between hospitals and are needed because of a lack of appropriate facilities in the referring hospital. This usually occurs within a pre-defined 'network' of specialist centres within a given geographical location (e.g. major trauma, specialist surgery, burns or children's intensive care).

Principles of safe transfer

The aim of any transfer is to move a patient to the most appropriate clinical setting for their treatment and ongoing care as safely as possible. This recognises that there is a risk associated with moving critically injured or ill patients and therefore adequate planning and preparation are required. The responsibility for the decision to transfer the critically injured and ill patient lies with the medical staff.

There are many potential adverse events or issues that can occur during patient transfer (Figure 66.1). To minimise these risks, many hospitals will have standardised policies and standards for patient transfer. The same level of planning is important for both intra- and inter-hospital transfers and is summarised in Figure 66.2. The first question that should be asked before any patient transfer is 'Is this transfer safe?'

Patient assessment and stabilisation

Planning and preparation for a transfer occurs concurrently with the ongoing management of the patient in the ED. The patient should be assessed using the 'ABCDE' principles (Chapter 4) to ensure that they are clinically safe for transfer. Because critically injured and ill patients are transferred for ongoing care, complete clinical stability will not be possible and the decision to transfer is based on the need to balance the risk of moving the patient with their clinical needs.

Preparation

Safe transfer includes preparation of the patient, equipment and personnel accompanying them. As well as making the patient clinically stable for transfer, the preparation of the patient includes securing all lines and tubes (chest drains, endotracheal tubes). Two intravenous access lines should be available and pumps and infusions should be reduced to essential medications only, to minimise the total equipment and risk of tangling of lines. For critically injured or ill patients, the minimum equipment levels are those relating to:

- Electrocardiogram (ECG) monitoring
- Non-invasive blood pressure
- Respiratory rate
- Arterial oxygen saturation (SaO_2)
- End-tidal carbon dioxide ($EtCO_2$) in ventilated patients
- Transfer bag – including equipment for manually supporting the airway
- Portable suction.

A minimum of two personnel are required for transfer. For critically injured or ill patients, this should include an anaesthetist or intensive care doctor trained in airway management and critical care. Inter-hospital transfers by road or air have additional attendants such as paramedics or technicians.

Communication and documentation

Appropriate communication is imperative across all stages of the transfer process. Patients and their relatives should be kept informed throughout the transfer.

The transfer personnel should agree on their roles and responsibilities before moving the patient. This includes equipment preparation, liaison with the receiving area and patient monitoring. It is usual for a verbal referral and acceptance of the patient to be made by medical staff; a separate nursing handover is useful if there are explicit issues. Specific computer referral systems and electronic letters exist to support referrals. It is particularly important for inter-hospital transfers that directions to the receiving department are clear and there is a means to contact the hospital en route.

Transfer checklists exist to ensure that the transferring personnel are adequately prepared (Figure 66.3). These can be used on both intra- and inter-hospital transfers. Inter-hospital transfers also require a means of documentation of the patient's condition and treatment during transfer.

Mode of transport

Most inter-hospital transfers are carried out by road ambulances. Emergency nurses transferring patients should listen to advice from the ambulance crew and agree responsibilities during the transfer for observations, monitoring and documentation. The ambulance crew will be familiar with the safety features of the vehicle and interventions during transfer should be kept to a minimum.

Air transfers, by helicopter or fixed-wing aircraft, are useful over long distances or in time-critical situations. They require specialist personnel trained in aeromedical care.

Transfer of critically ill children

Transfer of critically ill children is predominantly managed in the UK through a series of retrieval services whereby patients are 'retrieved' or collected by a specialist paediatric intensive care team from the referring hospital.

Training for transfer

All staff undertaking patient transfers should undergo appropriate training in the safe transfer of critically injured and ill patients. Training should include patient and equipment preparation, and instruction on local systems and organisational and network arrangements.

67 End of life care

Figure 67.1 Principles of breaking bad news

Preparation

- Confirm who will communicate the bad news
- Gather as much information as possible to respond to any questions
- Ensure a private room is available with access to tissues, drinking facilities and a phone
- Turn off bleeps and mobile phones

Communication

- Introduce yourself by name and profession
- Determine what the person already knows
- Use simple and direct language, free from jargon
- Be honest and sensitive
- Maintain eye contact
- Do not appear uncomfortable during periods of silence or distress

Planning and follow-up

- Identify who else should be notified and offer to do this
- Allow family and friends to view body if they wish
- Offer resources, including a bereavement booklet
- Document conversation in patient's record

Figure 67.2 Bereaved relatives' room

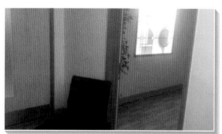
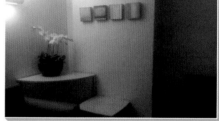
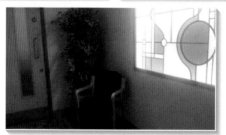

Figure 67.3 Reporting to the coroner in the UK

- The patient did not see a doctor during their last illness
- The patient did see a doctor during their last illness but the doctor is not able or available to certify the death
- The cause of death is unknown
- The death occurred during an operation or before recovery from an anaesthetic
- The death occurred at work or was due to industrial disease or poisoning
- The death was sudden and unexplained
- The death was unnatural (e.g. trauma, homicide)
- The death was due to violence or neglect
- The death occurred in other suspicious circumstances
- The death occurred in prison or police custody

Figure 67.4 Bereaved booklet information

- Contact details of ED, mortuary and bereavement office
- Deceased person's body (transfer, viewing, property)
- Coroner's role and responsibilities
- Organ and tissue donation
- Registering the death
- Brief information about funerals
- Useful numbers and resources

Emergency Nursing at a Glance, First Edition. Natalie Holbery and Paul Newcombe
© 2016 John Wiley & Sons, Ltd. Published 2016 by John Wiley & Sons, Ltd. Companion website: www.ataglanceseries.com/nursing/emergencynursing

While the primary goal of emergency departments (EDs) is to sustain life, there are some situations in which this goal needs to be revised. Some patients will present to an ED when their life-limiting condition may require symptom control rather than aggressive management. Other patients present following cardiac arrest or trauma, and may die within the ED.

Most deaths that occur in the ED are sudden and unexpected. Caring for patients and relatives at this time is often emotionally challenging for nurses and other ED professionals. ED nurses have a responsibility to care for the patient leading up to and after death, as well as to provide support for family and friends. A significant number of patients wish to die at home although the reality is that many present to an ED because of worsening symptoms and then die in hospital. Most common symptoms include pain, nausea and vomiting. Social issues such as the family being unable to cope with increasing care demands may also be a factor. The goals of end of life care should be determined by open communication with the patient and their family. Such decisions should be documented in the patient's medical record. Occasionally patients will have an 'advance decision' that should be followed if the team is aware of the document. This outlines decisions to refuse particular types of treatment. They commonly relate to life-saving interventions such as cardiopulmonary resuscitation (CPR).

End of life care

Treatment

As a patient nears end of life, a decision should be made regarding a ceiling of treatment. This should involve the patient and their family and outline decisions about fluids, nutrition, antibiotics, medication and CPR. Symptom control will be key and usually involves opioids and anti-emetics.

Do Not Attempt Resuscitation (DNAR)

As end of life approaches, a DNAR order is usually written. This is a legal document where the decision lies solely with the doctor. However, it is good practice for the doctor to discuss it with the patient, family and ED nurses. A DNAR order does not denote withdrawal of care, merely the avoidance of CPR, which is an invasive, undignified and often futile procedure.

Care after death

Breaking bad news

When a patient dies in an ED, notifying next of kin (NOK) becomes a priority. The NOK may be waiting in the ED or may need to be contacted by phone. In some situations the patient and/ or NOK details are unknown and police may need to be involved. Notifying family members of a death is ideally carried out face to face in a private room by a senior doctor and ED nurse who have been caring for the patient. This will ensure that any questions the family has are more easily answered. If breaking bad news has to be done over the phone, the clinician making the call should confirm that they are speaking with the NOK before following the principles of breaking bad news (Figure 67.1).

Environment

A dedicated, private room should be available in all EDs for family and friends following a death. Ideally the room should have tissues, a phone (with the ability to make external and mobile phone calls), comfortable and clean seating, and access to hot and cold drinks. In some EDs, the bereaved relatives' room has an adjoining viewing room (Figure 67.2).

Care of the deceased

Deceased patients should be continued to be cared for in a respectful and professional manner, respecting known wishes and religious and cultural beliefs whenever possible. Cannulas, drains and tubes should remain to avoid leakage. Jewellery should be removed and given to family, or labelled and stored safely according to local policy. Labels should be attached to the patient to assist identification in the mortuary. The body should then be wrapped according to local policy. This usually involves a sheet and plastic shroud. Transfer to the mortuary should be discreet, usually involving specially designed trolleys.

When there is an ongoing forensic investigation, the principles of evidence preservation should be followed (Chapter 38).

Coroner

The Coroner is responsible for determining cause of death when this is not known and a Medical Certificate of Cause of Death (MCCD) has not been generated. The Coroner may order a post-mortem to determine cause of death. In the UK there is a legal obligation to report certain deaths to the Coroner (Figure 67.3). Most deaths that occur in the ED are reported to the Coroner and include all children and infant deaths. When referred to a Coroner, all lines, drains and tubes are left in situ and capped off. The body should not be washed, including mouth care. Local guidelines should be followed because processes may vary between regions.

Organ donation

ED nurses should consider organ donation in all expected and actual deaths in the ED. Most organ donors in the UK die from traumatic brain injury, some of whom can be identified in the ED. The organ donation and transplantation team can be contacted for advice, usually via a regional organ donation specialist nurse.

Staff support

Regardless of experience, many ED nurses find end of life care an emotionally challenging experience. Many departments will have processes for debriefing following a sudden and unexpected death, and this should be offered to all staff involved in the patient's care, including those from the pre-hospital environment. This provides the team with the opportunity to learn from the event and give each other support. Most hospitals also have staff support services or occupational health departments that can assist with ongoing staff needs.

Resources

All EDs should have bereavement booklets to offer family and friends following a death in the ED. This should be produced in multiple languages, free from jargon and outline key contact details and 'next steps' (Figure 67.4).

Further reading/references

Chapter 1
NHS England (2015) *Urgent and Emergency Care Services in England.* Available at: http://www.nhs.uk/NHSEngland/AboutNHSservices/ Emergencyandurgentcareservices/Pages/urgent-care-overview .aspx

Chapter 2
Nixon, V. (ed.) (2013) *Professional Practice in Paramedic, Emergency and Urgent Care.* Chichester: Wiley Blackwell.
Willis, S. and Dalrymple, R. (eds) (2015) *Fundamentals of Paramedic Practice: A Systems Approach.* Chichester: Wiley Blackwell.

Chapter 3
Mackway-Jones, K., Marsden, J. and Windle, J. (eds) (2013) *Emergency Triage: Manchester Triage Group.* 3rd edition. Chichester: Wiley Blackwell.

Chapter 4
Resuscitation Council (UK) (2015) *A Systematic Approach to the Acutely Ill Patient (ABCDE Approach).* Available at: https://www .resus.org.uk/resuscitation-guidelines/a-systematic-approach- to-the-acutely-ill-patient-abcde/
Royal College of Physicians (2013) *Acute Care Toolkit 6: The Medical Patient at Risk: Recognition and Care of the Seriously Ill or Deteriorating Medical Patient.* Available at: https://www.rcplondon .ac.uk/resources/acute-care-toolkit-6-medical-patient-risk

Chapter 5
Royal College of Physicians (2015) *National Early Warning Score (NEWS).* Available at: https://www.rcplondon.ac.uk/resources/ national-early-warning-score-news

Chapter 6
College of Emergency Medicine (2014) *Management of Pain in Adults.* Available at: http://www.rcem.ac.uk

Chapter 7
Resuscitation Council (UK) (2011) *Airway Management and Ventilation.* Available at: https://lms.resus.org.uk/modules/m65-non- technical-skills/resources/chapter_7.pdf *(Kathy [note from author]: this is chapter 7 of the ALS Handbook and I'm not sure this should be an open access resource, but it appears to be currently)*

Chapter 8
Francis, C. (2011) *Respiratory Care.* Chichester: Blackwell.

Chapter 9
British Thoracic Society (2008) *Emergency Oxygen Use in Adult Patients Guideline.* Available at: https://www.brit-thoracic.org .uk/guidelines-and-quality-standards/emergency-oxygen-use- in-adult-patients-guideline/

Chapter 10
British Thoracic Society (2014) *Asthma Guideline.* Available at: https://www.brit-thoracic.org.uk/guidelines-and-quality- standards/asthma-guideline/
National Institute for Health and Care Excellence (NICE) (2010) *Chronic Obstructive Pulmonary Disease: Management of Chronic Obstructive Pulmonary Disease in Adults in Primary and Secondary Care (CG101).* Available at: https://www.nice .org.uk/guidance/cg101

Chapter 11
Jevon, P., Ewens, B. and Pooni, J.S. (2012) *Monitoring the Critically Ill Patient.* 3rd edition. Chichester: Wiley Blackwell.

Chapter 12
National Institute for Health and Care Excellence (NICE) (2013) *Intravenous Fluid Therapy In Adults In Hospital (CG174).* Available at: https://www.nice.org.uk/guidance/cg174

Chapter 13
Dellinger, R.P *et al.* (2012) *Surviving Sepsis Campaign: International Guidelines for Management of Severe Sepsis and Septic Shock: 2012.* Available at: http://www.survivingsepsis.org/ Guidelines/Pages/default.aspx
Resuscitation Council (UK) (2012) *Emergency Treatment of Anaphylactic Reactions: Guidelines for Healthcare Providers.* Available at: https://www.resus.org.uk/anaphylaxis/emergency- treatment-of-anaphylactic-reactions/
Royal College of Physicians (2014) *Acute Care Toolkit 9: Sepsis.* Available at: https://www.rcplondon.ac.uk/resources/acute- care-toolkit-9-sepsis

Chapter 14
Rowlands, A. and Sargent, A. (2014) *The ECG Workbook.* 3rd edition. Keswick: M&K Publishing.

Chapter 15
Aaronson, P.L., Ward, J.P.T. and Connolly, M.J. (2013) *The Cardiovascular System at a Glance.* 4th edition. Chichester: Wiley Blackwell.
Huff, J. (2011) *ECG Workout: Exercises in Arrhythmia Interpretation.* 6th edition. Philadelphia: Lippincott Williams & Wilkins.
Wesley, K. (2011) *Huszar's Basic Dysrhythmias and Acute Coronary Syndromes.* 4th edition. London: Mosby.

Chapter 16
Humphreys, M. (ed.) (2011) *Nursing the Cardiac Patient: Essential Skills for Nurses.* Chichester: Wiley Blackwell.

Kucia, A.M. and Quinn, T. (eds) (2010) *Acute Cardiac Care: A Practical Guide For Nurses*. Chichester: Wiley Blackwell.

Chapter 17

National Institute for Health and Care Excellence (NICE) (2014) *Acute Heart Failure: Diagnosing and Managing Acute Heart Failure (CG187)*. Available at: http://www.nice.org.uk/guidance/cg187

Riley, J. (2013) 'Acute decompensated heart failure: diagnosis and management', *British Journal of Nursing*, 22(22) pp. 1290–1295

Chapter 18

Resuscitation Council (UK) (2015) *Adult Advanced Life Support*. Available at: https://www.resus.org.uk/resuscitation-guidelines/

Chapter 19

Woodward, S. and Mestecky, A.M. (eds) (2011) *Neuroscience Nursing: Evidence-Based Practice*. Chichester: Wiley-Blackwell.

Chapter 20

Hickey, J.V. (2014) *The Clinical Practice of Neurological and Neurosurgical Nursing*. London: Lippincott, Williams and Wilkins.

Lindsay, K.W., Bone, I. and Fuller, G. (2010) *Neurology and Neurosurgery Illustrated*. 5th edition. Edinburgh: Churchill Livingstone.

Chapter 21

National Institute for Health and Care Excellence (NICE) (2008) *Stroke: Diagnosis and Initial Management of Acute Stroke and Transient Ischaemic Attack (TIA) [CG68]*. Available at: https://www.nice.org.uk/guidance/cg68

Chapter 22

National Institute for Health and Care Excellence (NICE) (2012) *The Epilepsies: The Diagnosis and Management of the Epilepsies in Adults and Children in Primary and Secondary Care [CG137]*. Available at: https://www.nice.org.uk/guidance/cg137

Chapter 23

National Institute for Health and Care Excellence (NICE) (2012) *Headaches: Diagnosis and management of headaches in young people and adults (CG150)*. Available at: https://www.nice.org.uk/guidance/cg150

Chapter 24

Cole, E., Lynch, A. and Cugnoni, H. (2006) 'Assessment of the patient with acute abdominal pain', *Nursing Standard*, 20 (39) pp. 67–75.

McArthur-Rouse, F. and Prosser, S. (eds) (2007) *Assessing and Managing the Acutely Ill Adult Surgical Patient*. Oxford: Blackwell.

Chapter 25

National Institute for Health and Care Excellence (NICE) (2012) *Acute Upper Gastrointestinal Bleeding: Management (CG141)*. Available at: https://www.nice.org.uk/guidance/cg141

Scottish Intercollegiate Guidelines Network (2008) *Management of Acute Upper and Lower Gastrointestinal Bleeding*. Available at: http://www.sign.ac.uk/guidelines/fulltext/105/

Chapter 26

National Institute for Health and Care Excellence (NICE) (2010) *Lower Urinary Tract Symptoms in Men: Assessment and Management (CG97)*. Available at: https://www.nice.org.uk/guidance/cg97

National Institute for Health and Care Excellence (NICE) (2010) *Scrotal Swellings. Clinical Knowledge Summaries (CKS)*. Available at: http://cks.nice.org.uk/scrotal-swellings#!topicsummary

National Institute for Health and Care Excellence (NICE) (2012) *Urinary Tract Infections in Adults (QS90)*. Available at: https://www.nice.org.uk/guidance/qs90

National Institute for Health and Care Excellence (NICE) (2013) *Pyelonephritis – Acute. Clinical Knowledge Summaries (CKS)*. Available at: http://cks.nice.org.uk/pyelonephritis-acute#!topic summary

Chapter 27

National Institute for Health and Care Excellence (NICE) (2013) *Acute Kidney Injury: Prevention, Detection and Management of Acute Kidney Injury up to the Point of Renal Replacement Therapy (CG169)*. Available at: https://www.nice.org.uk/guidance/cg169

Chapter 28

Joint British Diabetes Societies Inpatient Care Group (2012) *The Management of the Hyperosmolar Hyperglycaemic State (HHS) in Adults with Diabetes*. Available at: https://www.diabetes.org.uk/About_us/What-we-say/Specialist-care-for-children-and-adults-and-complications/

Joint British Diabetes Societies Inpatient Care Group (2013) *The Hospital Management of Hypoglycaemia in Adults with Diabetes Mellitus*. Available at: https://www.diabetes.org.uk/About_us/What-we-say/Specialist-care-for-children-and-adults-and-complications/

Joint British Diabetes Societies Inpatient Care Group (2013) *The Management of Diabetic Ketoacidosis in Adults*. 2nd edition. Available at: https://www.diabetes.org.uk/About_us/What-we-say/Specialist-care-for-children-and-adults-and-complications/

Chapter 29

National Institute for Health and Care Excellence (NICE) (2014) *Ectopic Pregnancy and Miscarriage [QS69]*. Available at: http://www.nice.org.uk/guidance/QS69

Chapter 30

Bateman, N. *et al.* (eds) (2014) *Oxford Desk Reference: Toxicology*. Oxford: Oxford University Press.

National Institute for Health and Care Excellence (NICE) (2012) *Poisoning or Overdose. Clinical Knowledge Summaries (CKS)*. Available at: http://cks.nice.org.uk/poisoning-or-overdose#!topicsummary

National Poisons Information Service (2015) *Toxbase*. Available at: https://www.toxbase.org/

Chapter 31

Royal College of Emergency Medicine (2013) *Paracetamol Overdose*. Available at: http://www.rcem.ac.uk/Shop-Floor/Clinical%20Guidelines/College%20Guidelines/Paracetamol%20Overdose/

Chapter 32

Public Health England (2014) *Carbon Monoxide: Properties, Incident Management and Toxicology*. Available at: https://www.gov.uk/government/publications/carbon-monoxide-properties-incident-management-and-toxicology

Chapter 33

National Confidential Enquiry into Patient Outcome and Death (NCEPOD) (2013) *Measuring the Units: A Review of Patients who Died with Alcohol-Related Liver Disease*. Available at: http://www.ncepod.org.uk/2013arld.htm

National Institute for Health and Clinical Excellence (NICE) (2010) *Alcohol-use Disorders: Diagnosis and Clinical Management of Alcohol-Related Physical Complications (CG100)*. Available at: https://www.nice.org.uk/guidance/cg100

Royal College of Emergency Medicine (2015) *Alcohol: A Toolkit for Improving Care*. Available at: http://www.rcem.ac.uk/ShopFloor/Clinical%20Guidelines/College%20Guidelines/

Chapter 34

Public Health England (no date) *Infectious Diseases*. Available at: https://www.gov.uk/topic/health-protection/infectious-diseases

World Health Organisation (no date) *Infectious Diseases*. Available at: http://www.who.int/topics/infectious_diseases/en/

Chapter 35

Public Health England (2014) *Notifications of Infectious Diseases (NOID)*. Available at: https://www.gov.uk/government/collections/notifications-of-infectious-diseases-noids

Chapter 36

Public Health England (2014) *Sexually Transmitted Infections (STIs): Surveillance, Data, Screening and Management*. Available at: https://www.gov.uk/government/collections/sexually-transmitted-infections-stis-surveillance-data-screening-and-management

Public Health England (2014) *Sexually Transmitted Infections (SMI S 6)*. Available at: https://www.gov.uk/government/publications/smi-s-6-sexually-transmitted-infections

Chapter 37

National Institute for Health and Care Excellence (NICE) (2014) *Domestic Violence and Abuse: How Services can Respond Effectively*. Available at: https://www.nice.org.uk/advice/lgb20/chapter/Introduction

Chapter 38

United Kingdom legislation *Sexual Offences Act (2003)*. Available at: http://www.legislation.gov.uk/ukpga/2003/42

Sexual Assault Referral Centre (SARC) Available at: http://www.solacesarc.org.uk/

Chapter 39

Callaghan, P. and Waldock, H. (eds) (2006) *The Oxford Handbook of Mental Health Nursing*. Oxford: Oxford University Press.

Callaghan, P., Playle, J. and Cooper, L. (eds.) (2011) *Mental Health Nursing Skills*. Oxford: Oxford University Press.

Chapter 40

Alderdice, J. *et al.* (2010) *Self-harm, Suicide and Risk: Helping People who Self-Harm. Royal College of Psychiatry Report CR158*. Available at: http://www.rcpsych.ac.uk/usefulresources/publications/collegereports/cr/cr158.aspx

Hart, C. (2014) *The Pocket Guide to Risk Assessment and Risk Management*. London: Routledge.

Chapter 41

Harrison, A. and Hart, C. (eds) (2006) *Mental Health Care for Nurses: Applying Mental Health Skills in the General Hospital*. Oxford: Blackwell.

Chapter 42

National Institute for Health and Care Excellence (NICE) (2010) *Dementia Quality Standard (QS1)*. Available at: https://www.nice.org.uk/guidance/qs1

National Institute for Health and Care Excellence (NICE) (2013) *Supporting People to Live Well with Dementia (QS30)*. Available at: https://www.nice.org.uk/guidance/qs30

Chapter 43

British Institute of Learning Disabilities http://www.bild.org.uk/

National Institute for Health and Care Excellence (NICE) (2015) *Challenging Behaviour and Learning Disabilities: Prevention and Interventions for People with Learning Disabilities whose Behaviour Challenges (NG11)*. Available at: https://www.nice.org.uk/guidance/ng11

Chapter 44

Department for Education (2015) *Working Together to Safeguard Children. A Guide to Inter-Agency Working to Safeguard qnd Promote the Welfare of Children*. Available at: https://www.gov.uk/government/publications/working-together-to-safeguard-children--2

Parliament of the United Kingdom (2004) *Children Act 2004*. Available at: http://www.legislation.gov.uk/ukpga/2004/31/contents

United Nations General Assembly (1989) *The United Nations Convention on the Rights of the child*. Available at: http://www.unicef.org.uk/UNICEFs-Work/UN-Convention/

Chapter 45

National Institute for Health and Care Excellence (NICE) (2009) *When to Suspect Child Maltreatment (CG89)*. Available at: https://www.nice.org.uk/guidance/cg89

National Institute for Health and Care Excellence (NICE) (2014) *Child maltreatment – recognition and management. Clinical Knowledge Summaries (CKS)*. Available at: http://cks.nice.org.uk/child-maltreatment-recognition-and-management

National Society for the Prevention of Cruelty to Children (NSPCC) (2015) *A Child's Legal Rights: Gillick Competency and Fraser Guidelines*. Available at: http://www.nspcc.org.uk/preventing-abuse/child-protection-system/legal-definition-child-rights-law/gillick-competency-fraser-guidelines/

Royal College of Nursing (2014) *Safeguarding Children and Young People – Every Nurse's Responsibility. RCN Guidance for Nursing Staff*. Available at: http://www.rcn.org.uk/development/practice/safeguarding/children_and_young_people

Chapter 46

Department of Health (2011) *Spotting the Sick Child*. Available at: https://www.spottingthesickchild.com

Chapter 47

National Institute for Health and Care Excellence (NICE) (2010) *Bacterial Meningitis and Meningococcal Septicaemia: Management of Bacterial Meningitis and Meningococcal Septicaemia in Children and Young People Younger than 16 Years in Primary and Secondary Care (CG102)*. Available at: https://www.nice.org.uk/guidance/cg102

National Institute for Health and Care Excellence (NICE) (2012) *Croup. Clinical Knowledge Summaries*. Available at: http://cks.nice.org.uk/croup#!topicsummary

National Institute for Health and Care Excellence (NICE) (2013) *Feverish Illness in Children: Assessment and Initial Management in Children Younger than 5 Years [CG160]*. Available at: https://www.nice.org.uk/guidance/cg160

Chapter 48

Resuscitation Council (UK) (2015) *Paediatric Advanced Life Support.* Available at: https://www.resus.org.uk/resuscitation-guidelines/

Chapter 49

National Institute for Health and Care Excellence (NICE) (2014) *Head Injury: Triage, Assessment, Investigation and Early Management of Head Injury in Children, Young People and Adults (CG176).* Available at: https://www.nice.org.uk/guidance/cg176

Chapter 50

Purcell, D. (2010) *Minor Injuries: A Clinical Guide.* 2nd edition. London: Churchill Livingstone Elsevier.

Chapter 51

Purcell, D. (2010) *Minor Injuries: A Clinical Guide.* 2nd edition. London: Churchill Livingstone Elsevier.

Chapter 52

Myers, B.A. (2011) *Wound Management: Principles and Practice.* 2nd edition. Upper Saddle River, NJ: Pearson Education.

Chapter 53

Khaw, P., Shah, P. and Elkington, A. (2004) *ABC of Eyes.* 4th edition. Hoboken, NJ: Wiley-Blackwell.

Chapter 54

Burton, M. (2000) *Hall and Colman's Diseases of the Ear, Nose and Throat.* 15th edition. London: Churchill Livingstone.

Chapter 55

Smith, J., Greaves, I. and Porter, K. (eds) (2010) *Oxford Desk Reference: Major Trauma.* Oxford: Oxford University Press.

Chapter 56

Smith, J., Greaves, I. and Porter, K. (eds) (2010) *Oxford Desk Reference: Major Trauma.* Oxford: Oxford University Press.

Chapter 57

National Institute for Health and Care Excellence (NICE) (2014) *Head Injury: Triage, Assessment, Investigation and Early Management of Head Injury in Children, Young People and Adults (CG17).* Available at: https://www.nice.org.uk/guidance/cg176
Smith, J., Greaves, I. and Porter, K. (eds) (2010) *Oxford Desk Reference: Major Trauma.* Oxford: Oxford University Press.

Chapter 58

Smith, J., Greaves, I. and Porter, K. (eds) (2010) *Oxford Desk Reference: Major Trauma.* Oxford: Oxford University Press.

Chapter 59

Smith, J., Greaves, I. and Porter, K. (eds) (2010) *Oxford Desk Reference: Major Trauma.* Oxford: Oxford University Press.

Chapter 60

Smith, J., Greaves, I. and Porter, K. (eds) (2010) *Oxford Desk Reference: Major Trauma.* Oxford: Oxford University Press.

Chapter 61

Smith, J., Greaves, I. and Porter, K. (eds) (2010) *Oxford Desk Reference: Major Trauma.* Oxford: Oxford University Press.

Chapter 62

British Burn Association http://www.britishburnassociation.org/
Smith, J., Greaves, I. and Porter, K. (eds) (2010) *Oxford Desk Reference: Major Trauma.* Oxford: Oxford University Press.

Chapter 63

Smith, J., Greaves, I. and Porter, K. (eds) (2010) *Oxford Desk Reference: Major Trauma.* Oxford: Oxford University Press.

Chapter 64

Smith, J., Greaves, I. and Porter, K. (eds) (2010) *Oxford Desk Reference: Major Trauma.* Oxford: Oxford University Press.

Chapter 65

NHS England (2015) *Core Standards for Emergency Preparedness, Resilience and Response.* Available at: https://www.england.nhs.uk/wp-content/uploads/2015/06/nhse-core-standards-150506.pdf
NHS England (2015) *Hazardous Materials (HAZMAT) and Chemical, Biological Radiological and Nuclear (CBRN).* Available at: http://www.england.nhs.uk/ourwork/eprr/hm/

Chapter 66

Association of Anaesthetists of Great Britain and Ireland (AAGBI) (2009) *Interhospital Transfer.* Available at: https://www.aagbi.org/sites/default/files/interhospital09.pdf

Chapter 67

Department of Health (2015) *Improvements to Care in the Last Days and Hours of Life.* Available at: https://www.gov.uk/government/publications/improvements-to-care-in-the-last-days-and-hours-of-life
National Institute for Health and Care Excellence (NICE) (2011) *End of Life Care for Adults (QS13).* Available at: https://www.nice.org.uk/guidance/qs13

Index

Emergency Nursing at a Glance, First Edition. Natalie Holbery and Paul Newcombe
© 2016 John Wiley & Sons, Ltd. Published 2016 by John Wiley & Sons, Ltd. Companion website: www.ataglanceseries.com/nursing/emergencynursing

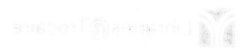